This book is dedicated to the faculty and staff of the State University of New York at Buffalo, School of Social Work. We are grateful for the education that provided the foundation for our academic careers. Thank you for teaching, mentoring, and investing in us.

CATHERINE AND LISA
MSW class of 1991
PhD class of 1999

HANDBOOK OF PREVENTIVE
INTERVENTIONS FOR ADULTS

Edited by

Catherine N. Dulmus
Lisa A. Rapp-Paglicci

WILEY

John Wiley & Sons, Inc.

This book is printed on acid-free paper. ∞

Limit of Liability/Disclaimer of Warranty: While the publisher and author have used their best efforts in preparing this book, they make no representations or warranties with respect to the accuracy or completeness of the contents of this book and specifically disclaim any implied warranties of merchantability or fitness for a particular purpose. No warranty may be created or extended by sales representatives or written sales materials. The advice and strategies contained herein may not be suitable for your situation. You should consult with a professional where appropriate. Neither the publisher nor author shall be liable for any loss of profit or any other commercial damages, including but not limited to special, incidental, consequential, or other damages.

This publication is designed to provide accurate and authoritative information in regard to the subject matter covered. It is sold with the understanding that the publisher is not engaged in rendering professional services. If legal, accounting, medical, psychological or any other expert assistance is required, the services of a competent professional person should be sought.

Designations used by companies to distinguish their products are often claimed as trademarks. In all instances where John Wiley & Sons, Inc. is aware of a claim, the product names appear in initial capital or all capital letters. Readers, however, should contact the appropriate companies for more complete information regarding trademarks and registration.

For general information on our other products and services please contact our Customer Care Department within the United States at (800) 762-2974, outside the United States at (317) 572-3993 or fax (317) 572-4002.

Wiley also publishes its books in a variety of electronic formats. Some content that appears in print may not be available in electronic books. For more information about Wiley products, visit our web site at www.wiley.com.

Library of Congress Cataloging-in-Publication Data:

Handbook of preventive interventions for adults / edited by Catherine N. Dulmus and Lisa
   A. Rapp-Paglicci.
    p.   cm.
   Includes bibliographical references and index.
   ISBN 0-471-56970-4 (cloth : acid-free paper)
    1. Medicine, Preventive—Handbooks, manuals, etc.   2. Mental health
services—Handbooks, manuals, etc.   3. Social service—Handbooks, manuals, etc.   I.
Dulmus, Catherine N.   II. Rapp-Paglicci, Lisa A.
   RA427.2.H365   2005
   362.198′97—dc22

          2004042296

Printed in the United States of America.

10 9 8 7 6 5 4 3 2

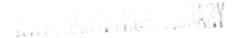

Contents ———————————

Part IV   Preventive Interventions for
Adult Social Problems

Part V   Conclusion

Preface

As we began to develop the idea for this book, it became obvious that although people were familiar with prevention, many conceptualized it primarily as geared for children and adolescents. Thus, we were faced with skepticism that prevention had a place in adult research and practice. Yet, adults are diagnosed with preventable disorders such as diabetes, hypertension, anxiety, and obesity at increased rates, with serious personal and societal costs. Developmental theorists have persuaded us to rethink adulthood as a series of continuing developmental stages, with differing tasks to be accomplished at each stage and with various risk factors at each stage that need addressing. With this in mind, it becomes obvious that prevention research and practice are very much applicable to adults at various stages of the life span and with varying conditions.

We need not continue to think of adulthood and aging as an inevitable time of illness and decline, because there are ways to prevent and reduce emotional, health, and social problems. Living longer should not be the only goal, but to live that longer life with optimal health and mental health. A focus on wellness and health is essential, as living to 80 while afflicted with Alzheimer's disease, high blood pressure, and marital distress is painful, debilitating, and costly. Our goal should be improved quality of life through healthier living, with adult prevention techniques and programs being our focus.

We thank Tracey Belmont and Isabel Pratt, our editors at John Wiley & Sons for recognizing the value of this project. Very few books are devoted solely to prevention, and no book thoroughly covered the various types of preventive interventions available for adults, until now. The intent of this book is to present the most effective and current preventive interventions and programs available on adult emotional, health, and social problems. The outstanding array of scholars and practitioners who authored chapters in this book did an exceptional job and we thank them. Each chapter provides an introduction; a summary of the problem;

data on trends and incidence; risk factors; interventions available on a universal, selective, and indicated levels; and future research directions.

As this handbook indicates, it is no longer necessary for individuals, families, and communities to endure an array of physical, emotional, and social problems. We now have the knowledge base to prevent many of these problems. Policy makers, administrators, and practitioners must increase their awareness of effective preventive interventions for adults and make available these tactics instead of waiting for problems to occur. As life expectancy increases and medical costs rise, individuals and society can no longer afford not to take a preventive approach to health and wellness in adulthood.

CATHERINE N. DULMUS
LISA A. RAPP-PAGLICCI

About the Editors ———————————————————

Catherine N. Dulmus, PhD, is an associate professor in the College of Social Work at the University of Tennessee. She received her baccalaureate in Social Work from Buffalo State College in 1989, a master's degree in Social Work from the State University of New York in 1991, and a PhD in Social Welfare from the State University of New York at Buffalo in 1999. Dr. Dulmus's research focuses on child mental health, prevention, and violence. She is coeditor of *Best Practices in Mental Health: An International Journal,* coeditor of *The Journal of Evidence-Based Social Work: Advances in Practice, Programming, Research, and Policy,* and associate editor of *Stress, Trauma, and Crisis: An International Journal,* and sits on the editorial board of the *Journal of Human Behavior in the Social Environment.* In 2002, she was awarded an excellence in teaching citation from the University of Tennessee. Prior to obtaining her PhD, Dr. Dulmus practiced in the fields of mental health and school social work.

Lisa A. Rapp-Paglicci, PhD, is an associate professor at the University of South Florida, Lakeland, School of Social Work. She received her baccalaureate in Psychology from LeMoyne College in 1989, a master's degree in Social Work from the State University of New York at Buffalo in 1991, and a PhD in Social Welfare from the State University of New York at Buffalo in 1999. Her research focuses on juvenile violence, prevention, and at-risk youth. Dr. Rapp-Paglicci serves on the editorial boards of the *Journal of Human Behavior in the Social Environment* and *Journal of Evidence-Based Social Work: Advances in Practice, Programming, Research, and Policy.* She received the 1999–2000 Outstanding Teaching award from the Greenspun College of Urban Affairs. Her previous social work practice experience encompassed work with juvenile offenders and children and youth with mental illness.

Contributors

Robert D. Abbott, PhD
Professor
University of Virginia School of Medicine
Division of Biostatistics and
   Epidemiology
Charlottesville, Virginia

Laura E. Bedard, PhD
Director of Undergraduate Studies
   and Internships
Florida State University
School of Criminology and
   Criminal Justice
Tallahassee, Florida

Gina C. Belleau, MS
Research Associate
Pacific Health Research Institute
Honolulu, Hawaii

Thomas Broffman, PhD
Assistant Professor
Eastern Connecticut State University
Social Work Program
Willimantic, Connecticut

Patricia Brownell, PhD
Associate Professor
Fordham University
Graduate School of Social Services
New York, New York

Graham A. Colditz, MD, DrPH
Professor of Medicine
Harvard Medical School
Harvard Center for Cancer Prevention
   and Channing Laboratory
Boston, Massachusetts

Shelley Craig, MSW
Doctoral Student
Florida International University
School of Social Work
Miami, Florida

J. David Curb, MD
President, CEO and Medical Director
Pacific Health Research Institute
Honolulu, Hawaii

Cindy Davis, PhD
Assistant Professor
The University of Tennessee
College of Social Work
Nashville, Tennessee

Jorge Delva, PhD
Associate Professor
The University of Michigan
School of Social Work
Ann Arbor, Michigan

Catherine N. Dulmus, PhD
Associate Professor
The University of Tennessee
College of Social Work
Knoxville, Tennessee

Tonya Edmond, PhD
Assistant Professor
Washington University
George Warren Brown School of
    Social Work
St. Louis, Missouri

Gretchen Ely, PhD
Assistant Professor
The University of Kentucky
College of Social Work
Lexington, Kentucky

Sondra J. Fogel, PhD, MSSW, ACSW
Associate Professor
University of South Florida
School of Social Work
Tampa, Florida

Andres G. Gil, PhD
Associate Professor and Associate
    Director
Community-Based Intervention
    Research Group
College of Health and Urban Affairs
Florida International University
Miami, Florida

Bert Hayslip Jr., PhD
Professor
University of North Texas
Department of Psychology
Denton, Texas

Carolyn Hilarski, PhD
Assistant Professor
Rochester Institute of Technology
School of Social Work
Rochester, New York

Matthew O. Howard, PhD
Professor of Social Work and
    Psychiatry
The University of Michigan
School of Social Work and Department
    of Psychiatry
Ann Arbor, Michigan

Jeffrey M. Jenson, PhD
Professor
The University of Denver
Graduate School of Social Work
Denver, Colorado

Mary Ann Leitz, PhD, RN
Assistant Professor
Tarleton State University
Tarleton, Texas

William D. Lemley, RN
Neonatal Intensive Care Unit
Columbus Regional Medical Center
Columbus, Ohio

Mayte Lopez-Sandrin, MD
Division of Endocrinology, Diabetes,
    and Metabolism
University of Miami
Miami, Florida

Robert J. Maiden, PhD
Professor
Alfred University
Department of Psychology
Alfred, New York

Andrea K. McCarter, MSSW
Doctoral Student
The University of Tennessee
College of Social Work
Knoxville, Tennessee

Kaye McGinty, MD
Assistant Professor
East Carolina University
Brody School of Medicine
Greenville, North Carolina

Karen McGuffee, JD
Assistant Professor
University of Tennessee, Chattanooga
College of Arts and Sciences
Criminal Justice Department-Legal
    Assistant Studies Program
Chattanooga, Tennessee

MaryAnn Overcamp-Martini, PhD
Assistant Professor
University of Nevada Las Vegas
School of Social Work
Las Vegas, Nevada

John H. Pierpont, PhD
Associate Professor
East Carolina University
School of Social Work
Greenville, North Carolina

Lisa A. Rapp-Paglicci, PhD
Associate Professor
The University of South Florida
    at Lakeland
School of Social Work
Lakeland, Florida

Dominique E. Roe-Sepowitz, MSW
Doctoral Student
Florida State University
School of Social Work
Tallahassee, Florida

William S. Rowe, DSW
Director and Professor
University of South Florida
School of Social Work
Tampa, Florida

Jay S. Skyler, MD
Director, Division of Endocrinology,
    Diabetes, and Metabolism
University of Miami
Miami, Florida

Karen M. Sowers, PhD
Dean and Professor
The University of Tennessee
College of Social Work
Knoxville, Tennessee

Cynthia J. Stein, MD, MPH
Instructor of Medicine
Harvard Medical School
Harvard Center for Cancer Prevention
    and Channing Laboratory
Boston, Massachusetts

Matthew T. Theriot, PhD
Assistant Professor
The University of Tennessee
College of Social Work
Knoxville, Tennessee

Barbara Thomlison, PhD
Professor and Director, Institute for
    Children and Families at Risk
Florida International University
School of Social Work and Stempel
    School of Public Health
Miami, Florida

Bruce A. Thyer, PhD
Dean and Professor
Florida State University
School of Social Work
Tallahassee, Florida

Jonathan G. Tubman, PhD
Graduate Director
Community-Based Intervention Research
    Group
College of Arts and Sciences
Florida International University
Miami, Florida

Michael G. Vaughn, MS
Doctoral Candidate
Washington University
George Warren Brown School of
    Social Work
St. Louis, Missouri

Thomas M. Vogt, MD, MPH, FAHA
Director
Kaiser Permanente Center for Health
    Research Hawaii
Honolulu, Hawaii

Bradley J. Willcox, MD
Investigator
Pacific Health Research Institute
Honolulu, Hawaii

PART I

Introduction

Chapter 1

PREVENTION ACROSS THE ADULT LIFE SPAN

LISA A. RAPP-PAGLICCI AND CATHERINE N. DULMUS

Individuals are living longer, but in many cases, their quality of life is impeded due to preventable emotional, physical, and/or social problems. Adults continue to be diagnosed with physical and mental illnesses such as diabetes, hypertension, anxiety, and obesity, at a time when social problems such as partner violence and economic instability are escalating. In many cases, these illnesses and social problems have serious personal and societal costs. Some of these problems can be prevented.

Prevention tactics are now more prevalent, but the focus continues to be toward children and adolescents, while adults are neglected. However, prevention is appropriate, possible, and necessary across the entire life span. Developmental theorists have persuaded us to rethink adulthood as a series of continuing developmental stages with differing tasks to be accomplished and various risk factors that need to be addressed at each stage. With this in mind, it becomes obvious that prevention research and practice is not only applicable, but essential for adults at various stages of the life span.

Research studies have begun to identify the myriad of prevention techniques targeted toward young, middle, and older adults at varying problem stages utilizing micro, mezzo, and macro level approaches. Although these techniques and programs will not be difficult to implement, changing our attitudes regarding prevention and the aging process may be a far greater challenge.

PREVENTION RECONSTRUCTION

The Institute of Medicine (1994) defines *prevention* as those interventions that occur before the initial onset of the disorder, with preventive research and interventions being limited to the processes that occur before there is a diagnosable disorder or problem. The treatment of such disorders is defined as *maintenance*. We support this approach since, unlike the public health model, this approach is pure prevention focusing on interventions to prevent the onset of a disorder or problem. Gordon's model of prevention addresses prevention from this perspective (Gordon, 1983, 1987). Gordon's model of preventive interventions is broken down into three areas: universal, selective, and indicated. *Universal preventive interventions* are defined as interventions for disorders or problems that are targeted to the general public or a whole population group that has not been identified on the basis of individual risk. *Selective preventive interventions* are those interventions that are targeted to individuals or a subgroup of the population who are at high risk of developing a specific disorder or problem at some point in their lifetime. *Indicated preventive interventions* are defined as those interventions that are targeted to high-risk individuals who do not meet the specific criteria for a mental or medical disorder, but who otherwise are identified as having minimal but detectable signs or symptoms of a specific disorder or who have a biological marker indicating predisposition for the disorder (Institute of Medicine, 1994). Thus, a risk reduction model to prevention complements Gordon's approach to prevention.

RISK REDUCTION MODEL

A risk reduction model is a promising approach to prevention that identifies risk factors and matches them to empirically tested interventions (Institute of Medicine, 1994). Risk factors are those characteristics, variables, or hazards that, if present for a given individual, make it more likely that this individual, rather than someone selected from the general population, will develop a particular disorder (Werner & Smith, 1982). Risk groups could be identified on the basis of biological, psychological, or social risk factors that are known to be associated with the onset of a specific disorder. Once identified, individuals or subgroups of the population at risk for developing a particular disorder could be targeted with selective preventive interventions (Institute of Medicine, 1994).

It is likely that both biogenetic factors and social conditions may jointly operate to heighten the risk status of an individual (Garmezy, 1993). We know that manifestations of problematic development in vulnerable adults are as varied as the risk factors to which they are exposed (Hauser, Vieyra, Jacobson, & Wertlieb, 1985). Psychosocial development from early childhood through adolescence and into adulthood is shaped by a myriad of specific events, ongoing circumstances, and inherent strengths and vulnerabilities of the individual (Hauser et al., 1985). Certain events and circumstances are especially likely to adversely affect this development. Cowen and Work (1988) state, "negative psychological effects of multiple stressful life events and circumstances cumulate like lead poisoning" (p. 591). These situations vary widely. If risk factors can be decreased or in some way altered, and/or if protective factors can be enhanced, the likelihood would decrease of at-risk individuals eventually developing a specific disorder or problem (Dulmus & Rapp-Paglicci, 2000).

RESILIENT CHILDREN BECOME RESILIENT ADULTS

Children who are exposed to risk factors associated with development of particular disorders, yet maintain their mental and/or physical health, are of particular interest to researchers. Children who despite exposure to identified stressors obtain competence are referred to in the literature as "resilient," "invulnerable," or "ego-resistant." Resilience is defined as "the tendency to rebound or recoil," "to return to a prior state," "to spring back," "the power of recovery." Garmezy (1993) defines a competence item as one that measures successes and achievement in meeting the major adaptational expectations or requirements of people in society. Rutter (1981) defines resilience as a phenomenon stating, "as shown by the young people who 'do well' in some sense in spite of having experienced a form of 'stress,' which in the population as a whole is known to carry a substantial risk of an adverse outcome."

Arnold (1990) reports that the way children respond to stress may either promote growth and a sense of efficacy or cause behavioral, social, academic, or psychosomatic problems. Children exposed to stress that increases the risk of an adverse outcome are said to be "vulnerable" to that outcome, therefore resilience is defined in terms of two concepts—vulnerability and competence: Children who are vulnerable to an adverse outcome yet achieve competence are resilient. Cowen and Work (1988) state, "knowledge about the effects of multiple, chronic stressful life events and circumstances on children and in vivo factors that shield them against serious psychological problems are key building blocks that undergird efforts to understand the nature and determinants of invulnerability and develop preventive interventions to promote wellness in profoundly stressed children."

Fortunately, the majority of children exposed to various forms of adversity grow up to enjoy productive, normal lives (Hauser et al., 1985). It is only a minority of children-at-risk who experience serious difficulties in their personality and physical development (Garmezy, 1981).

Resilient children may hold the key that can change the present focus on pathology to one of health and wellness in children and adults alike. Cowen and Work (1988) report the primary goal of intervention would be to provide the adjustment enhancing skills and conditions that many profoundly stressed children fail to acquire in their natural life experiences and, thus, to disrupt the inevitable maladaptive spiral in which they are caught. Certainly, the same approaches could be taken with adults. Garmezy (1993) states, "once we have identified the biological, psychological, and sociocultural mechanisms that activate resilient behavior and the developmental processes that are integral to the operation of these mechanisms, we will then be in a better position to generate scientifically sturdy programs for intervention that may enable us to develop methods for enhancing resilient behavior in children disadvantaged by status and stress." These intervention programs would need to utilize empirical measures so outcomes could be tracked and evaluated.

PROMOTING RESILIENCY

Garmezy (1993) states, "The central element in the study of resilience lies in the power of recovery and in the ability to return once again to those patterns of adaptation and competence that characterized the individual prior to the pre-stress period." Practitioners, policy makers, and researchers must look for protective factors that promote health and resiliency and presumably compensate for risk elements that are inherent in the lives and in the environments of many underprivileged children. Focus on those elements in person, family, and community that may be conducive in the development of adaptive or maladaptive behaviors.

How then do we promote resilient outcomes? It is clear that there is usually no comprehensive intervention at a single point that accomplishes comprehensive goals of prevention for a lifetime. The ultimate goal to achieve optimal prevention should be to build the principles of prevention into the ordinary activities of everyday life and into the community structures to enhance development over the entire life span. Risk factors that occur in multiple domains—home, work, peer group, or neighborhood—require interventions in all of them.

The more that is known about etiology, the greater the chance to target preventive interventions to intervene in causal chains. The Institute of Medicine (1994) reports,

> Because it appears that most risk and protective factors are not specific to a single disorder, the most fruitful approach for preventive interventions at this time may be to use a risk reduction model that includes the enhancement of protective factors and to aim at clusters or constellations of populations, but the interventions will be aimed at those causal and malleable risk factors that appear to have

a role in the expression of several mental disorders. Identification of relative and attributable risks associated with various clusters could greatly facilitate prevention intervention research. (p. 128)

FURTHER RESEARCH

Further research on the process of adaptation will lead to a better understanding of normal and pathological development and will have direct relevance for refining existing intervention and prevention programs. Understanding the processes by which some individuals remain confident and develop supportive relationships in the midst of adversity is crucial to the development of effective prevention and intervention strategies (Rutter, 1990).

As researchers, it is imperative that we continue to build on the literature. Cicchetti and Garmezy (1993) state, "currently the popularity of resilience as a construct has exceeded the research output associated with it. As such, resilience is at risk for being viewed as a popularized trend that has not been verified through research and thereby is in danger of losing credibility within the scientific community. To prevent this, it is imperative that theorists in the area of resilience devote equal effort to advancing the construct empirically." There is an urgent need to develop standardized and validated measures of resiliency. Researchers must continue to do empirical research in the area of resiliency and assist practitioners in the development and implementation of resiliency enhancement programs not only for children, but for adults as well. The need for preventative strategies is imperative.

PREVENTIVE INTERVENTION

A more rewarding approach to prevention, given current knowledge of etiology, lies in the identification of risk factors and the design of interventions aimed at reducing these risks in vulnerable individuals (Fraser & Galinsky, 1997). The economic, as well as the clinical and sociomedical arguments for primary mental health care prevention are growing (Murray, 1992). The lack of educational campaigns aimed at prevention from the mental health sector though, reflects the absence of consensus on etiology of the more prevalent minor affective disorders, and the wide range of biological, personality, educational, social, and behavioral factors that influence susceptibility (Murray, 1992).

It is imperative to formulate preventive interventions not only for the individual and the family, but also for the community. Social issues such as poverty, inadequate housing and health care, and violence negatively affect adults and their families. Rappaport (1992) states, "we find it more attractive to blame people, rather than social institutions for problems in living." He further states,

> In the United States, the National Institute of Mental Health has been forced to deal with the governments individual responsibility social agenda that since 1980 has forced prevention policies to become less concerned with social conditions and more focused on specific disorders. Prevention defined as interventions to prevent diagnosable mental disorders by searching for causal agents in individuals will always be supported by governments.

It is crucial to have preventionists who also have an interest in preventive social change and a focus on a community mental health perspective that addresses the social factors putatively underlying individuals emotional distress (Baker, 1982). Albee (1982) states, "Efforts at prevention require the ideological decision to line up with the humanists who believe in social change, in the effectiveness of consultation, in education, in the primary prevention of human physical and emotional misery and in the maximization of individual competence."

OVERVIEW OF BOOK

It is time to promote a purely preventative approach to adults' physical and mental health. The *Handbook of Preventive Interventions for Adults* brings together outstanding scholars to summarize the empirical literature related to a variety of disorders and to provide guidelines for preventive interventions relative to each level of Gordon's model. This Handbook challenges practitioners and policy makers to approach adults with a prevention mind-set to best promote optimal health and mental health. Such an approach will subsequently improve quality of life for many adults, while at the same time decrease societal financial costs for an aging population.

REFERENCES

Albee, G. W. (1982). Preventing psychopathology and promoting human potential. *American Psychologist, 37,* 143–150.

Arnold, E. L. (1990). *Childhood stress.* New York: Wiley.

Baker, F. (1982). Effects of value systems on service delivery. In H. C. Schulberg & M. Killilea (Eds.), *The modern practice of community mental health.* San Francisco: Jossey-Bass.

Cicchetti, D., & Garmezy, N. (1993). Milestones in the development of resilience. *Development and Psychopathology, 5*(4), 497–502.

Cowen, E. L., & Work, W. C. (1988). Resilient children, psychological wellness, and primary prevention. *American Journal of Community Psychology, 16*(4), 591–607.

Dulmus, C. N., & Rapp-Paglicci, L. A. (2000). The prevention of mental disorders in children and adolescents: Future research and public policy recommendations. *Families in Society, 81*(3), 294–303.

Fraser, M. W., & Galinsky, M. J. (1997). Toward a resilience-based model of practice. In M. W. Fraser (Ed.), *Risk and resilience in childhood* (pp. 195–215). Washington, DC: National Association of Social Workers Press.

Garmezy, N. (1981). Children under stress: Perspectives on antecedents and correlates of vulnerability and resistance to psychopathology. In A. I. Rabin, J. Aronoff, A. Barclay, & R. A. Zucker (Eds.), *Further explorations in personality* (pp. 196–270). New York: Wiley.

Garmezy, N. (1993). Children in poverty: Resilience despite risk. *Psychiatry Interpersonal and Biological Processes, 56*(1), 127–136.

Gordon, R. (1983). An operational classification of disease prevention. *Public Health Reports, 98,* 107–109.

Gordon, R. (1987). An operational classification of disease prevention. In J. A. Steinberg & M. M. Silverman (Eds.), *Preventing mental disorders* (pp. 20–26). Rockville, MD: Department of Health and Human Services.

Hauser, S. T., Vieyra, M. B., Jacobson, A. M., & Wertlieb, D. (1985). Vulnerability and resilience in adolescence: Views from the family. *Journal of Early Adolescence, 5*(1), 81–100.

Institute of Medicine. (1994). *Reducing risks for mental disorders: Frontiers for preventive intervention research.* Washington, DC: National Academy Press.

Murray, J. (1992). Prevention and the identification of high risk groups. *International Review of Psychiatry, 4,* 281–286.

Rappaport, J. (1992). The dilemma of primary prevention in mental health services: Rationalize the status quo or bite the hand that feeds you. *Journal of Community and Applied Social Psychology, 2,* 95–99.

Rutter, M. (1981). Stress, coping and development: Some issues and some questions. *Journal of Child Psychology and Psychiatry, 22,* 323–256.

Rutter, M. (1990). Psychosocial resilience and protective mechanisms. In A. Rolf, A. S. Masten, D. Cicchetti, K. H. Nuechterlein, & S. Weintraub (Eds.), *Risk and protective factors in the development of psychopathology* (pp. 181–214). New York: Cambridge University Press.

Werner, E. E., & Smith, R. S. (1982). *Vulnerable but invincible: A longitudinal study of resilient children and youth.* New York: McGraw-Hill.

PART II

Preventive Interventions for Adult Emotional and Mental Problems

Chapter 2

ANXIETY

DOMINIQUE E. ROE-SEPOWITZ, LAURA E. BEDARD, AND
BRUCE A. THYER

Anxiety disorders are the most common, frequently occurring, so-called mental disorders in the United States (we say "so-called" because there are compelling reasons to doubt the notion that these conditions have their etiology in the "mind" of individuals). Differing from everyday stress and anxiousness caused by stimuli such as examinations, new jobs, and morning traffic, anxiety disorders are pervasive and chronic and may need professional care to alleviate or cure them. Over 19 million Americans between the ages of 18 and 54 are estimated to meet the formal diagnostic criteria for one or more anxiety disorders (National Institute of Mental Health [NIMH], 1999). Anxiety disorders can be the result of life stressors and events, learning, parental upbringing, illness-induced stress, genetic endowment and other biological conditions, and the inability to cope with and manage all of those factors at once. Mental health problems such as anxiety present particular problems during adulthood, including contributing to high rates of suicide, relationship problems, and difficulty functioning in society. Some specific events during adulthood (having children, divorcing, and expectations about success) can contribute to the development of an anxiety disorder.

Some anxiety is helpful, keeping persons alert and aware of their environment; too much anxiety, however, fatigues a person and can lead to diminished functioning. Anxiety disorders are linked by extreme or pathological anxiousness as the principal disturbance. The term *anxiety disorder* is formally given to pathological disturbances of affect, thinking, behavior, and physiological activity (U.S. Surgeon General, 1999). This subsumes emotional responses such as intense fear and feelings of dread and physical symptoms of shortness of breath, cold hands and feet, perspiration, lightheadedness or dizziness, rapid heart rate, trembling, restlessness, and muscle tension (U.S. Surgeon General, 1999). Anxiety disorders are characterized by an excessive or inappropriate state of fear, apprehension, and uncertainty (NIMH, 1999).

TYPES OF ANXIETY DISORDERS

There are several specific types of anxiety disorders, including the following.

Phobias

The underlying element in all phobias is an *irrational fear* of something. They can range in intensity from mild to traumatic, but "in all cases there is a sense of predictability which accompanies them" (Clark & Wardman, 1985, p. 13). The following are general definitions of several common phobias.

Specific Phobia

Formerly known as "simple phobia," specific phobia is persistent fear of an object or situation. According to the *Diagnostic and Statistical Manual of Mental Disorders* text revision (*DSM;* American Psychological Association, 2000), there are five subtypes of specific phobia: animal type (generally with childhood onset; examples include fear of snakes, dogs, or insects), natural environment type (fear of storms, heights, weather), blood-injection injury type (fear cued by seeing blood), situational type (fear cued by a situation such as crossing a bridge, driving, being in enclosed places), and other (e.g., fear of clowns, claustrophobia, fear of choking). Exposure to the stimulus causes intense fear and stimulates avoidance behavior by the individual. The fears are excessive and unreasonable. Most specific phobias begin during childhood and eventually disappear. They are more common in women than in men.

Social Phobia

Also called "social anxiety disorder," social phobia is diagnosed when a person's shyness and social avoidance becomes so severe and intense that it causes impairment or dysfunction. The anxiety-evoking stimulus involves being observed, judged, or evaluated by others. Social phobia is one of the most common anxiety disorders and can become worse over time if not treated (Thyer, 2002; Thyer, Tomlin, Curtis, Cameron, & Nesse, 1985). Social phobia is defined by the *DSM* as "marked or persistent fear of social or performance situations in which embarrassment may occur" (American Psychiatric Association, 2000, p. 450). Situations that are often feared by people with social phobia are speaking in public, participating in sports, being in public places, meeting new people, talking to an authority figure, using public lavatories when others are present, and musical or other performances. Clinical presentations may be different across cultures. By some criteria, social phobia is the third most prevalent mental health care problem in the world.

Agoraphobia

The word *agoraphobia* literally translates as "fear of the marketplace" (Clark & Wardman, 1985, p. 8) and refers to a generalized fear of being in public places. More specifically, agoraphobia is "anxiety about being in places or situations from which escape might be difficult (or embarrassing) or in which help may not be available in the event of having a panic attack or panic-like symptoms" (American Psychiatric Association, 2000, p. 432). This anxiety usually leads to the individual avoiding situations in which the anxiety may arise. In severe cases, individuals are unable to leave their comfort zone and often self-isolate to the point of being housebound.

General Anxiety Disorder

This disorder is characterized by excessive anxiety or worry accompanied by at least three of the following: restlessness, fatigue, lack of concentration, muscle tension, irritability, and lack of sleep. General Anxiety Disorder can manifest in physical symptoms such as trembling, twitching, muscle aches, and soreness as well as diarrhea and vomiting. The intensity and worry individuals report is grossly out of proportion to the real risk. This disorder frequently occurs with mood disorders and other anxiety disorders and is more common in women than in men.

Panic Disorder

Panic Disorder is characterized by panic attacks, which are described as a "rush of fear or discomfort that reaches a peak in less than 10 minutes" (Antony & Swinson, 2000, p. 12). These attacks are accompanied by physical symptoms such as a racing heart, shortness of breath, sweating, shaking, chest pain, faintness, and hot flashes or chills. Panic attacks often occur in the absence of any specific stimuli but can be brought on by stressful events such as an exam or a public speaking event. According to the *DSM* (American Psychiatric Association, 2000), there are three subtypes of Panic Disorder: unexpected (occur without warning or a precipitating event), situationally bound (occur in a particular situation, e.g., with phobia exposure), and situationally predisposed (these fall somewhere in between the two previous). Panic attacks are often disabling. Panic Disorder is estimated to impact more than 4% of Americans (Datilio, 2001).

Obsessive Compulsive Disorder

The *DSM* defines Obsessive Compulsive Disorder (OCD) as "recurrent obsessions or compulsions that are severe enough to be time consuming (more than 1 hour a day) or cause marked distress or significant impairment" (American Psychiatric Association, 2000, p. 458). OCD usually presents with both obsessive thoughts and compulsive behaviors, although individuals may suffer from only one. The obsessions are characterized by persistent thoughts, images, or impulses that cause marked anxiety or stress; for example, the thought of germs contaminating one's hands, ruminating over whether one locked the door, or the urge to blurt out an obscenity. The compulsive behaviors are often associated with the obsessions: with the thought of germs comes excessive hand washing, even to the point where the skin is extremely chafed. Adults with OCD usually realize that these actions are inappropriate, unreasonable, and excessive. If they do not come to this realization, the illness is referred to as OCD with poor insight.

Posttraumatic Stress Disorder

In Posttraumatic Stress Disorder (PTSD), a person who has experienced a traumatic situation that involved actual or threatened death or serious bodily harm responds with trauma-related symptoms of intense fear, helplessness, or horror. Events can include, but are not limited to, crime victimization, wartime events, or serious accident. Symptoms can include distressing dreams about the event, feeling as if the event is recurring, stress surrounding the anniversary of the event, flashbacks, or avoiding activities associated with the event. In addition, the individual may have difficulty concentrating, may have insomnia, may display outbursts of anger, may be unable to recall the traumatic event, and may display a lack of interest in activities. PTSD is common among victims of rape and personal assault and those who serve in active combat. Sometimes the victim is unable to make the connection between the traumatic event and current struggles.

PREVENTION

There has been much research on the diagnosis and treatment of adult anxiety disorders but little attention paid to prevention. Anxiety disorders can be prevented provided the person has access to treatment or prevention information in the early stages of the disorder (Leighton, 1987). Delay in treatment and a lack of information about anxiety disorders and management contribute to the development of a diagnosable anxiety disorder.

The primary problem with attempting to prevent anxiety disorders is that individuals often try to camouflage their disorder instead of getting treatment. They may hide their symptoms from friends, family members, and coworkers, leading to a delay in professional treatment and intervention for perhaps many years, or until they are so uncomfortable and the symptoms so overwhelming that they are functionally impaired (Craske & Zucker, 2001).

Anxiety prevention programs have slowly grown in numbers, but few have been empirically supported. Three types of prevention programs are discussed in this chapter: universal, selective, and targeted. Programs aimed toward preventing the entire population or a community from feeling stressed or anxious about life events are monumental undertakings. This type of program is called a *universal* preventive intervention. *Selective* interventions are aimed at a population known to be at risk for anxiety problems or at higher risk than the average person, such as adults who have been exposed to violence at home or in the community. Preventive interventions aimed at adults who are already showing signs and symptoms of anxiety disorders are called *targeted.*

TRENDS AND INCIDENCE

The cost of anxiety disorders to the United States is more than $42 billion a year, with more than $22 billion attributed to repeat medical care costs in a search for relief from symptoms that look like physical illness (Greenberg, Sisitsky, & Kessler, 1999). People with anxiety disorders are three to five times more likely to go to the doctor and six times more likely to be hospitalized for psychiatric disorders. About one in seven adults in the United States and Britain are affected by anxiety disorders each year (Brown, 2003; see Table 2.1 on page 18).

RISK FACTORS

The predictors and risk factors for anxiety disorders have been well studied. A combination of biological, psychological-behavioral, and social-environmental factors determines if an individual will develop an anxiety disorder (Substance Abuse and Mental Health Services Administration [SAMHSA], 2003). The Anxiety Disorders Association of America suggests that anxiety disorders develop from a complex combination of risk factors, including genetics, brain chemistry, personality, and life events.

Table 2.1   Disorder Distribution among U.S. Adults

Disorder	Number (in Millions)	Percentage	Gender
	Total U.S. Population Affected		
Generalized Anxiety Disorder	4	2.8	Women are twice as likely as men to be afflicted.
Obsessive Compulsive Disorder	3.3	2.3	Equally afflicts men and women.
Panic Disorder	2.4	1.7	Women are twice as likely as men to be afflicted.
Posttraumatic Stress Disorder	5.2	3.6	Women are more likely than men to be afflicted.
Social phobia	5.3	3.7	Equally afflicts men and women.
Specific phobia	6.3	4.4	Women are twice as likely as men to be afflicted.
Total all/any phobia	14.8	10.3	

Source: Retrieved February 15, 2004, from www.adaa.org/mediaroom/index.cfm.

Life stressors and events may include severe or life-threatening trauma either during adulthood or childhood that contributes to the stress level of an individual (see Thyer, 1993). Stressors may include maltreatment during childhood, exposure to violence in or external to the home, violent relationships during adulthood, and being exposed to violence or trauma in personal or work environments. Some events can result in distress and dysfunction that, if not treated or managed, manifests as a mental illness, such as an anxiety disorder (U.S. Surgeon General, 1999).

For a substantial proportion of individuals who meet the criteria for an anxiety disorder, a clear biological or psychosocial etiology cannot be established. *Women* are at twice the risk for anxiety disorders compared to men, with the exception of OCD and possibly social anxiety. Possible explanations for this discrepancy include hormonal differences, cultural pressures, and a higher rate of reporting anxiety. Anxiety disorders appear to have a genetic factor and run in families. Many other factors influence an individual, including social, home, and peer relationships, but genetics plays a strong role.

EFFECTIVE UNIVERSAL PREVENTIVE INTERVENTIONS

The following interventions group all anxiety disorders together and attempt to prevent them for the entire population or community.

National Institute of Mental Health Anxiety Disorders Education Program

This program was developed by the NIMH Communications and Public Liaison Office. The purpose of the program was to educate and increase awareness among the public and health care providers about anxiety disorders and their "realness," and to convey the message that these conditions can be effectively diagnosed and treated. The primary goal of the program was to improve the lives of people with anxiety disorders. A six-pronged approach was used to disseminate information:

- A toll-free information line (800-ANXIETY) to receive free printed materials.
- A web site about anxiety disorders (www.nimh.nih.gov/anxiety).
- Radio and television public service announcements.
- Printed and audiovisual materials discussing diagnosis, treatment, and referral information about anxiety disorders.
- Print media outreach.
- Partnerships with community mental health, health, and civic organizations that provide public and professional education and research at the local level.

National Anxiety Disorders Screening Day: May 1

The purpose of this day is to destigmatize anxiety disorders, educate the public, and help people with anxiety disorders connect with service providers to obtain treatment. This has been a federal education and prevention program since 1994.

National Campaign on Anxiety and Depression Awareness 2004

This program is a year-long campaign to educate the public about the signs and symptoms of anxiety and depressive illnesses and guide affected individuals to treatment networks. The campaign includes public service announcements, print media releases, promotion of films about mental health issues, visits to communities, colleges, and universities, and a web site and toll-free number. Individuals found to have signs and symptoms of anxiety and depressive illness will be referred to a registered mental health provider to receive a free telephone or in-person mental health screening.

Anxiety Web Sites

A number of web sites that describe anxiety disorders, their features and symptoms, resources for more education and diagnosis, and methods of prevention are available with simple searches on the Internet. The following is a list of prevention-specific sites:

- www.panicanxietydisorder.org.au/4_Prevention.htm
- eMedicine.com: www.emedicine.com/aaem/topic26.htm
- Anxiety Disorders Association of America: www.adaa.org
- The Anxiety Panic Internet Resource: www.algy.com/anxiety/index.html
- Obsessive-Compulsive Foundation: www.ocfoundation.org/indright.htm

EFFECTIVE SELECTIVE PREVENTIVE INTERVENTIONS

The following interventions attempt to prevent all types of anxiety disorders for individuals identified as at risk.

Exercise Training Studies

The purpose of exercise programs were examined and found to be more beneficial for those with stressful lifestyles regarding anxiety reduction and management. Low to moderate stress management was achieved by participating in aerobic exercise including walking and jogging from a minimum of 5 weeks to 1 year.

Stress Management Training Program

Timmerman, Emmelkamp, and Sanderman (1998) developed a training protocol addressing issues that may cause increased stress in an individual's life: changing an unhealthy lifestyle, relaxation training, problem-solving training, and social skill training. Individuals randomly selected from a single community were chosen to participate after a screening to determine that they did not have serious mental health complaints but had an increased chance of developing one if exposed to stress. Participants were assigned to either a treatment or a control group. The treatment group, which followed the training protocol, reported more assertiveness, more satisfaction with social support, fewer daily hassles, less trait anxiety, and less distress.

Stress Inoculation Training for Step-Couples

Fausel (1995) designed this program to assist step-couples dealing with the stress of mourning the loss of their first families as well as learning how to cope and negotiate new relationships. The technique used Stress Inoculation Training in a three-phase program of behavioral and imaginal rehearsal, self-monitoring and instruction, cognitive restructuring, problem solving, didactic teaching, Socratic discussion, relaxation training, self-reinforcement, and environmental manipulation. Results of the program found that 62% of the 51 step-couples participating had reduced their stress scores.

Stress Management Exploratory Cognitive-Behavioral College Course

College students elected to take this course due to their interest in stress management and anxiety (Schiraldi & Brown, 2001). The course was based on the components of Stress Inoculation Training. The students were taught skills to reduce anger, prevent anxiety and depression, and improve self-esteem. The course lasted 15 weeks and pre- and posttests showed significant reductions in anxiety and depression and improvement in self-esteem.

Toastmasters International

This organization offers basic public speaking and communication skills along with methods to diminish fear and anxiety related to public speaking and leadership roles. The meetings feature learning how to develop presentations, lead teams and conduct meetings, give and receive constructive evaluations, and improve listening skills. The program is self-paced and meetings are offered around the world at many locations and times. There is a nominal fee for membership. See www.toastmasters.org for more information.

EFFECTIVE INDICATED PREVENTIVE INTERVENTIONS

Prevention Program for Panic Disorders, Brief Prevention Program for Recent Assault Victims, Video Intervention Program for Rape Survivors, Critical Incident Stress Debriefing, and Agoraphobics in Motion Self-Help Group are programs supported by empirical research studies.

Prevention Program for Panic Disorders

This program involved attending a 1-day prevention workshop group and monthly contact for 6 months (Gardenswartz & Craske, 2001). The workshop was based on cognitive-behavioral treatment techniques and focused on education about panic, strategies to control panic, information about agoraphobia, and exposure to overcome physical sensations and fears. Participants were selected to attend the workshop or to go on a wait-list (comparison group) if they reported they had at least one panic attack in the previous year and had at least moderate anxiety sensitivity but did not have diagnosed Panic Disorder. Outcomes showed that workshop participants were less likely to develop Panic Disorder in comparison to those wait-listed.

Prevention Workshop for College Students

First-year college students ($n = 231$) identified to be at risk for depression and anxiety were assigned to treatment or control groups over a 3-year period (Seligman, Schulman, & DeRubeis, 1999). The intervention was done three times over the 3-year period. The treatment group participated in 16 hours of meetings over 8 weeks as well as completing homework assignments led by a trainer and a cotrainer. The content of the treatment was based on cognitive-behavioral techniques; specific topics included:

> the cognitive theory of change, identifying automatic negative thoughts and underlying beliefs, marshaling evidence to question and dispute automatic negative thoughts and irrational beliefs, replacing automatic negative thoughts with more constructive interpretations, beliefs, and behaviors, behavioral activation strategies, interpersonal skills, stress management, and generalizing these skills to new and relevant situations. (para. 20)

The workshop participants showed fewer episodes of Generalized Anxiety Disorder and fewer anxiety symptoms than the control group.

Brief Prevention Program for Recent Assault Victims

This program targeted recent female victims of sexual and nonsexual assault (Foa, Hearst-Ikeda, & Perry, 1995). The treatment group ($n = 10$) received four sessions of cognitive-behavioral interventions, while a control group received repeated assessments only. Education about common reactions to assaults was provided along with a mixture of cognitive-behavioral techniques, including video narration, relaxation techniques, cognitive distortion recognition and discussion, imaginal exposure, and cognitive restructuring. Two months after the assault, the treatment group demonstrated significantly fewer PTSD symptoms. After five and a half months, the treatment group participants were significantly less depressed and had significantly fewer severe symptoms of re-experiencing the event compared to those in the assessment-only group.

Video Intervention Program for Rape Survivors

The purpose of this prevention program was to decrease the anxiety of recent sexual assault victims during the forensic exam and prevent PTSD (Resnick, Acierno, Holmes, Kilpatrick, & Jager, 1999). Recent sexual assault victims who had been forcibly penetrated orally, anally, or vaginally within the previous 72 hours were randomly assigned to a treatment ($n = 13$) or a control group ($n = 33$). The treatment group watched a 17-minute video prior to the sexual assault forensic exam. The video was created to reduce distress during the exam as well as provide education about preventing PTSD, substance abuse, depression, and Panic Disorder. The video described the forensic exam and instructed viewers on how to recognize and implement techniques to reduce avoidance. Mood control and controlling anxiety levels were also discussed and modeled along with exposure exercises. Results indicated that distress during the forensic exam was reduced for the treatment group.

Critical Incident Stress Debriefing

Critical incident stress debriefings (CISDs) are single-session group debriefings designed to be used with primary and secondary victims of crisis and trauma (victims of crime or terrorism, emergency service workers, police officers; Mitchell, 1983, 1988). Sessions incorporate a seven-step structured group discussion: introduction of team members, process, and expectations from group; group members describing their role in the incident (without identifying their related feelings); discussion of each member's thoughts and reactions; discussion of emotional reactions; reframing the event; teaching about normal reactions and basic stress management; and summary of the discussions.

CISDs have been used worldwide in response to the psychological needs of victims and service providers. Twenty years after the debriefings were introduced, few studies have found evidence that the method produces positive outcomes (decreasing PTSD symptoms and diagnoses), with some studies showing negative outcomes (Rose, Bisson, & Wessely, 2003). Caution should be used when considering this intervention to address posttraumatic stress symptoms due to the potential to cause harm (see Lewis, 2003, for a comprehensive review of the evidence). At present, CISD is not recommended as a preventive program.

Agoraphobics in Motion Self-Help Group

Agoraphobics in motion (AIM) was founded over 20 years ago by an individual suffering from agoraphobia and Panic Disorder as an educational, supportive, and therapeutic (nonprofessional) program. Usually at each meeting (held in community-based locations), guest speakers make a presentation about some aspect of an anxiety disorder. Field trips facilitate gradual reentry into feared situations. The organization has a web site, an Internet message board, a newsletter, and a pen pal program (for the housebound). Its message is that recovery is possible. AIM is but one example of numerous consumer-based self-help groups available for individuals who suffer from crippling anxiety, regardless of whether they have been formally diagnosed or whether they receive professional care. See www.aim-hq.org.

PRACTICE AND POLICY IMPLICATIONS

The anxiety literature has focused on assessment and treatment but has neglected the development and validation of prevention models for adult anxiety disorders. A limited number of studies have empirically tested prevention programs for individuals at risk for the development of an anxiety disorder, as well as for the general public. However, none of these programs can be said to rise to the level of an evidence-based preventive intervention. This renders direct practice and policy implications more speculative than empirical.

It does seem clear that the widespread failure to effectively educate the public about anxiety disorders tends to promote ignorance and stigma around this significant mental health problem. The social and financial costs associated with the anxiety disorders are considerable and rising, justifying some additional efforts at prevention. Their prevalence justifies an increased focus as well on the provision of specialized training for health care providers, ideally at the level of graduate education, and less optimally through evidence-based continuing education programs. Attention must be given to the cost-effectiveness of prevention programs, especially those involved in primary prevention aimed at the general public and funded by taxpayers' dollars. Compelling evidence is required regarding the numbers needed to be reached through such programs and the associated reduction in the development of anxiety disorders and their psychosocial sequelae (including functional impairments) relative to the costs incurred. Is a billion-dollar prevention program that effectively prevents five persons from developing OCD worth it? How about 500, or even 5,000 cases? For prevention programs in the anxiety disorders (as well as in all other fields) to be seen as justifiable, relatively unambiguous data are required to show that the public receives value for money, in addition to being helpful to small numbers of individuals. As yet, no compelling theory exists for either the etiology of the anxiety disorders or the possible efficacy of prevention programs. While these lacunae do not prohibit the development of effective prevention efforts, they do tend to inhibit advances in the field. We have a long way to go.

REFERENCES

American Psychiatric Association. (2000). *Diagnostic and statistical manual of mental disorders* (4th ed., text rev.). Washington, DC: Author.

Antony, M., & Swinson, R. (2000). *Phobic disorders and panic in adults: A guide to assessment and treatment.* Washington, DC: American Psychological Association.

Brown, P. (2003, September 6). In the shadow of fear. *New Scientist,* p. 30.

Clark, J., & Wardman, W. (1985). *Agoraphobia: A clinical and personal account.* Oxford, England: Pergamon Press.

Craske, M. G., & Zucker, B. G. (2001). Prevention of anxiety disorders: A model for intervention. *Applied and Preventive Psychology, 10,* 155–175.

Datilio, F. M. (2001). Crisis intervention techniques for panic disorders. *American Journal of Psychotherapy, 55,* 388–405.

Fausel, D. F. (1995). Stress inoculation training for step couples. *Marriage and Family Review, 21,* 137–155.

Foa, E. B., Hearst-Ikeda, D., & Perry, K. J. (1995). Evaluation of a brief cognitive-behavioral program for the prevention of chronic PTSD in recent assault victims. *Journal of Consulting and Clinical Psychology, 6,* 948–955.

Gardenswartz, C. A., & Craske, M. G. (2001). Prevention of panic disorders. *Behavior Therapy, 32,* 725–737.

Greenberg, P. E., Sisitsky, T., & Kessler, R. C. (1999). The economic burden of anxiety disorders in the 1990s. *Journal of Clinical Psychiatry, 60,* 427–435.

Leighton, A. H. (1987). Primary prevention of psychiatric disorders. *Acta Psychiatrica Scandinavica, 76,* 7–13.

Lewis, S. J. (2003). Do one-shot preventive interventions for PTSD work: A systematic research synthesis of psychological debriefings. *Aggression and Violent Behavior, 8,* 329–343.

Long, C., & Van Stavel, R. (1995). Effects of exercise training on anxiety: A meta-analysis. *Journal of Applied Sport Psychology, 7,* 167–189.

Mitchell, J. T. (1983). When disaster strikes: The critical incident stress debriefing process. *Journal of Emergency Medical Services, 8,* 36–39.

Mitchell, J. T. (1988). Development and functions of a critical incident stress debriefing team. *Journal of Emergency Medical Services, 13,* 43–46.

National Institute of Mental Health. (1999). *Anxiety disorder research: Fact sheet.* Bethesda, MD: Department of Health and Human Services, National Institute of Health.

Resnick, H., Acierno, R., Holmes, M., Kilpatrick, D. G., & Jager, N. (1999). Prevention of post-rape psychopathology: Preliminary findings of a controlled acute rape treatment study. *Journal of Anxiety Disorders, 13,* 359–370.

Rose, S., Bisson, J., & Wessely, S. (2003). A systematic review of single-session psychological interventions (debriefing) following trauma. *Psychotherapy and Psychosomatics, 72,* 176–184.

Schiraldi, G. R., & Brown, S. L. (2001). Primary prevention for mental health: Results of an exploratory cognitive-behavioral college course. *Journal of Primary Prevention, 22,* 55–67.

Seligman, M. E. P., Schulman, P., & DeRubeis, R. J. (1999). The prevention of depression and anxiety. *Prevention and Treatment, 2.* Retrieved January 22, 2004, from http://journals.apa.org/prevention/volume2/pre0020008a.html.

Substance Abuse and Mental Health Services Administration. (2003). *Science-based prevention programs and principles.* Rockville, MD: Department of Health and Human Services.

Thyer, B. A. (1993). Childhood separation anxiety disorder and adult-onset agoraphobia: Review of evidence. In C. G. Last (Ed.), *Anxiety across the lifespan: A development perspective on anxiety and the anxiety disorders* (pp. 128–147). New York: Springer.

Thyer, B. A. (2002). Treatment plans for clients with social phobia. In A. R. Roberts & G. I. Greene (Eds.), *Social workers' desk reference* (pp. 346–352). New York: Oxford University Press.

Thyer, B. A., Tomlin, P., Curtis, G. C., Cameron, O. G., & Nesse, R. (1995). Diagnostic and gender differences in the expressed fears of anxious patients. *Journal of Behavior Therapy and Experimental Psychiatry, 16,* 111–115.

Timmerman, I. G. H., Emmelkamp, P. M. G., & Sanderman, R. (1998). The effects of a stress-management training program in individuals at risk in the community at large. *Behaviour Research and Therapy, 36,* 863–875.

U.S. Surgeon General's Report on Mental Health. (1999). *Mental health: A report of the Surgeon General: Executive summary.* Rockville, MD: U.S. Department of Health and Human Services.

Chapter 3

COGNITIVE LOSS

BERT HAYSLIP JR. AND ROBERT J. MAIDEN

For almost 2 decades, cognitive aging researchers have subscribed to a view that suggests aging-related decrements in functioning are not inevitable, and consequently, can be compensated for via interventions designed to improve intellectual-cognitive functioning. Such a view reflects a "decrement with compensation" perspective on cognitive aging (Kramer & Willis, 2002), wherein declines in functioning are minimized or eliminated completely via efforts by the individual or others or via a change in the environment in which the older individual is embedded. Such a view also reflects a "levels of intervention" approach to minimizing or preventing cognitive loss (Danish, 1981), where efforts to alter functioning could be directed to the individual, one's family and friends or coworkers, one's immediate environment (home, work, neighborhood), or society at large. It also reflects an approach to cognitive aging emphasizing the continued plasticity (see Baltes & Danish, 1980) of older persons so that, despite their age, individuals are equally amenable to change and receptive to interventions designed to minimize or prevent cognitive loss.

Our discussion emphasizes the importance of the distinction between primary, secondary, and tertiary prevention (Baltes & Danish, 1980) and a pluralism of approaches to dealing with age-related cognitive losses in the domains of intellectual functioning, memory, and everyday competence. In this context, *primary prevention* reflects actions to prevent the occurrence of cognitive loss; such actions might be initiated in young adulthood or midlife. *Secondary prevention* emphasizes the early treatment of an existing problem to reduce its intensity of duration. *Tertiary prevention* is rehabilitative in nature; efforts to intervene are directed to returning the individual to a normal level of functioning. In these respects, prevention and intervention are not only preemptive or restorative in nature, but they also help to generate new knowledge about the process of cognitive aging, with some criterion or goal (i.e., optimal, productive, or successful aging) in mind. *Pluralism* (see Baltes, 1997) reflects the assumption that such losses may be alleviated or prevented altogether via any number of diverse methods that are, for our purposes here, psychosocial or biomedical in nature.

Important to our discussion are the distinctions by Gordon (1983, 1987), which overlap with those just discussed, between *universal* preventive interventions, targeting the general public or those not deemed to be at risk for decline; *selective* preventive interventions, targeting those at risk for experiencing cognitive decline at some time in the future; and *indicated* preventive interventions, focusing on high-risk individuals who have yet to experience decline but nevertheless have minimal or detectable signs of such loss or who may be biologically predisposed toward experiencing declines in cognitive functioning. In these respects, universal interventions at multiple levels that are geared to educating persons about what has been deemed healthy, productive, or successful aging (Morrow, Howell, Hinterlong, & Sherraden, 2001; Rowe & Kahn, 1998; Valliant, 2002) are quite relevant.

Selective interventions targeting persons who are depressed (see Blazer, 2002; Gallo, Rebok, Tennstedt, Wadley, & Horgas, 2003), in poor cardiovascular health, or suffering from either preclinical dementia (see Peterson, 2003) or Alzheimer's disease can either minimize the rate of decline or lessen its future severity. Such efforts are also salient for those individuals who are not aging well, cognitively speaking (i.e., persons who have some impairment), but who have yet to manifest symptoms of dementia. Such persons may have learned a variety of compensatory techniques to mask what might otherwise be debilitating declines in intellect, memory function, or everyday competence. It is to the picture of age-related change in these domains of cognition that we now turn.

TRENDS AND INCIDENCE: AGE-RELATED CHANGES IN COGNITIVE FUNCTIONING

Understanding the nature of age-related growth and decline in learning, memory, and intelligence is key to the development of interventions designed to either minimize decline or enhance functioning. Moreover, recognizing the selective and/or differential nature of such changes is key to the development of an accurate, nonstereotypical view of age-related changes in cognitive functioning.

Learning and Memory

Critical to the distinction between universal, selective, and indicated prevention, it is important to distinguish between normal, maturational changes in memory skills that are independent of disease, termed *age-associated memory*

impairments (Crook et al., 1986), and pathological changes in memory, for example, those due to Alzheimer's disease or multi-infarct dementia (Cherry & Smith,
1998). As age differences in memory depend on the nature of the memory system
and associated processes, what it is that one is trying to remember, and how one
assesses memory (Cherry & Smith, 1998), there are great individual differences
among adults in the nature of their memory skills (Powell, 1994).

Reflecting the distinction between sensory, primary, secondary, and tertiary
memory (see Craik, 2000), there appear to be few clear age differences or age
changes regarding sensory memory, which is preattentive in nature and whose
content dissipates rapidly (Kausler, 1994). Indeed, it may be difficult to demonstrate that sensory memory even exists for elderly adults who may be experiencing serious sensory or attentional deficits. Although its capacity is small,
primary memory plays an important role in the control and assimilation of information (Craik, 2000), serving more as a temporary holding and organizing
reservoir, and is essentially passive in nature (Craik, 2000). When material to be
remembered exceeds primary memory, it enters the secondary (or working)
memory store, whose capacity is less limited. Working memory reflects the simultaneous processing of two tasks, one of which must be stored while the other
is being actively processed (e.g., having to remember a guest's name at a party
while being introduced to someone else).

In general, there seems to be, at best, a moderate age decrement in primary
memory, reflected in simple, relatively effortless, overlearned performance
(Craik, 2000; Kausler, 1994). In contrast, age differences favor young adults in
complex tasks, which often tap secondary or working memory (Craik, 2000).
These decrements have been attributed to the inefficient use of attentional resources, the slower processing of information, or a lack of inhibitory processes
that would otherwise screen out unwanted information (see Salthouse, 1993). Tertiary or long-term memory, whose storehouse is in theory limitless and permanent, refers to recall of remote events or extended recall for recent events.
Although age differences in tertiary memory do exist, they tend to favor older
adults (Smith, 1996). Deficits with age in tertiary memory are difficult to
demonstrate, however, given the confounding of the age of the individual and the
age (datedness) of that which is to be recalled (Botwinick, 1984).

As opposed to memory structures, an approach emphasizing memory
processes explains *how* material is transferred from one memory store to another. *Registration* is a prerequisite for further processing information, and thus
older adults who suffer from sensory loss are at a disadvantage. Important in
this respect, *encoding* refers to the process of giving meaning to information
after it has been registered, and *storage* suggests that information, having been
encoded in some form, is then organized in a hierarchic (general-to-specific)
pattern. Older adults are less likely to spontaneously organize or use verbal or

visual mediators, and they store information less efficiently (Kausler, 1994). *Retrieval* reflects the "getting out" of the information that has been registered, encoded, and stored. Research suggests that retrieval (i.e., the provision of meaningful cues) is essential to both secondary and tertiary memory performance (Craik, 2000). These age effects parallel the distinctions between episodic memory (context-specific detail) and semantic memory (knowledge apart from the context in which such knowledge was acquired; Craik, 2000). Generally speaking, age deficits in learning and memory tasks are greatest when such tasks require effortful processing, reflecting the demands on working memory (Park, 2000). Indeed, age deficits in executive processing have been linked to memory strategy implementation and recall performance (Bryan, Luszcz, & Pointer, 1999).

Learning and Memory in Everyday Life

Memory difficulties obviously manifest themselves in everyday life. In this context, *practical memory* refers to use of one's skills to cope with everyday demands, and the use of memorial skills is influenced by beliefs about and estimates of memory, termed *metamemory* (Dixon, 1989). Related to metamemory is (1) memory self-efficacy—the confidence one has in one's memory skills; (2) memory management—the strategies and techniques one employs to make best use of one's memory; (3) memory remediation—the efforts one makes to improve memory; and (4) memory fears—concerns about memory loss that affect one personally (Reese, Cherry, & Norris, 1998). Reese et al. found older persons reported that they could remember important dates (birthdays, anniversaries) but not names, used external memory aids most often, wanted to improve their memory for names and for verbal information, and linked the loss of their independence to memory failures. Such findings may be a function of their greater knowledge of and attention to memory aging (Reese, Cherry, & Copeland, 2000).

It is worth noting that in interpreting what we know about normal memory function and aging, some older persons who have been included in such work are in fact suffering from preclinical dementia, whose impairments are not typically detected by conventional screening tools, where such losses may precede diagnosis by at least 10 years (Slivinski, Hofer, Hall, Buschke, & Lipton, 2003).

Age-Related Changes in Intelligence

Early cross-sectional studies found an age decline in overall Wechsler Adult Intelligence Scale (WAIS) performance (see Botwinick, 1984), and longitudinal studies typically display increases in WAIS performance with age (see Schaie,

1996). The most common picture is what is termed a "classic aging pattern in intelligence" (Botwinick, 1984), where a decline in performance scores, relative to stability in verbal scores, is seen.

Utilizing Thurstone's theory of primary mental abilities (PMA; i.e., spatial ability [visualizing figures in space], perceptual speed, numerical ability, verbal relations, word fluency, memory, and induction [predicting the next letter or number in a sequence of letters or numbers]), Schaie conducted perhaps the most extensive studies of adult intellectual development to date (see Schaie, 1979), beginning with a series of cross-sectional and longitudinal studies that began in 1956. Data from the first cross-sectional study conducted in 1956 suggested that different types of abilities demonstrated diverse age-related peaks of functioning. Schaie found PMA reasoning to peak most early, versus space, verbal fluency, word fluency, and number, which all peaked later. Moreover, longitudinal (1956–1963) findings suggested that age-related changes in intelligence were minimal until persons reached their sixties. Schaie's data suggested that cohort differences were more important in explaining the cross-sectional or longitudinal age effects found for many abilities than was chronological age (Schaie & Willis, 1996), where findings also indicated that in early adulthood and in very late adulthood, age effects on abilities within cohorts might also be substantial. Schaie's analyses suggested positive cohort effects, that is, more favorable performance for successively younger cohorts, for verbal meaning, space, and reasoning. For PMA number, cohort effects were minimal, while for word fluency, cohort effects were slightly negative, where younger cohorts scored more poorly. Thus, different cohorts age intellectually in unique ways. As Schaie's data also indicate that declines in ability are largely restricted to those 70 or older, such declines, when they exist, are restricted to the very old and are more apparent for the mechanics of intellect (fluid ability, working memory, speed of processing) than for its pragmatics (crystallized knowledge, wisdom; Baltes, 1997; Singer, Verhaeghen, Ghisletta, Lindenberger, & Baltes, 2003).

In this respect, the distinction between crystallized (Gc) and fluid (Gf) abilities (Horn & Hofer, 1992; Horn & Null, 1997) reflects the fact that Gc is determined by purposeful, "acculturational" learning provided by societal institutions, such as the home environment or the school (and, by implication, the work environment). In contrast, Gf fluctuates with the demands made in novel situations and is determined by idiosyncratic, largely self-determined causal learning influences (Horn, 1978). Gf generally increases and then declines over the life span, whereas Gc generally increases or remains stable over the adult years (Horn & Hofer, 1992; Horn & Null, 1997). In this respect, Ackerman (2000) has investigated domain-specific knowledge, an attribute of Gc in young and middle-aged persons. With increased age, scores on 10 of 18 knowledge domains increased, and such scores were positively related to Gc.

Considerable variation can be observed both within and across individuals in Gf and Gc functioning due to effort, fatigue, or anxiety (Hayslip, 1989), personality-related interests (Ackerman, 1996), or attentional lapses (Horn, 1978). Generally speaking, age declines in intelligence are seen in terms of the speed, capacity, or efficiency of central processing resources (e.g., working memory, attention, processing speed; Salthouse, 1998).

Everyday Intelligence and Aging

In 1957, Demming and Pressy developed tests "with content and tasks more natural or 'indigenous' to adult life" (p. 144) in response to the inadequacy of then current tests to measure adult abilities. They found that people scored progressively lower on traditional tests of intelligence across the life span, but the reverse pattern was evidenced on their "indigenous" tests. Recently, however, the adaptive aspects of everyday intelligence have been emphasized, such as the skills one uses in shopping, map reading, cooking, reading schedules and ads, and understanding directions (Deihl, 1998; Willis, 1996). Allaire and Marsiske (2002) differentiated well- and ill-defined measures of everyday skill (defined in terms of the amount of means-end information provided for solution) and found that while the former were more strongly related to basic measured cognitive abilities, both sets of everyday skills predicted everyday instrumental functioning (IADLs).

Among community-residing elderly persons, 20% to 30% report having difficulty with at least one of the seven domains of independent living (Fillenbaum, 1985, 1990), though to a certain extent, these estimates vary by age, gender, and the nature of the IADL considered, whose frequency of performance does vary (Fillenbaum, 1985; Stone & Murtaugh, 1990). Indeed, Schaie and Willis (1996) have found IADL performance to decline over time. Overall, although estimates of some degree of IADL disability range from 5% to 15% among community-residing elderly (Jette, 1995), there remains that proportion of the elderly population who either do not accurately report the extent of their difficulty with IADLs or do not volunteer for survey research.

For many elderly individuals, the loss of everyday competence may stem from a variety of sources; notable among these is the presence of disease (Jette, 1995; Willis, 1991). In addition, an awareness of losses in everyday competence is a prerequisite for conscious, deliberate efforts at compensation (Backman & Dixon, 1992). Older persons whose self-esteem is closely linked to their ability to remain independent may be especially prone to anxiety about the loss of everyday living skills. Such persons, paradoxically, have already invested greater effort into maintaining their skills as a function of their concern about losing such skills (Hayslip, 1988). For older individuals, the management of anxiety about the loss of their everyday living skills may represent a means of compensating for declines. Significantly, depression is as common a determinant or correlate of disability and deficits in everyday skills as are impaired cognitive skills (Gallo et al., 2003; Kemp & Mitchell, 1992). In this respect, Rothermund and Brandstadter (2003) found that while older persons were successful in their efforts to compensate for declines in functional skills up to age 70, thereafter, while equally contented with their level of functional performance, they downgraded their expectations for performance as a function of the success of their efforts to compensate for such declines. In effect, older persons had adapted to changes in their skills by adopting more lenient standards for performance, wherein low performance expectations are set a priori, protecting the individual from failure.

Clearly, belief systems and associated behaviors may undermine individual efforts to maintain everyday competence. Acknowledging the powerful role of age stereotypes (i.e., that with aging comes dependence) and personal goals (i.e., to avoid becoming dependent on others by maintaining independent living skills) is critical to successful efforts in enhancing skill levels in later life (Bieman-Copland, Bouchard-Ryan, & Cassano, 1998).

RISK FACTORS AFFECTING COGNITION IN ADULTHOOD

Given the magnitude of individual differences with age (Nelson & Dannefer, 1992), it should not be surprising that there are a number of factors influencing the extent to which declines in cognition accompany increased age. Indeed, Baltes and Lindenberger (1997) assert that sensory abilities are the bedrock on which intelligence rests, and older persons who are in poor physical and mental health tend to perform more poorly on a measure of fluid ability (M. Perlmutter & Nyquist, 1990). Zelinski, Crimmins, Reynolds, and Seeman (1998) found high blood pressure, strokes, and diabetes to adversely influence intelligence later in life (see also Brady, Spiro, McClinchey-Berroth, Milberg, & Gaziano, 2001; Fahlander et al., 2000).

Personality processes may also impact cognitive performance, so that persons who have adaptive personalities either age better intellectually, or intelligence may permit more flexibility in adulthood. In one study, older persons who were more anxious about their intellectual skills had higher Gc scores, utilizing defense mechanisms that protect them from feelings of self-worthlessness and failure and a loss of control over their real-life environments (Hayslip, 1988).

Likewise, older individuals with positive self-efficacy expectations who perceive difficult tasks as challenges and see failure as related to their effort and under their control, function more effectively (Artistico, Cervone, & Pezzuli, 2003), and age better cognitively (Albert et al., 1995). Indeed, lessened self-efficacy is related to more negative perceptions of one's functional skills among older persons (Seeman, Unger, McAvay, & deLeon, 1999). In this respect, the activation of negative self-stereotypes can directly undermine cognitive functioning (Hess, Auman, Colcombe, & Rahhal, 2003; Levy, 2003). However, decrements in perceived changes (consistent underestimates of) in one's ability over time may also contribute to declines in intelligence (Schaie, Willis, & O'Hanlon, 1994); such changes may be a function of the negative age stereotypes older persons encounter as they age. Indeed, Levy, Hausdorff, Hencke, and Weir (2000) found that older persons subliminally exposed to positive age stereotypes exhibited a more adaptive cardiovascular response (blood pressure, heart rate) to stress than those exposed to negative age stereotypes.

Considering risk factors associated with age-related cognitive declines underscores the fact that individual differences in rates of cognitive change are extremely powerful (Christensen et al., 1999; Wilson et al., 2002). Such variability is a function of cardiovascular health (Zelinski et al., 1998), depression (Christensen et al., 1999), and level of education (Albert et al., 1995; Cagney & Lauderdale, 2002). Schooler, Mulatu, and Oates (1999) suggest that a cognitively challenging work situation during adulthood may be beneficial; persons in such environments increase their level of cognitive functioning to a greater extent than do those who are not embedded in challenging, complex environments that require the active engagement of their skills (see also Schooler & Mulatu, 2001).

SELECTIVE PREVENTIVE INTERVENTIONS: ENHANCING LEARNING AND MEMORY IN ADULTHOOD

For the most part, efforts to impact memory function among older adults are properly considered examples of selective preventive intervention strategies. Older persons recall the fewest correct words when they are not given sufficient time to respond, referred to as task pacing (Canestrari, 1968); increasing the time available to search and retrieve a correct response lessens age differences in learning and memory (Monge & Hultsch, 1971). In addition, encouraging and training adults in the use of verbal and visual mediators seems to help memory encoding (Canestrari, 1968). In this respect, Robertson-Tchabo, Hausman, and Arenberg (1976) had success with the method of loci, where the learner is asked to associate each familiar loci with words to be recalled. Unfortunately, in the long term (3 years after training), older learners frequently abandon the method of loci even though it has been effective (Anschultz, Camp, Markley, & Kramer, 1987), though the evidence for the durability of memory training is inconsistent (see Pushkar & Arbuckle, 1998, for a review; Scogin & Bienias, 1988). Likewise, specific instructions to organize the material, for example, using the alphabet or creating categories, can enhance learning and memory, as has the provision of cues to aid in the retrieval of information to be recalled (see Bieman-Copland et al., 1998).

A meta-analysis of a variety of memory training studies concluded that such training was indeed effective (see Verhaeghen, 2000), but that no form of training was superior to any other. Rasmusson, Rebok, Bylsma, and Brandt (1999) concluded that any form of mnemonically stimulating activity, rather than specific memory strategy training, is most effective with healthy older persons, and Woolverton, Scogin, Shackelford, Black, and Duke (2001) found that more intensive, less target-specific forms of memory training were most effective. Troyer (2001) found that educating older persons about memory in concert with the provision of memory strategies was effective in increasing memory knowledge and memory performance.

Helping older adults learn to manage their anxiety about failure is also very important (Hayslip, 1989; Wetherell, Reynolds, Gatz, & Pedersen, 2002). Moreover, if one is depressed, becoming fatigued makes the learning and retention of new material particularly difficult (Hayslip, Kennelly, & Maloy, 1990). Rasmusson et al. (1999) found that although older persons who completed three memory training programs did report fewer depressive symptoms and better memory performance, the two effects were independent of one another (see also Hill & Vandervoort, 1992). Older adults exposed to negative stereotypes regarding memory and aging performed more poorly in a recall task, and those who valued their memory ability most were most affected in this respect (Hess et al., 2003).

Designing tasks and environments that make fewer demands on the effortful processing of information also constitutes an important type of preventive intervention to either minimize age-related deficits in working memory or maintain functioning over time. Thus, "environmental support" for many older persons who are experiencing minimal or unmeasurable memory decline is a key form of universal prevention that can and should be utilized by older persons, their families, and practitioners. For example, altering the environment physically (reducing glare, reducing sensory overload by limiting background noise, and arranging furniture to facilitate interaction) can be helpful (Bieman-Copland et al., 1998).

As age-related changes in memory are relative to the nature of the information to be learned and recalled and the abilities and motives of the individual, the choice and design of preventive or remedial interventions directed at older adults must be flexible. In his review of memory training with older persons, Verhaeghen (2000) concludes that the effects of most types of such interventions are robust yet narrow in scope, vary by individual difference characteristics, and are of long duration. Thus, there is both good news and bad news regarding memory training effects—a trade-off between specificity of training effects and duration, as well as such effects varying by persons.

SELECTIVE PREVENTIVE INTERVENTIONS: OPTIMIZING INTELLIGENCE IN ADULTHOOD

On the assumption that declines in intelligence with age are not irreversible, a series of cognitive training studies growing out of project ADEPT (Baltes & Willis, 1982) demonstrated that the fluid ability (Gf) performance of older persons can be enhanced via cognitive skill training, emphasizing as criteria a hierarchical pattern of training transfer and its maintenance over time (see review by Verhaeghen, 2000). Indeed, Schaie and Willis (1986) have demonstrated that training can reverse 14-year declines in PMA performance. Over a 7-year interval, older persons trained to enhance their intellectual performance exceeded their original levels.

In his review of plasticity and cognitive aging intervention studies, Verhaeghen (2000) concluded that ability training's effects are fairly durable, and that such ability-specific training (figural relations, inductive reasoning, spatial orientation) in some cases provides greater benefit than does practice alone. However, practice alone also produces substantial gains in performance (Hayslip, 1989; Verhaeghen, 2000). Hayslip utilized both ADEPT induction training and stress inoculation to change Gf performance, finding that (1) induction training and stress inoculation were both effective, (2) the range of training transfer was very narrow, and (3) training effects for the stress inoculation intervention seemed to vary with the difficulty of the task and persons' willingness to access the anxiety-coping techniques they had been taught to use. Hayslip, Maloy, and Kohl (1995) found that booster sessions were necessary to maintain the 3-year effects of specific rule-based training, and that such persons still performed worse on measures of fluid ability than did those who received anxiety-reduction training. Collectively, practice and anxiety-reduction training seems to activate skills that already exist rather than develop new skills (as might be assumed with ability-specific training). While the durability of cognitive interventions or practice is critical (Verhaeghen, 2000), subject to either (1) reinforcement by others for utilizing previously learned skills or for the exercise of one's skills via practice or (2) experience with everyday problems requiring the use of such skills (see Pushkar, Arbuckle, Conway, Chaikelson, & Maag, 1997), the long-term effects of any training may or may not be evident.

UNIVERSAL PREVENTION: USE IT OR LOSE IT?

Whether the benefits of such practice are equivalent to the "use it or lose it" mentality that pervades many laypersons' beliefs about their skills is dubious. In these respects, although Hultsch, Hertzog, Small, and Dixon (1999) found limited support for the fact that a cognitively engaged lifestyle buffers persons' decline, they also found that persons who involve themselves in intellectually challenging activities experience less cognitive change over time, as did Gold et al. (1995), based on a 40-year longitudinal study. Similarly qualified evidence for the impact of mental and physical activity on cognition was found by MacKinnon, Christensen, Hofer, Korten, and Jorm (2003), and limited evidence for the positive impact of everyday activity involvement on adult cognition has also been found by Aarsten, Smits, Van Tilburg, Knipscheer, and Deeg (2002). Masunaga and Horn (2001) found that purposeful and well-designed practice, that is, expertise, was effective in this respect, yet the results of Salthouse, Berish, and Miles (2002) clearly do not support the benefits of cognitive activity as a hedge against decline. Moreover, Pushkar et al. (1997) found no support for the hypothesis that competence, but not engaging in difficult everyday activities, predicted well-being.

UNIVERSAL AND SELECTIVE PREVENTIVE INTERVENTIONS: EVERYDAY COGNITION

In light of the discussion of the antecedents of declines in everyday cognition, Deihl (1998) cites preliminary findings based on a sample of older rehabilitation patients that suggest persons who are unaware of their deficits have greater deficits in their independent living skills. Viewed recursively (Willis, 1996), enhanced self-efficacy can be both a determinant and a consequence of improvements in everyday skill. From both a universal and a selective preventive perspective, the use of interventions that affect either the extent to which individuals over- or underestimate their need for assistance with IADLs, react to the presence of an IADL-related disability, or influence the extent to which individuals are amenable to remediation, are valuable. In this respect, Jette (1995) and Schulz and Martire (1999) discuss counseling as a buffer to influence (reduce) the risk of disability. Social, behavioral, psychological, and environmental factors are defined as risk variables in predisposing some individuals and not others to disability, and intra-individual factors such as specific psychosocial attributes and coping skills (e.g., positive or negative affect, control beliefs, cognitive adaptive strategies) are identified as mediating factors influencing the process of disablement (Jette, 1995). To the extent that disability can be prevented, postponed, or remediated, there is also the advantage of saving health care costs (see Deihl, 1998) and the more efficient use of social and rehabilitative services for those who require outside assistance to maintain an independent or semi-independent lifestyle.

While interventions directed to changing the physical environment (e.g., relying on a microwave in lieu of actually preparing a meal) or the social environment (e.g., by home delivery of precooked meals) may be helpful, interventions directed at the individual are also important. Krause (1997) has stressed that everyday competence needs to be understood not only in terms of physical health status and cognitive functioning, but also in terms of the perceptions and behaviors of others (or, in this case, one's perceptions of others' perceptions and behavior) as well as the elder's self-perceptions. Indeed, there is much support for a model of everyday competence that has as its foundation basic cognitive abilities and emphasizing the domain specificity of both basic cognitive abilities and everyday skills (Allaire & Marsiske, 1999; Schaie & Willis, 1996). Allaire and Marsiske, for example, found a strong and consistent pattern of relationships between psychometric skills, inductive reasoning, working memory, basic knowledge, and parallel everyday cognitive measures.

In contrast to this perspective, there is indeed evidence to indicate that older adults are anxious or concerned about their ability to perform everyday tasks critical to independent living. Hayslip, Servaty, and Ward (1996) and Hayslip, Servaty, Ward, and Blackburn (1995) surveyed nearly 400 community-residing elderly who rated 100 task examples along the dimensions of worry, intellectual vitality, everyday relevance, and competence, and found that such ratings were related to measures of intellectual self-efficacy, needs for cognitive stimulation and activity, self-rated everyday cognitive difficulties, locus of control, and anxiety. This suggests that older persons worried more about their ability to perform everyday tasks, ascribed more everyday importance (functionality) to such tasks, deemed them to be more critical to their intellectual health and vitality, and, surprisingly, felt more competent in their ability at present to complete such tasks well. All of these judgments were contrasted with "nonecological" measures of short-term memory, Gc, and Gf. This suggests that older persons are concerned about losing those skills that are intact at present, setting the stage for universal, if not selective, preventive interventions. Hayslip et al. (1996) also found that there are substantial relationships between worry, vitality, competence, functionality, and performance on the ETS Basic Reading Skills test.

Significantly, everyday functionality was *negatively* related to Gf performance. Self-rated worry was also negatively related to generalized self-efficacy, need for cognitive stimulation, and intellectual self-efficacy, and positively related to state anxiety and everyday cognitive failures. In contrast, self-rated everyday competence was positively related to measures of self-efficacy and negatively related to anxiety and everyday cognitive failures.

More direct evidence regarding the relationship between anxiety and everyday skill has been gathered by Hayslip, Elias, Barta, and Henderson (1998). They found that older persons who had greater concerns about their current and future levels of everyday functioning scored more poorly on a variety of measures assessing everyday cognition and reported more everyday cognitive failures. Such persons also were more depressed, were more state anxious, and had less intellectual self-efficacy. For persons with higher self-rated everyday task efficacy, these relationships were in the opposite direction. In a separate study of 30 VA outpatients (Hayslip et al., 2000), these relationships were essentially replicated: Persons with more everyday task concerns and less everyday task self-efficacy performed more poorly, were more state anxious, and reported more everyday cognitive failures.

The most direct evidence for the impact of anxiety-reduction training on everyday skill in older persons has been gathered by Hayslip, Galt, et al. (1998), who contrasted five-session (1½ hours/session) stress inoculation training with a waiting list control condition regarding impact on everyday skill. Hayslip, Galt, et al. found that the extent to which persons concerned about present and future declines in everyday functioning were anxious, depressed, or self-efficacious interacted with the efficacy of stress inoculation versus benefiting from practice. It was also found that for persons who were younger, male, less healthy, and less highly educated, training gains were greater (Hayslip, Galt, et al., 1998).

Regarding stress inoculation, some findings (Hayslip, Galt, et al., 1998) indicated that persons who, for example, are more depressed or preoccupied with decline may not utilize the cognitive restructuring and relaxation techniques as effectively as they might and therefore do not evidence the same degree of everyday skill improvement. For such persons, more intensive training, a longer training program, or the provision of booster or supplemental training may be beneficial. In contrast, these results in part also suggest that some persons paradoxically may be more attuned to the possibility of decline in their everyday skills and perhaps have taken steps to deal with such feelings. These persons may benefit more from such training. Interestingly, there was some limited evidence to suggest that persons in the training group gained to a greater extent regarding an index of everyday self-efficacy (being able to teach others) relative to controls, and that gains in generalized self-efficacy were greater in the training group. In a separate analysis of the VA outpatient data, persons in a stress inoculation training group tended to be more likely to evidence immediate (1-week) gains in everyday skill than did waiting list controls. Project ACTIVE, a large-scale research effort funded by the National Institute on Aging (NIA), which explored the impact of a variety of *cognitive* interventions (e.g., cognitive skills training, speeded performance, memory training) on everyday cognition, found *no short-term impact whatsoever* on older persons' everyday competence as a function of the three types of cognitive interventions (Ball et al., 2002).

INDICATED PREVENTIVE INTERVENTIONS

Camp and his colleagues have demonstrated that after as few as two brief training sessions, memory-impaired elderly persons could remember the name of a staff person using the spaced retrieval technique. Camp, Bird, and Cherry (2000) provided an extensive review of research detailing the potential of spaced retrieval for persons with dementia. This technique initially involves presenting the client with the name to be learned and the client's repeating the name, and subsequently progressively varying the recall interval with every correct answer. The advantages of this technique are that clients can experience immediate success at remembering and that it is less cognitively demanding than other, more elaborate memory-enhancement techniques such as the method of loci. Several studies targeting similarly constructed memory interventions with persons suffering from Alzheimer's disease have reported some success (e.g., Arkin, 2000; Cherry, 1999; Dixon, Hopp, Cohen, DeFrias, & Bachman, 2003), as have studies focusing on persons with mild cognitive impairment (Rapp, Brenes, & Marsh, 2002).

BIOMEDICAL APPROACHES TO COGNITIVE IMPAIRMENT: UNIVERSAL PREVENTION

Among the possible sources of cognitive loss associated with normal aging are biomedical problems such as hypertension and cardiovascular disease (CVD) and neurodegenerative diseases such as Alzheimer's disease and vascular dementia. Researchers and medical professionals have proposed a variety of biological interventions to block or minimize the cognitive losses that are frequently associated with getting older (see Winett, 1995).

Blood Pressure and Cardiovascular Disease

As discussed earlier, there is an association between the physiological factors of hypertension and CVD and cognitive loss (see Hertzog, Schaie, & Gribbon,

1978), though the exact biological mechanism that produces these decrements in cognitive functioning is unknown. Several authors (Botwinick, 1984; Hertzog et al., 1978) have conjectured that the causal mechanism is hypoxia as a result of reduced blood flow to the brain. These speculations foreshadowed a host of studies examining the relationship of oxygenation, increased blood flow, and cognitive functioning in the relatively healthy aged. Oxygenation is considered to be critical for older people as they require more blood flow and higher oxygen metabolism levels (Jennings, Nebes, & Yovetich, 1990) than younger adults do in performing cognitive tasks.

Researchers have not only examined the impact of exercise or aerobics on cognitive features, but have looked at other factors that increase blood flow or oxygen to the brain such as the daily intake of antioxidants, for example, vitamins E and C, nutrition (e.g., folic acid; Martin, Cherubini, Andres-Lacueva, Paniagua, & Joseph, 2002), and nonsteroidal anti-inflammatory drugs (NSAIDs; e.g., aspirin, ibuprofen, and Celebrex) in lessening or preventing cognitive loss. Initially, there were favorable findings (Rowe & Kahn, 1998) for the effects of NSAIDs, vitamins, and nutrition, but these were considerably dampened by follow-up studies that failed to find any effect on cognitive functioning (Aisen et al., 2003; Farlow, 2003; Martin et al., 2002). There is considerable research showing that moderate to rigorous exercise increases cognitive functioning (see Buchner, Beresford, Larson, LaCroix, & Wagner, 1992, for a review). For example, Rowe and Kahn (1998) found that older adults who engaged in strenuous physical activity as a normal part of their daily lives, such as in maintaining their homes, gardening, and performing home repairs, were more likely to retain optimal levels of cognitive functioning. However, this leaves us with the proverbial question: Which came first, the chicken or the egg? As Buchner et al. (1992, p. 276) put it: "Does exercise make people smarter, or do smarter people simply exercise more?" While the former cannot be ruled out, there is support for the latter. We tend to see the same pattern as found in the case of NSAIDs, vitamins, and nutrition: Early, promising studies demonstrating that exercise improved cognition (e.g., Clarkson-Smith & Hartley, 1989) tended to be overshadowed and contradicted by better-controlled later studies that revealed little or modest cognitive gains, at best (Emery & Gatz, 1990; Madden, Blumentahl, Allen, & Emery, 1989). Yet, one cannot ignore the fact that studies continue to be published that demonstrate improved cognitive functioning and, perhaps even more amazing, increased neuronal growth (Hawkins, Kramer, & Capaldi, 1992) as result of vigorous exercise.

Researchers have critically examined the studies that failed to show cognitive improvements and found them to be flawed as well. For example, Buchner et al. (1992) suggested that the exercise programs used in the studies were too short and that more rigorous and prolonged exercise programs would result in benefits in improved cognitive functioning. Hill, Storandt, and Malley (1993) found that participants in the control group showed a marked and significant decline in their intellectual functioning, in contrast to no change for the participants in the experimental group. Thus, in support of exercise programs, Hill et al. (p. 16) proposed, "The possibility emerges that the exercise training might have acted to remediate normal memory declines with aging." In this context, another confound or moderating variable is the time of measurement error: Exercise is "in the air" and fashionable. Thus, participants in these studies may have already been exercisers or took it upon themselves to begin exercise programs, thereby making it more difficult to interpret results. Furthermore, how cognitive functioning and exercise are operationalized or measured varies from study to study (Buchner et al., 1992; Hawkins et al., 1992; Hill et al., 1993). Future research needs to further clarify this issue.

Neurodegenerative Diseases: Indicated Prevention

Indicated preventive interventions to treat cognitive loss linked to neurological diseases have also been studied. Initial studies were positive and generated considerable enthusiasm, only to be dampened by later, better designed and controlled studies. For example, Rowe and Kahn (1998) reported several studies that showed the preventive effects of the female hormone estrogen on cognition and memory in older women who are believed to be more likely than men to develop Alzheimer's disease, controlling for the fact they live longer than men (Evans & Manning, 2004). The authors proposed that estrogen empowers brain cells by boosting chemical functioning, stimulating cell growth, and protecting against toxins. However, these studies tended to involve small sample sizes or the samples were not carefully matched. Although one major study did find a connection between hormone use and lower rates of Alzheimer's disease in women, it was confounded by sample selection and there was no placebo group. Other large-scale studies have not found estrogen to be effective (see Farlow, 2003; Mulnard et al., 2000). In one study, women were randomly receiving estrogen and progestin or a placebo; contrary to expectations, women in the experimental group developed high rates of breast cancer and were much more likely to have strokes (Shumaker et al., 2003) than the women in the placebo group. Because of these unanticipated side effects, the study was discontinued, although an offshoot of the project is continuing to look at the effects of estrogen alone on Alzheimer's disease (see Mortimer, 2003).

Because of the grave risk of undesirable side effects, the current emphasis has shifted to indicated prevention, aimed at targeted individuals in the early stages of a disease involving cognitive impairment. New medications are being developed to slow down or prevent the ravages of neurological diseases such as strokes, Parkinson's disease (although, as yet, there is no FDA-approved medication to treat its cognitive features), and Alzheimer's disease (Tariot, Farlow, et al., 2003). The medications showing the most promise at indicated prevention are focused on dementia, particularly Alzheimer's disease (see Evans & Manning, 2004). Alzheimer's disease has no known cure, but recent clinical studies have shown that medications can slow down its progress and stabilize cognitive functioning, particularly with respect to memory loss. Several medications have been approved by the FDA, such as tacrine (Cognex), rivastigmine (Exelon), and galantamine (Reminyl); the most successful is the anticholinesterase inhibitor donepezil (Aricept), approved in 1996. Double-blind clinical trials have shown that although donepezil does not reverse the memory loss from Alzheimer's disease, it can slow down or forestall the progress of the disease and vascular dementia (Pratt & Perdomo, 2002) for up to a year or two. Patients taking donepezil show stability on measures of cognitive functioning such as the Mini-Mental Status Examination as compared to placebo groups.

Donepezil treats the deficiency of cholinergic transmissions in the hippocampus, which is believed to cause memory loss (Bartus, Dean, Beer, & Lippa, 1982). In effect, it maintains memory by increasing the levels of acetylcholine that is available at the synapse of neurons in the hippocampus, much as SSRIs and Paxil do for the neurotransmitter serotonin in treating depression. Recently, because of its tendency to increase levels of acetylcholine, it has been discovered that donepezil may be even more effective in blunting memory loss for individuals diagnosed with preclinical Alzheimer's disease or who have high-risk factors for Alzheimer's (Farlow, 2003). Donepezil is generally considered the preferred medication to treat early to moderate Alzheimer's disease at the indicated prevention level.

Recently, however, a new drug called memantine (Namenda) was approved by the FDA to treat moderate to severe Alzheimer's disease either singly or with donepezil (Farlow et al., 2003). Memantine works through a different mechanism from the cholinesterase inhibitors. Winblad and Poritis (1999) explain that the neurotransmitter glutamate protects neurons from calcium overloads that produce memory loss; when glutamate is at low levels, it allows calcium in large quantities to enter a neuron, disrupting its function and eventually causing the cell to wither and die. Normally, magnesium draws the calcium from the cell. This biochemical process allows the cell to be ready to respond to the next signal. However, the low levels of glutamate displace the magnesium levels, thereby disrupting the cell's functioning. Memantine acts like magnesium normally would and is not affected by the low levels of glutamate. It restores the normal biochemical balance which lets calcium enter the cell so normal transmission between the cells can be reestablished.

Double-blind clinical trials (Reisberg et al., 2003; Tariot et al., 2000) typically use a variety of cognitive outcome measures; Tariot et al. reported that on a cognitive global measure, 64% to 68% of patients in the memantine groups remained stable or improved after 5 months, compared to 47% of those in the placebo group. Furthermore, more patients in the memantine groups scored seven or more points higher on a 70-point cognitive status scale as compared to the placebo group (see also Reisberg et al., 2003). Unfortunately, though very promising, this medication only decreases the slope of advanced Alzheimer's disease, as both groups displayed memory loss from their pretest scores. Moreover, once the medication is discontinued, the experimental group's slope soon matches the placebo group's, indicating no permanent or lasting effect has occurred. This suggests that medical professionals need to intervene at the selective preventive level before Alzheimer's disease becomes symptomatic.

FUTURE DIRECTIONS: PERSONAL PROFILES AND TARGETING HIGH-RISK POPULATIONS

Because medications such as donepezil and memantine have serious side effects, not to mention their being expensive, it is unlikely that they will be distributed to the general public. However, several recent studies have shown that individuals can be identified at high risk for a disorder or illness before they show the signs or symptoms of the disease (see Mortimer, 2003); that is, selective prevention is called for. For example, in the well-known nun study (Snowden, 2001; Snowden et al., 1996), looking at 678 nuns from the ages of 75 to 102 who agreed to donate their brain to science upon their death, the authors were able to measure idea density (i.e., number of ideas present in every 10 words) on the basis of autobiographies written 50+ years earlier. They found that idea density in the writings predicted with a high degree of accuracy those individuals who later developed the symptoms of Alzheimer's disease, as well as the extent to which persons with the disease deteriorated over time.

Besides verbal measures, state-of-the-art medical technology can also be utilized to identify early precursors of Alzheimer's disease. For example, brain scans can provide evidence of early shrinkage of the hippocampus, increased beta amyloid plaques, and changes in brain blood flow (Evans & Manning, 2004) that are also predictive of Alzheimer's (Gosche, Mortimer, Smith, Marksbery, & Snowden, 2002). Once identified, high-risk individuals could be treated with a variety of medications, diet, and, when appropriate, exercise programs. High-risk individuals may also be vaccinated against developing the amyloid plaques associated with Alzheimer's disease. Although recent clinical trials had to be halted (Schenk et al., 1999) because 15% of the individuals vaccinated developed a fatal form of encephalitis, scientists believe that soon there will be a safer vaccine available (Mortimer, 2003). In targeting high-risk individuals for these types of treatment, medical professionals must be very careful. Single measures do not furnish enough accuracy. The most effective screening approach must include multiple predictors to be safer and more accurate (Mortimer, 2003).

Practice and Policy Implications

Our discussion of the many types of interventions available to the practitioner to either prevent or minimize cognitive loss suggests that a broad and flexible view should be taken in considering their efficacy. Intervening either cognitively or psychosocially at the level of the individual, the immediate environmental context (societally or culturally), and the biomedical level can be effective in either alleviating declines after they have appeared or enhancing functioning among those persons who have yet to experience measurable declines in their cognitive abilities. Moreover, not all persons will benefit from a given intervention, regardless of the level at which it is targeted or the ability or skill to which it is directed. Also, the short-term benefits to persons may not be paralleled in the long-term everyday context in which new skills are learned, or that in which previously held skills are reactivated.

At the societal level, sadly, it remains true that older persons' efforts to maintain their skills or acquire new ones are undermined by cultural stereotypes suggesting that cognitive aging is downhill. Consequently, altering both younger and older persons' expectations of themselves, cognitively speaking, is critical. From a public health perspective, goals that remain to be achieved include improving awareness of the distinctions between normal and pathological cognitive aging, embedding programs in everyday environments aiming to alter attitudes about the aging of one's skills, and providing basic information about and access to both structured and everyday activities that enhance self-esteem and the use of one's skills. Soon perhaps, persons will be as aware of the importance of taking care of their cognitive skills as they are about Alzheimer's disease, cancer, stroke, depression, vitamin supplements, eating a balanced diet, and exercise.

As pointed out by MacKinnon et al. (2003), there are limits to what individuals can accomplish regarding the prevention of decline. Some factors, such as a lack of education, visual and auditory impairments, and genetic predisposition to illness, are not modifiable, whereas others, such as being intellectually engaged as a young adult, are not attainable by older persons. Yet, everyday activities that are challenging and enriching have the potential to enhance cognitive functioning and improve persons' self-esteem and well-being, which may have indirect benefits on future cognitive activities and opportunities. In this respect, mental aerobics training (Paggi & Hayslip, 1999) and the provision of exemplary cognitive tasks and exercises (Hogan, in press) may hold promise to enhance the cognitive vitality, resilience, and mental skills of older persons. Interventions that have direct policy implications by increasing persons' access to social services, providing income and medical care supports, and funding programs that enhance social involvement and integration are all crucial in this respect (see MacKinnon et al., 2003; Pushkar & Arbuckle, 1998). Helping persons make good choices regarding lifestyle, both early and later in life, may also ultimately improve cardiovascular functioning and therefore make such persons less likely to experience decline. Encouraging everyday activities such as reading, solving crossword puzzles, putting jigsaw puzzles together, solving anagrams, returning to school to pursue a degree, enrolling in self-improvement courses (i.e., Elderhostel), or providing Internet-based access to new learning opportunities can all have beneficial effects in this regard.

Enriched environments (created by others or by oneself) can potentially lead to a greater number of neuronal interconnections, alter brain metabolism, and improve immune system functioning (Berkman, 2000; Katzman, 1995). We saw earlier that many of the biomedical primary interventions failed to ease or prevent cognitive loss, with the possible exception of moderate to strenuous exercise regimens (the jury is still out on this). Yet, in the very near future, medical professionals will be prescribing medications or vaccinating profiled individuals who possess a number of features prestaging the development of Alzheimer's disease or other dementias (such as Parkinson's disease) before they become symptomatic, holding the greatest promise of treating cognitive loss before it occurs. Within the next 2 decades, as researchers refine their tools and improve the medications as never before, a greater proportion of older adults may be able to live out their remaining years with their memory and cognitive skills intact.

We end this review by reinforcing the importance of recognizing the vast individual differences in the extent and rate of cognitive decline. Some persons experience very little loss; they are models for others who are yet to be old as well as those who are older and have experienced some cognitive decline. Many older persons have found ways of compensating for the declines they have experienced or have developed new skills on their own. They need no intervention; they are and always have been resilient, self-starting individuals, and they have attended to their health, lifestyle, and interpersonal relationships to lead satisfying and productive lives. Just as practitioners and researchers have much to offer in the form of cognitive training and remediation, so, too, do professionals have much to learn from the special older people who have triumphed over illness, adversity, and loss to maintain their skills well into later life.

REFERENCES

Aarsten, M. J., Smits, C., Van Tilburg, T., Knipscheer, K., & Deeg, D. (2002). Activity in older adults: Cause or consequence of cognitive functioning? A longitudinal study on everyday activities and cognitive performance in older adults. *Journals of Gerontology: Psychological Sciences, 57B,* P153–P162.

Ackerman, P. (1996). A theory of adult intellectual development: Process, personality, interests, and knowledge. *Intelligence, 22,* 227–257.

Ackerman, P. (2000). Domain-specific knowledge as the "dark matter" of adult intelligence: Gf/Gc, personality and interest correlates. *Journals of Gerontology: Psychological Sciences, 55B,* P69–P84.

Aisen, P. S., Schafer, K. A., Grundman, M., Pfeiffer, E., Sano, M., Davis, K. L., et al. (2003). Effects of Rofecoxib or Naproxen vs. placebo on Alzheimer disease progression: A randomized controlled trial. *Journal of the American Medical Association, 4,* 2865–2867.

Albert, M. S., Jones, K., Savage, C. R., Berkman, L., Seeman, T., Blazer, D., et al. (1995). Predictors of cognitive change in older persons: MacArthur studies of successful aging. *Psychology and Aging, 10,* 578–589.

Allaire, J. C., & Marsiske, M. (1999). Everyday cognition: Age and intellectual ability correlates. *Psychology and Aging, 14,* 627–645.

Allaire, J. C., & Marsiske, M. (2002). Well- and ill-defined measures of everyday cognition: Relationship to older adults' intellectual ability and functional status. *Psychology and Aging, 17,* 101–115.

Anschultz, L., Camp, C. J., Markley, R. P., & Kramer, J. J. (1987). A three-year follow-up on the effects of mnemonic training in elderly adults. *Experimental Aging Research, 13,* 141–143.

Arkin, S. M. (2000). Alzheimer memory training: Students replicate learning successes. *American Journal of Alzheimer's Disease, 15,* 152–162.

Artistico, D., Cervone, D., & Pezzuli, L. (2003). Perceived self-efficacy and everyday problem solving among young and older adults. *Psychology and Aging, 18,* 68–79.

Backman, K., & Dixon, R. A. (1992). Psychological compensation: A theoretical framework. *Psychological Bulletin, 112,* 259–283.

Ball, K., Berch, D. B., Helmers, K. F., Jobe, J. B., Leveck, M. D., Marsiske, M., et al. (2002). Effects of cognitive training interventions with older adults: A randomized controlled trial. *Journal of the American Medical Association, 288,* 2271–2281.

Baltes, P. B. (1997). On the incomplete architecture on human ontogeny. *American Psychologist, 52,* 366–379.

Baltes, P. B., & Danish, S. (1980). Intervention in life span development: Issues and concepts. In R. R. Turner & H. W. Reese (Eds.), *Life-span developmental psychology: Intervention* (pp. 49–78). New York: Academic Press.

Baltes, P. B., & Lindenberger, U. (1997). Emergence of a powerful connection between sensory and cognitive functions across the lifespan: A new window on the study of cognitive aging? *Psychology and Aging, 12,* 12–21.

Baltes, P. B., & Willis, S. L. (1982). Plasticity and enhancement of intellectual functioning in old age: Penn State's Adult Development and Enrichment Program (ADEPT). In F. I. M. Craik & S. E. Trehub (Eds.), *Aging and cognitive processes* (pp. 353–389). New York: Plenum Press.

Bartus, T. R., Dean, L. R., III, Beer, B., & Lippa, S. A. (1982). The cholinergic hypothesis of geriatric memory dysfunction. *Science, 217,* 408–417.

Berkman, L. F. (2000). Which influences cognitive function: Living alone or being alone? *Lancet, 9212,* 1315–1319.

Bieman-Copland, S., Bouchard-Ryan, E., & Cassano, J. (1998). Responding to the challenges of late life: Strategies for maintaining and enhancing competence. In D. Pushkar, W. M. Bukowski, A. E. Schwartzman, D. M. Stack, & D. R. White (Eds.), *Improving competence across the life span: Building interventions based on theory and research* (pp. 141–157). New York: Plenum Press.

Blazer, D. (2002). *Depression in late life.* New York: Springer.

Botwinick, J. (1984). *Aging and behavior* (3rd ed.). New York: Springer.

Brady, C. B., Spiro, A., III, McClinchey-Berroth, R., Milberg, W., & Gaziano, J. M. (2001). Stroke risk, predicts verbal fluency decline in healthy old men: Evidence from the normative aging study. *Journals of Gerontology: Psychological Sciences, 56B,* P340–P347.

Bryan, J., Luszcz, M. A., & Pointer, S. (1999). Executive function and processing resources as predictors of adult age differences in the implementation of encoding strategies. *Aging, Neuropsychology, and Cognition, 6,* 273–287.

Buchner, D. M., Beresford, S. A., Larson, E. B., LaCroix, A. Z., & Wagner, E. H. (1992). Effects of physical activity on health status in older adults II: Intervention studies. *Annual Review of Public Health, 13,* 469–488.

Cagney, K. A., & Lauderdale, D. S. (2002). Education, wealth, and cognitive function in older adults. *Journals of Gerontology: Psychological Sciences, 57B,* P163–P172.

Camp, C. J., Bird, M. J., & Cherry, K. (2000). Retrieval strategies as a rehabilitation aid for cognitive loss in pathological aging. In R. D. Hill, L. Bachman, & A. S. Neely (Eds.), *Cognitive rehabilitation in old age* (pp. 224–248). New York: Oxford University Press.

Canestrari, R. E. (1968). Age changes in acquisition. In G. A. Talland (Ed.), *Human aging and behavior* (pp. 169–187). New York: Academic Press.

Cherry, K. E. (1999). Effects of a target object orientation task on recall in older adults with probable Alzheimer's disease. *Clinical Gerontologist, 20,* 39–63.

Cherry, K. E., & Smith, A. D. (1998). Normal memory aging. In M. Hersen & V. van Hasselt (Eds.), *Handbook of clinical gerontology* (pp. 87–110). New York: Plenum Press.

Christensen, H., MacKinnon, A. J., Korten, A. E., Jorm, A. F., Henderson, A. S., Jacomb, P., et al. (1999). An analysis of diversity in the cognitive performance of elderly community dwellers: Individual differences in change scores as a function of age. *Psychology and Aging, 14,* 365–379.

Clarkson-Smith, L., & Hartley, A. A. (1989). Relationships between physical exercise and cognitive ability in older adults. *Psychology and Aging, 4,* 183–189.

Craik, F. I. M. (2000). Age-related changes in human memory. In D. Park & N. Schwarz (Eds.), *Cognitive aging: A primer* (pp. 75–92). Philadelphia: Taylor & Francis.

Crook, T. H., Bartus, R. T., Ferris, S. H., Whitehouse, P., Cohen, G. D., & Gershon, S. (1986). Age-associated memory impairment: Proposed diagnostic criteria and measures of clinical change [Report of an NIMH work group]. *Developmental Neuropsychology, 2,* 261–276.

Danish, S. (1981). Life span development and intervention: A necessary link. *Counseling Psychologist, 9,* 40–43.

Deihl, M. (1998). Everyday competence in later life: Current status and future directions. *Gerontologist, 38,* 422–433.

Demming, J., & Pressy, S. (1957). Tests indigenous to the adult and older years. *Journal of Counseling Psychology, 4,* 144–148.

Dixon, R. (1989). Questionnaire research on metamemory and aging: Issues of structure and function. In L. Poon, D. Rabin, & B. Wilson (Eds.), *Everyday cognition in adulthood and late life* (pp. 394–415). New York: Cambridge University Press.

Dixon, R. A., Hopp, G., Cohen, A., DeFrias, C., & Bäckman, L. (2003). Self-reported memory compensation: Similar patterns in Alzheimer's disease and very old adult samples. *Journal of Clinical and Experimental Neuropsychology, 25,* 382–390.

Emery, C. F., & Gatz, M. (1990). Psychological and cognitive effects of an exercise program for community-residing adults. *Gerontologist, 30,* 184–188.

Evans, J. M., & Manning, C. (2004, February). *Dealing with dementia: Diagnosis, treatment, and behavior management considerations.* Paper presented at the Association for Gerontology in Higher Education, Richmond, VA.

Fahlander, K., Waklin, A., Fastbom, J., Grut, M., Forsell, Y., Hill, R. D., et al. (2000). The relationships between signs of cardiovascular deficiency and cognitive performance in old age: A population-based study. *Journals of Gerontology: Psychological Sciences, 55B,* P259–P265.

Farlow, M. R. (2003, December). Alzheimer's disease: Treatment update. *CNS News Special Edition,* 35–38.

Fillenbaum, G. G. (1985). Screening the elderly: A brief instrumental activities of daily living measure. *Journal of the American Geriatrics Society, 33,* 698–706.

Fillenbaum, G. G. (1990). *Multidimensional functional assessment of older adults.* Hillsdale, NJ: Erlbaum.

Gallo, J. J., Rebok, G. W., Tennstedt, S., Wadley, V. G., & Horgas, A. (2003). Linking depressive symptoms and functional disability in late life. *Journal of Aging and Mental Health, 7,* 469–480.

Gold, D. P., Andres, D., Etezadi, J., Arbuckle, T. Y., Schwartzman, A. E., & Chailkelson, J. (1995). Structural equation model of intellectual change and continuity and predictors of intelligence in older men. *Psychology and Aging, 10,* 294–303.

Gordon, R. (1983). An operational classification of disease prevention. *Public Health Reports, 98,* 107–109.

Gordon, R. (1987). An operational classification of disease prevention. In J. A. Steinberg & M. M. Silverman (Eds.), *Preventing mental disorders* (pp. 20–26). Rockville, MD: Department of Health and Human Services.

Gosche, K. M., Mortimer, J. A., Smith, C. D., Marksbery, W. R., & Snowden, D. A. (2002). Hippocampal volume as an index of Alzheimer neuropathology: Findings from the nun study. *Neurology, 58,* 1476–1482.

Hawkins, H. L., Kramer, A. F., & Capaldi, D. (1992). Aging, exercise, and attention. *Psychology and Aging, 7,* 643–653.

Hayslip, B. (1988). Personality-ability relationships in aged adults. *Journals of Gerontology: Psychological Sciences, 43B,* P74–P84.

Hayslip, B. (1989). Alternative mechanisms for improvements in fluid ability among aged persons. *Psychology and Aging, 4,* 122–124.

Hayslip, B., Elias, J., Barta, J., & Henderson, C. (1998, April). *Perceptions of everyday skill and everyday task performance in older adults.* Paper presented at the Biannual Cognitive Aging Conference, Atlanta, GA.

Hayslip, B., Galt, C., Lambert, P., Kelly, K., Elias, J., Barta, J., et al. (1998, November). *The impact of anxiety reduction training on everyday skill among older adults.* Paper presented at the annual scientific meeting of the Gerontological Society of America, Philadelphia.

Hayslip, B., Kennelly, K., & Maloy, R. (1990). Fatigue, depression, and cognitive performance among aged persons. *Experimental Aging Research, 16,* 111–115.

Hayslip, B., Maloy, R. M., & Kohl, R. (1995). Long-term efficacy of fluid ability interventions with older adults. *Journals of Gerontology: Psychological Sciences, 59B,* P141–P149.

Hayslip, B., Ratliff, L., Galt, C., Lane, B., Lane, M., Radika, L., et al. (2000, April). *Perceptions of everyday skill and everyday task performance in older adults: A replication.* Paper presented at the biannual Cognitive Aging Conference, Atlanta, GA.

Hayslip, B., Servaty, H., & Ward, A. (1996, April). *Perceptions of everyday and psychometric intelligence and ability performance among older adults.* Paper presented at the sixth annual Cognitive Aging Conference, Atlanta, GA.

Hayslip, B., Servaty, H., Ward, A., & Blackburn, J. (1995, November). *Toward a definition of everyday cognition in later life.* Paper presented at the annual scientific meeting of the Gerontological Society of America, Los Angeles.

Hertzog, C., Schaie, K. W., & Gribbon, K. (1978). Cardiovascular disease and changes in intellectual functioning from middle to old age. *Journals of Gerontology, 33B,* P872–P883.

Hess, T. M., Auman, C., Colcombe, S. J., & Rahhal, T. A. (2003). The impact of stereotype threat on age differences in memory performance. *Journals of Gerontology: Psychological Sciences, 58B,* P3–P11.

Hill, R. D., Storandt, M., & Malley, M. (1993). The impact of long-term exercise training on psychological function in older adults. *Journals of Gerontology: Psychological Sciences, 48,* 12–17.

Hill, R. D., & Vandervoort, D. (1992). The effects on state anxiety on recall performance in older learners. *Educational Gerontology, 18,* 597–605.

Hogan, M. J. (in press). Exemplary exercises for older adults. *International Journal of Aging and Human Development.*

Horn, J. L. (1978). Human ability systems. In P. Baltes (Eds.), *Life-span development and behavior* (Vol. 1, pp. 211–256). New York: Academic Press.

Horn, J. L., & Hofer, S. (1992). Major abilities and development during the adult period. In R. Sternberg & C. Berg (Eds.), *Intellectual development* (pp. 44–99). New York: Cambridge University Press.

Horn, J. L., & Null, J. (1997). Human cognitive capabilities: Gf-Gc theory. In D. Flanagan & J. Genshaft (Eds.), *Contemporary intellectual assessment* (pp. 53–91). New York: Guilford Press.

Hultsch, D., Hertzog, C., Small, B., & Dixon, R. (1999). Use it or lose it: Lifestyle as a buffer of cognitive decline in aging? *Psychology and Aging, 14,* 245–263.

Jennings, J. R., Nebes, R. D., & Yovetich, N. A. (1990). Aging increases the energetic demands of episodic memory: A cardiovascular analysis. *Journal of Experimental Psychology—General, 119,* 77–91.

Jette, A. (1995). Disability trends and transitions. In R. Binstock & L. George (Eds.), *Handbook of aging and social sciences* (pp. 94–117). San Antonio, TX: Academic Press.

Katzman, R. (1995). Can late life leisure activities delay the onset of dementia? *Journal of the American Geriatrics Society, 43,* 583–584.

Kausler, D. (1994). *Learning and memory in normal aging.* San Diego, CA: Academic Press.

Kemp, B. J., & Mitchell, J. (1992). Functional assessment in geriatric mental health. In J. E. Birren, R. B. Sloane, & G. D. Cohen (Eds.), *Handbook of mental health and aging* (pp. 672–698). New York: Academic Press.

Kramer, A. F., & Willis, S. L. (2002). Enhancing the cognitive vitality of older adults. *Current Directions in Psychological Science, 5,* 173–177.

Krause, N. (1997). Commentary: The social context of competence. In S. L. Willis, K. W. Schaie, & M. Hayward (Eds.), *Societal mechanisms for maintaining competence in old age* (pp. 83–93). New York: Springer.

Levy, B. R. (2003). Mind matters: Cognitive and physical effects of aging self-stereotypes. *Journals of Gerontology: Psychological Sciences, 58B,* P203–P211.

Levy, B. R., Hausdorff, J. M., Hencke, R., & Weir, J. Y. (2000). Reducing cardiovascular stress with positive self-stereotypes of aging. *Journals of Gerontology: Psychological Sciences, 55B,* P205–P213.

MacKinnon, A., Christensen, H., Hofer, S. M., Korten, A. E., & Jorm, A. F. (2003). Use it and still lose it? The association between activity and cognitive performance established latent growth techniques in a community sample. *Aging, Neuropsychology, and Cognition, 10,* 215–229.

Madden, D. J., Blumentahl, J. A., Allen, P. A., & Emery, C. F. (1989). Improving aerobic capacity in healthy older adults does not necessarily lead to improved cognitive performance. *Psychology and Aging, 4,* 307–320.

Martin, A., Cherubini, A., Andres-Lacueva, C., Paniagua, M., & Joseph, J. (2002). Effects of fruits and vegetables on levels of vitamins E and C in the brain and their associations with cognitive performance. *Journal of Nutrition, Health, and Aging, 6,* 392–404.

Masunaga, H., & Horn, J. L. (2001). Expertise and age-related changes in components of intelligence. *Psychology and Aging, 16,* 293–311.

Monge, R. H., & Hultsch, D. (1971). Paired-associate learning as a function of adult age and the length of the anticipation and inspection intervals. *Journals of Gerontology, B26,* P157–P162.

Morrow, N., Howell, N., Hinterlong, J., & Sherraden, M. (2001). *Productive aging: Concepts and challenges.* Baltimore: Johns Hopkins University Press.

Mortimer, J. A. (2003). *Early detection and prevention: The future of geriatrics.* Washington, DC: Association for Gerontology in Higher Education.

Mulnard, R. A., Cotman, C. W., Kawas, C., Van-Dyck, C. H., Sano, M., Doody, R., et al. (2000). Estrogen replacement therapy for treatment of mild to moderate Alzheimer disease: A randomized controlled trial. *Journal of the American Medical Association, 283,* 1007–1015.

Nelson, E. A., & Dannefer, D. (1992). Aged heterogeneity: Fact or fiction? The fate of diversity in gerontological research. *Gerontologist, 32,* 17–23.

Paggi, K., & Hayslip, B. (1999). Mental aerobics: Exercises for the mind in later life. *Educational Gerontology, 25,* 1–12.

Park, D. C. (2000). The basic mechanisms accounting for age-related decline in cognitive function. In D. C. Park & N. Schwarz (Eds.), *Cognitive aging: A primer* (pp. 3–22). Philadelphia, PA: Taylor & Francis.

Perlmutter, M., & Nyquist, L. (1990). Relationships between self-reported physical and mental health and intelligence performance across adulthood. *Journals of Gerontology: Psychological Sciences, 45B,* P145–P155.

Peterson, R. C. (2003). *Mild cognitive impairment: Aging to Alzheimer's disease.* New York: Oxford University Press.

Powell, D. (1994). *Profiles in cognitive aging.* Cambridge, MA: Harvard University Press.

Pratt, R. D., & Perdomo, C. A. (2002). Donepezil improves cognitive function in patients with vascular dementia: Results from Study 307, a 24-week, randomized, double-blind, placebo-controlled trial. *Neurology, 58,* A61–A62.

Pushkar, D., & Arbuckle, T. (1998). Interventions to improve cognitive, emotional, and social competence in late maturity. In D. Pushkar, W. M. Bukowski, A. E. Schwartzman, D. M. Stack, & D. R. White (Eds.), *Improving competence across the life span: Building interventions based on theory and research* (pp. 159–178). New York: Plenum Press.

Pushkar, D., Arbuckle, T., Conway, M., Chaikelson, J., & Maag, U. (1997). Everyday activity parameters and competence in older adults. *Psychology and Aging, 12,* 600–609.

Rapp, S. R., Brenes, G., & Marsh, A. P. (2002). Memory enhancement training for older adults with mild cognitive impairment: A preliminary study. *Journal of Aging and Mental Health, 6,* 5–11.

Rasmusson, D. X., Rebok, G. W., Bylsma, F. W., & Brandt, J. (1999). Effects of three types of memory training in normal elderly. *Aging, Neuropsychology, and Cognition, 6,* 656–661.

Reese, C., Cherry, K., & Copeland, A. L. (2000). Knowledge of normal versus pathological memory in younger and older adults. *Aging, Neuropsychology, and Cognition, 7,* 1–8.

Reese, C., Cherry, K., & Norris, L. (1998). *Practical memory concerns of older adults.* Unpublished manuscript [Doctoral thesis], Louisiana State University.

Reisberg, B., Doody, R., Stoffler, A., Schmitt, F., Ferris, S., & Mobius, H. J. (2003). Memantine in moderate-to-severe Alzheimer's disease. *New England Journal of Medicine, 348,* 1333–1341.

Robertson-Tchabo, E., Hausman, C., & Arenberg, D. (1976). A classical mnemonic for older learners: A trip that works! *Educational Gerontology, 1,* 215–216.

Rothermund, K., & Brandstadter, J. (2003). Coping with deficits and losses in later life: From compensatory action to accommodation. *Psychology and Aging, 18,* 896–905.

Rowe, J. W., & Kahn, R. L. (1998). *Successful aging.* New York: Pantheon Books.

Salthouse, T. A. (1993). Attentional blocks are not responsible for age-related slowing. *Journals of Gerontology: Psychological Sciences, 48B,* P263–P270.

Salthouse, T. A. (1998). Cognitive and information processing perspectives on aging. In I. Nordhus, G. Vandenbos, S. Berg, & P. Fromholt (Eds.), *Clinical gerontology* (pp. 49–60). Washington, DC: American Psychological Association.

Salthouse, T. A., Berish, D., & Miles, J. (2002). The role of cognitive stimulation on the relations between age and cognitive functioning. *Psychology and Aging, 17,* 548–557.

Schaie, K. W. (1979). The primary mental abilities in adulthood: An exploration in the development of psychometric intelligence. In P. Baltes & O. Brim (Eds.), *Life-span development and behavior* (Vol. 2, pp. 68–115). New York: Academic Press.

Schaie, K. W. (1996). Intellectual development in adulthood. In J. Birren & K. Schaie (Eds.), *Handbook of the psychology of aging* (pp. 266–286). San Diego, CA: Academic Press.

Schaie, K. W., & Willis, S. L. (1986). Can decline in adult intellectual functioning be reversed? *Developmental Psychology, 22,* 223–232.

Schaie, K. W., & Willis, S. L. (1996). Psychometric intelligence and aging. In F. Blanchard-Fields & T. Hess (Eds.), *Perspectives on cognitive change in adulthood and aging* (pp. 293–324). New York: McGraw-Hill.

Schaie, K. W., Willis, S. L., & O'Hanlon, A. (1994). Perceived intellectual change over seven years. *Journals of Gerontology: Psychological Sciences, 49B,* P108–P118.

Schenk, D., Barbour, R. R., Dunn, W., Gordon, G., Grajeda, H., Guido, T., et al. (1999, July 8). Immunization with amyloid-beta attenuates Alzheimer-disease-like pathology in the PDAPP mouse. *Nature, 400*(6740), 173–177.

Schooler, C., & Mulatu, M. (2001). The reciprocal effects of leisure time activities and intellectual functioning in older people: A longitudinal analysis. *Psychology and Aging, 16,* 466–482.

Schooler, C., Mulatu, M., & Oates, G. (1999). The continuing effects of substantively complex work on intellectual functioning. *Psychology and Aging, 14,* 483–505.

Schulz, R., & Martire, L. M. (1999). Intervention research with older adults: Introduction, overview, and future directions. In R. Schulz, G. Maddox, & M. P. Lawton (Eds.), *Annual Review of Gerontology and Geriatrics* (Vol. 19, pp. 1–16). New York: Springer.

Scogin, F., & Bienias, J. (1988). A three-year follow-up of older adult participants in a memory-skills training program. *Psychology and Aging, 3,* 334–337.

Seeman, T. E., Unger, J. B., McAvay, G., & deLeon, C. (1999). Self-efficacy beliefs and perceived declines in functional ability: MacArthur studies of successful aging. *Journals of Gerontology: Psychological Sciences, 54B,* P214–P222.

Shumaker, S. A., Legault, C., Rapp, S. R., Thal, L., Wallace, R. B., Ockene, J. K., et al. (2003). Estrogen plus progestin and the incidence of dementia and mild cognitive impairment in postmenopausal women: The women's health initiative memory study: A randomized controlled trial. *Journal of the American Medical Association, 289,* 2651–2662.

Singer, T., Verhaeghen, P., Ghisletta, P., Lindenberger, U., & Baltes, P. (2003). The fate of cognition in very old age: Six-year longitudinal findings in the Berlin Aging Study. *Psychology and Aging, 18,* 318–331.

Slivinski, M. J., Hofer, S. M., Hall, C., Buschke, H., & Lipton, R. B. (2003). Modeling memory decline in older adults: The importance of preclinical dementia, attrition, and chronological age. *Psychology and Aging, 18,* 658–671.

Smith, A. D. (1996). Memory. In J. E. Birren & K. W. Schaie (Eds.), *Handbook of the psychology of aging* (pp. 236–250). San Diego, CA: Academic Press.

Snowden, D. A. (2001). *Aging with grace: What the Nun Study teaches us about leading longer, healthier, and more meaningful lives.* New York: Bantam Press.

Snowden, D. A., Kemper, S. J., Mortimer, J. A., Greiner, L. H., Wekstein, D. R., & Markesbery, W. R. (1996). Linguistic ability in early life and cognitive function and Alzheimer's disease in late life: Findings from the Nun Study. *Journal of the American Medical Association, 275,* 528–532.

Stone, R., & Murtaugh, C. (1990). The elderly population with chronic functional disability: Implications for home care eligibility. *Gerontologist, 30,* 491–496.

Tariot, P. N., Farlow, M., Grossberg, G. T., Gergel, I., Graham, S., & Jin, J. (2003). Memantine/donepezil dual therapy is superior to placebo/donepezil therapy for treatment of moderate to severe Alzheimer's disease. *Neurology, 60,* 4–12.

Tariot, P. N., Solomon, P. R., Morris, J. C., Kershaw, P., Lilienfield, S., & Ding, C. (2000). A 5-month, randomized, placebo-controlled study of galantamine in AD. *Neurology, 54,* 2269–2276.

Troyer, A. K. (2001). Improving memory knowledge, satisfaction, and function via an education and intervention program for older adults. *Aging, Neuropsychology, and Cognition, 8,* 256–268.

Valliant, G. E. (2002). *Aging well: Surprising guideposts to a happier life.* Boston: Little, Brown.

Verhaeghen, P. (2000). The interplay of growth and decline: Theoretical and empirical aspects of plasticity of intellectual and memory performance in normal old age. In

R. D. Hill, L. Bachman, & A. S. Neely (Eds.), *Cognitive rehabilitation in old age* (pp. 3–22). New York: Oxford University Press.

Wetherell, J. L., Reynolds, C. A., Gatz, M., & Pedersen, N. L. (2002). Anxiety, cognitive performance, and cognitive decline in normal aging. *Journals of Gerontology: Psychological Sciences, 57B,* P246–P255.

Willis, S. (1996). Everyday competence in elderly persons: Conceptual issues and empirical findings. *Gerontologist, 36,* 595–601.

Willis, S. L. (1991). Cognition and everyday competence. In K. W. Schaie & M. P. Lawton (Eds.), *Annual Review of Gerontology and Geriatrics* (Vol. 11, pp. 80–109). New York: Springer.

Wilson, R. S., Beckett, L. A., Barnes, L. L., Schneider, J. A., Bach, J., Evans, D. A., et al. (2002). Individual differences in rates of change in cognitive abilities of older persons. *Psychology and Aging, 17,* 179–193.

Winblad, B., & Poritis, N. (1999). Memantine in severe dementia: Results of the 9M-best study (benefit and efficacy in severely demented patients during treatment with memantine). *International Journal of Geriatric Psychiatry, 14,* 135–146.

Winett, R. (1995). A framework for health promotion and disease prevention programs. *American Psychologist, 50,* 341–350.

Woolverton, M., Scogin, F., Shackelford, J., Black, S., & Duke, L. (2001). Problem-targeted memory training for older adults. *Aging, Neuropsychology, and Cognition, 8,* 241–255.

Zelinski, E., Crimmins, E., Reynolds, S., & Seeman, T. (1998). Do medical conditions affect cognition in older adults? *Health Psychology, 17,* 504–512.

Chapter 4

SUICIDE

JOHN H. PIERPONT AND KAYE McGINTY

Although the National Save-a-Life Foundation was established in 1906, suicide prevention began in earnest in the United States only a half-century later, in the 1960s (Wallace, 2001). In his lucid and concise history of suicide prevention and suicidology in the United States, Wallace describes the fortuitous confluence of societal and professional events that eventuated in what is now the familiar place of suicidology in the mental health landscape. The progressive, community-oriented approach to domestic policy and programming that began with President Kennedy's "New Frontier" continued in President Johnson's "Great Society." The Community Mental Health Centers Act of 1963 (CMHCA), followed by the Economic Opportunity Act of 1964, which called for "maximum feasible participation" by grassroots stakeholders, were indicative of a political and popular milieu favoring government-supported, community-level strategies for addressing social problems (see Day, 2003). This was also the era in which the volunteer movement found its stride in the United States, having been significantly influenced by the Samaritans in England (Wallace, 2001). In 1968, at the first meeting of the American Association of Suicidology, it was said that "the lay volunteer was probably the most important single discovery in the 50-year history of suicide prevention" (Schneidman, 1988, p. 11).

The community-level approach to social problem solving found its way into the helping professions in the 1960s as preventive psychiatry, community psychology, and social work each contributed to the nascent community mental health movement. As Presidents Kennedy and Johnson were addressing social ills that beset the nation, many mental health professionals began to show more interest in environmental factors associated with the mental health of the nation than with psychopathology. In 1964, Gerald Caplan's landmark work *Principles of Preventive Psychiatry* provided both rationale and direction for mental health practitioners. Preventive psychiatry emphasizes removing or ameliorating environmental factors thought to contribute to mental illness. Thus, its focus is on prevention in the general population.

Eric Lindemann's (1944) work on crisis intervention, though written in the 1940s, was not widely applied until it was given political and economic impetus through the community mental health movement in the 1960s (Wallace, 2001). The appeal of crisis intervention was twofold. First, it was theoretically compatible with community mental health, that is, with a preference for community-based treatment over hospitalization when possible. Second, it provided an in-community treatment approach compatible with the CMHCA funding requirement that mental health centers provide emergency services (Wallace, 2001). Events of the 1960s, including the move toward community mental health, set the stage for current-day suicide prevention efforts. It was the community mental health movement that

> helped shape the direction that the suicide prevention movement would take. . . . The growth in community mental health helped to provide a model with which a suicide prevention program could be established. Attacking the problem at the community level, rather than in hospitals, demonstrated a greater appreciation for the social and cultural forces that were operating. (p. 247)

Today, suicide is recognized as one of the nation's most serious public health problems. In 1999, in response to a conference attended by leading suicidologists in Reno, Nevada, in October 1998, Surgeon General David Satcher issued a call to action to prevent suicide, which at the time was the eighth leading cause of death in the United States. In a special hearing before a subcommittee of the Senate Committee on Appropriations on February 8, 2000, Dr. Satcher emphasized the importance of awareness, intervention, and methodology: " 'Awareness' signifies our commitment to broaden the public's awareness of suicide and its risk factors. 'Intervention' means we will enhance services and programs, both population-based and clinical care to reduce suicide . . . 'methodology' compels us to advance the science of suicide prevention" (U.S. Government Printing Office, 2000, p. 4). In May 2001, the surgeon general unveiled the first step in a National Strategy for Suicide Prevention (NSSP), saying, "Suicide has stolen lives and contributed to the disability and suffering of hundreds of thousands of Americans each year. . . . There are few who escape being touched by the tragedy of suicide in their lifetimes" (Substance Abuse and Mental Health Services Administration [SAMHSA], 2004a). SAMHSA of the U.S. Department of Health and Human Services sponsors the NSSP. Cosponsors include the Association for Suicide Prevention, the American Association of Suicidology, and the Suicide Prevention and Advocacy Network (SAMHSA, 2004a). The NSSP continues to serve as a blueprint for addressing suicide prevention and intervention, including universal, selected, and indicated intervention efforts. In 2002, the Institute of Medicine's Committee on Pathophysiology and Prevention of Adolescent and Adult Suicide issued its report, *Reducing Suicide: A National Imperative* (Goldsmith, Pellmar, Kleinment, & Bunney, 2002). This study represents the most comprehensive investigation to date on suicide in the United States.

It is in the nature of an essay such as this to focus on academic concerns: historical background, risk factors, statistics regarding incidence, program specifications, and so on. However, we must not lose sight of the terribly high cost of this subject in human terms. Annually, suicide steals as many as 30,000 lives and causes untold suffering for countless survivors. Therefore, it is important to note that useful distinctions may be made among "pain," "suffering," and "unnecessary suffering." Just as we experience simple pain when we hit our thumb with a hammer or stub a toe, we may also experience pain, though of a different sort, when one of our children is injured or sick or when we experience estrangement from family or friends. Our pain may become suffering when an illness or injury is severe or when we face the loss of a loved one. Muñoz, Ying, Perez-Stable, and Miranda (1993) suggest that "unnecessary suffering" occurs when, through extreme emotional reactions, people add to the pain or suffering caused by injury or illness. Pain and suffering are inevitable; unnecessary suffering is not. It is the unnecessary suffering—unbearable and avoidable—that is the target of the preventive interventions discussed in this chapter.

INCIDENCE AND TRENDS

The epidemiology of suicide is usually discussed in terms of incidence rate rather than prevalence rate (Lester, 2001). Incidence describes the rate of completed suicides over a period of time, and prevalence describes the number of suicides at a particular point in time. In 2000, the incidence rate for suicide in the United States was 10.7 deaths per 100,000 people in the population (Centers for Disease Control [CDC], 2003a). According to a recent report by the Institute of Medicine (IOM), approximately 30,000 people complete suicide in the United States each year (Goldsmith et al., 2002); the CDC (2003a) reported 29,350 completed suicides in 2000. The IOM further reported that as many as 650,000 people annually receive treatment after a suicide attempt; in contrast, the CDC (2003b) reported that in 2000, over 264,000 people were treated in hospital emergency departments for nonfatal self-inflicted injuries, of which approximately 60% (158,000) were suicide attempts, and Roy (2001) states that "there are no national, population-based data on attempted suicide" (p. 109). Clearly there is no concensus regarding incidence and prevalence of attempted suicide. Problems associated with collecting data pertinent to suicide are discussed below.

Suicide is the eleventh leading cause of death in the United States and fourth among persons between the ages of 18 and 65. Although women are more likely to attempt suicide, men are four times more likely to complete suicide (CDC, 2003b). The suicide rate is especially high for White males over 75 years of age (Goldsmith et al., 2002), and it is the leading cause of violence-related deaths among persons age 18 to 85 (CDC, 2003a). In the year 2000, 84% of all completed suicides among persons age 65 and older occurred among men, and "the ten year period, 1980–1990, was the first decade since the 1940s that the suicide rate for older residents rose instead of declined" (CDC, 2003b). Between 1980 and 1998, "the largest relative increases in suicide rates occurred among those 80 to 84 years of age. The rate for men in this age group increased 17% (from 43.5 per 100,000 to 52.0)" (CDC, 2003b, para. No. 8).

Each year twice as many people die from suicide as from HIV/AIDS, and among teenagers and young adults, suicide takes more lives than cancer, heart disease, AIDS, pneumonia, influenza, and chronic lung disease combined (SAMSHA, 2004b).

On average each year, three people die from suicide for every two who die from homicide (U.S. Government Printing Office, 2000). In 2001, there were 10,736 more deaths due to suicide than homicide (CDC, 2003a), and the IOM reports that "over the last 100 years suicides have out-numbered homicides by at least 3 to 2. Almost 4 times as many Americans died by suicide than in the Vietnam War during the same time period" (Goldsmith et al., 2002, p. 17). In 2001, the number of firearms-related suicides exceeded the number of firearms-related homicides by 64% (CDC, 2003b).

Although Whites accounted for 90% of all suicides in 1999, between 1979 and 1992 the suicide rate for Native Americans (Alaska Natives and American Indians) was 1.5 times the national rate, and "there was a disproportionate number of suicides among young male Native Americans during this period, as males 15–24 accounted for 64% of all suicides by Native Americans" (CDC, 2003b). Among young persons, suicide rates have increased steadily over the past half-century. The incidence of suicide among adolescents and young adults nearly tripled between 1952 and 1995, and from 1980 to 1997 the suicide rate for young persons between the ages of 15 and 19 rose by 11% (CDC, 2003b). In 1999, the surgeon general reported that the rate of suicide among African American males had increased by 105% between 1980 and 1996, and that nearly all of this increase was associated with the availability of firearms (U.S. Public

Health Service, 1999). Although suicide is rare among young children, for those age 10 to 14 the rate of suicide increased 105% in the 17 years between 1980 and 1997 (CDC, 2003b).

It is important to note that statistics on death by suicide tend to be less accurate than those for other causes of death, in large part because it requires determining intent. This difficulty leads to significant underreporting of completed suicides, which, combined with the lag of approximately 3 years between the event year and the release of national data, compromises the accuracy of suicide incidence, rates, and trends (Potter, 2001). Further, the absence of timely, accurate data makes it impossible to efficiently and effectively target certain malleable risk factors, for example, suicide contagion. Suicide may also be underreported due to the stigma attached to it or out of concern for survivors. For example, U.S. Army officials reported in January 2004 that 18 soldiers in the Iraq war had committed suicide, which was considered "on the high end" of suicides seen in past combat settings. Amid concern that the Department of Defense might be underreporting the incidence of suicide by American service personnel in Iraq, in March 2004 the Army revised the number to include soldiers who completed suicide after returning home from combat. As of March 2004, the number stood at 29 (National Public Radio [NPR], 2004).

RISK FACTORS

Suicidologists recognize that suicidal behavior is multidetermined; that is, there are multiple factors in several domains associated with each completed suicide (see Goldsmith et al., 2002; Potter, 2001; U.S. Public Health Service, 1999). However, we lack an integrated understanding of the independent and interactive influence of the psychological, biological, social, and environmental factors associated with suicide risk (Goldsmith et al., 2002). In his discussion of suicide prevention in the context of public health, Potter describes an ecological model in which individual motivation and behavior occur in the context of social systems involving family, friends, employers, and others, all of whom live in the immediate and larger community environments. Each individual and system in an ecological environment is affected by cultural, social, and economic factors, and each in turn affects and is affected by the others. Thus, a phenomenon such as suicide has multiple individual and environmental risk factors, "and their combination may vary by age, gender, and ethnicity" (U.S. Public Health Service, 1999, p. 9).

Community risk factors include high poverty and unemployment rate (see Stack, 2001). An individual's biology (see van Praag, 2001) and even temperament may predispose him or her toward suicide (Goldsmith et al., 2002). Other personal risk factors are the presence of mental illness, including alcoholism and comorbidity of mental illness with alcoholism; advanced age; family history of suicide; a worldview (perhaps based on cultural, spiritual, or religious beliefs) that promotes or allows suicide as an acceptable act; hopelessness, including hopelessness resulting from social isolation and physical illness; and readily available lethal means, especially firearms (U.S. Public Health Service, 1999).

As one would expect, having made a previous suicide attempt is a significant risk factor, as approximately 40% of persons attempting suicide have a history of one or more previous attempts (Roy, 2001). On March 7, 2004, the body of writer and actor Spalding Gray was found in New York's East River. Gray was widely known to have suffered from anxiety and depression, which became more severe as he became older. In his monologues, he frequently referred to his mother's suicide and his inability to be angry with her because she was "psychotic," and, for her, suicide "made sense." In 2002, he had a very serious automobile accident that left him more depressed than he had been previously. After being hospitalized for depression twice in 2002, he attempted suicide by jumping from a bridge (NPR, 2004). Certainly, Gray's tragic death exemplifies the increased potential for suicidality associated with multiple risk factors. Gray's mother's suicide, his depression and anxiety, serious physical injury, advancing age, a worldview in which suicide "makes sense," the availability of means, and a previous attempt were each risk factors. In combination they were, clearly, overwhelming.

A thorough discussion of all of the risk factors associated with suicidality would require a volume in itself. Readers desiring a more comprehensive treatment of suicide risk factors are referred to Goldsmith et al. (2002) and Lester (2001). For purposes of discussing preventive interventions, we limit ourselves to three risk factors present in Potter's ecological environment: mental illness, advanced age, and easy access to lethal means. Of course, not all risk factors can be ameliorated by preventive interventions, and the presence of risk factors does not necessarily mean a person is or will become suicidal. However, knowledge of risk factors may increase others' awareness and make it possible to intervene effectively when intervention is called for.

Mental Illness

Over 90% of completed suicides in the United States are associated with mental illness and/or substance abuse (including alcohol abuse). However, fully 10% of persons completing suicide have no known psychiatric diagnosis. Significantly, more than 95% of all persons diagnosed with psychiatric disorders do not complete suicide (Goldsmith et al., 2002). Despite this, Roy (2001) suggests that virtually every psychiatric disorder increases the risk of suicidality, with the exceptions of dementia and mental retardation. Those psychiatric disorders that appear to put persons at greatest risk are Major Depression, Alcoholism, Bipolar Disorder, Drug Dependence, Schizophrenia, and Panic Disorder (Roy, 2001).

Suicidality and psychiatric disorders associated with it have overlapping symptomatology. However, they do not always respond to treatment similarly. For example, in some individuals, medication may reduce depression without a concomitant reduction in suicidality. Likewise, psychotherapy may reduce suicidality without reducing depression, feelings of hopelessness, a sense of meaninglessness, and so on (Goldsmith et al., 2002). Although not a psychiatric disorder in itself, hopelessness is strongly associated with suicidality.

"Over 30 years of research confirms the relationship between hopelessness and suicide across diagnoses. Hopelessness can persist even when other symptoms of an associated disorder, such as depression, have abated" (p. 2). It is for good reason that Goldsmith et al. opine that "the relationship between suicide and mental illness is a conundrum" (p. 2).

Advanced Age

The risk for suicide increases with age and the highest incidence rates are among persons age 65 and older (CDC, 2003b). Older persons constitute approximately 13% of the population, and they account for 18% of all suicides. Depression is the most significant risk factor among older Americans (National Institute of Mental Health [NIMH], 2004). Suicidality is higher for those who are widowed or divorced than for those who are married. In a 1992 survey, the suicide rate for widowed and divorced men was 2.7 times the rate for married men. Interestingly, the rate for widowed and divorced men was 1.4 times higher than for men who had never married, and 17 times that for married women. The suicide rate for widowed and divorced women was 1.8 times the rate for married women and 1.4 times the rate for women who had never married (CDC, 2003b).

The CDC (2003b) reports that risk factors for older persons are different from those associated with younger ages. The elderly are more likely to use more lethal methods than are young people, and it is probably for this reason that they make fewer attempts for each completed suicide. Older adults are also more likely than younger to experience depression, have more physical illnesses, and to be socially isolated. The elderly are also more likely to have seen a health care provider shortly before their suicide (CDC, 2003b; NIMH, 2004; U.S. Public Health Service, 1999) and "thus represent a missed opportunity for intervention" (U.S. Public Health Service, 1999, p. 3).

Availability of Firearms

Surgeon General Satcher has attributed nearly 100% of the dramatic increase in the suicide rate among young Black males to the availability of firearms and singles out "easy access to lethal weapons, especially guns" as an important risk factor (U.S. Public Health Service, 1999). The CDC reports that in 2000, 57% of all completed suicides involved the use of a firearm. In that year, 79.5% of males and 37% of females age 65 and older who completed suicide used a firearm. In 2001, firearms-related suicide was the leading cause of violence-related deaths among persons of both sexes and all races, accounting for 16,412 deaths. In contrast, firearms accounted for 10,502 homicides in 2001.

In addition to other environmental risk factors, such as poverty and having a family member who completed suicide, easy access to means, especially firearms, is a serious family- and community-level risk factor and is known to be associated with increased risk for completed suicide (see Potter, 2001). Goldsmith et al. (2002) report that "the presence of a gun in the home is highly predictive of its use for completed suicide" (p. 282). However, the use of a gun to complete suicide is very infrequent when there is no gun in the home. The recent study by the IOM (Goldsmith et al., 2002) also emphasizes that higher incidence of firearms in the home is associated with greater risk for suicide, and lower incidence of firearms in the home is associated with reduced risk of suicide. Significantly, substitution of one means for another to complete suicide is not inevitable. Reducing availability of firearms lowers risk because means substitution does not invariably occur (Goldsmith et al., 2002).

EFFECTIVE UNIVERSAL PREVENTIVE INTERVENTIONS

Over a decade ago, Muñoz et al. (1993) produced a vignette addressing the complex issues surrounding the development and implementation of universal preventive interventions aimed at severe depression, a leading risk factor associated with suicidality. By analogy, the vignette may be used to address virtually any suicide risk factor, and it addresses in a succinct yet compelling fashion several important issues pertaining to prevention. The vignette and subsequent discussion, quoted at length, provide a useful starting point to begin our discussion of universal preventive interventions for suicide.

> Suppose . . . that an effective prevention intervention for depression were developed which significantly reduces the occurrence of depressive episodes for at least a ten year period. Suppose further, that it could be applied throughout the

life span and worked reasonably well for both genders. Two projects are put forward, and only one can be funded: the first targets elderly men in nursing homes; the second targets 18- to 24-year-old women pregnant with their first child.

Even if the risk for depression were the same in both populations, the repercussions of depressive episodes within the next 10 years would be much greater for the women about to begin their childbearing years. When focusing on the individuals themselves, the decisions and the achievements of the next ten years are going to have a major effect on the women's lives for much longer than the decisions and achievements of the men in the nursing home. Going beyond the individuals themselves, there are sufficient data now to indicate that maternal depression can have serious repercussions on the welfare of their children. . . . The choices to be made are real. The difficulty of making these choices is also very real. One runs into the quagmire of labeling one person's life as more important, or at least more influential than another's. Do these differences make one less worthy than another for societal support?

One possible way to reduce the difficulty involved in making this type of decision is to make preventive interventions as universal as possible, and so inexpensive as to make it unreasonable to deny their implementation. Whether such universal and inexpensive interventions can be sufficiently effective to have a major impact on the incidence . . . of depression remains to be seen. (Muñoz et al., 1993, pp. 53–55)

Of course, the hypothesized interventions do not represent the reality of treatment for depression or prevention of suicide. We have no interventions that are equally effective for both genders, at various points during the life span, lasting for 10 years, and so on. For our purposes, it is instructive to note that serious moral questions accompany decisions regarding whom to treat with insufficient resources and that universal preventive interventions seem to represent a viable alternative to the quagmire such decisions necessarily create. Certainly there can be no question that preventing suicidality would be far more humane than attempting to treat an individual once he or she has become suicidal. The remaining difficulty, recognized by Muñoz and his colleagues, is whether such universal preventive interventions can be effective. We return to this question later.

Universal preventive interventions address one or more conditions in an entire population, such as a school, community, state, or nation. Universal measures to prevent suicide are intended to reach every person in a given population by

removing barriers to care, enhancing knowledge of what to do and say to help suicidal individuals, increasing access to help, and strengthening protective processes like social support and coping skills. Universal interventions include programs such as public education campaigns, school-based "suicide awareness" programs, means restriction, education programs for the media on reporting practices related to suicide, and school-based crisis response plans and teams. (Goldsmith et al., 2002, p. 274)

In recent years, increasing rates of suicidality among young people have engendered an increase in emphasis on prevention programs targeting that population, especially school-based programs (see Goldsmith et al., 2002). Given the scope of this volume, we limit our discussion to programs targeting adults and refer the reader interested in suicide prevention among adolescents to the discussion by McCarter, Sowers, and Dulmus (2004) in the companion volume, *Handbook of Preventive Interventions for Children and Adolescents* (Rapp-Paglicci, Dulmus, & Wodarski, 2004).

Media Campaigns

Media campaigns have the potential to influence very large numbers of people and for this reason are among the most important universal preventive interventions. Electronic and print media have the ability to inform a variety of audiences simultaneously with "stories about suicide [that] inform readers and/or viewers about the likely causes of suicide, warning signs, trends in suicide rates, and recent advances in treatment" (CDC, 2003b).

The American Foundation for Suicide Prevention (AFSP), founded in 1987, was the first national nonprofit foundation established for the purpose of funding education, research, and treatment programs for suicide prevention (AFSP, 2004a). In addition to policy statements on suicide prevention, assisted suicide, and gun control, the AFSP offers extensive resources to the media to improve coverage of stories pertaining to suicide and the study of suicide. Working in conjunction with the American Association of Suicidology and the Annenberg Public Policy Center, the AFSP presented background information and recommendations to the National Press Club in Washington, DC. These recommendations primarily were made in an effort to prevent suicide contagion or "copycat" suicides. Suicide contagion, also referred to as suicide imitation or modeling, may occur "in several circumstances, such as in the case of temporal clusters of suicides in a particular community or culture . . . suicide among family members . . . and suicide following exposure to a media presentation of a real or fictional suicide" (Goldsmith et al., 2002, p. 277). On its Web page, in a box titled "Suicide Contagion Is Real," the AFSP (2004b) displays the following information:

Between 1984 and 1987, journalists in Vienna covered the deaths of individuals who jumped in front of trains in the subway system. The coverage was extensive and dramatic. In 1987, a campaign alerted reporters to the possible negative effects of such reporting, and suggested alternate strategies for coverage. In the first six months after the campaign began, subway suicides and non-fatal attempts dropped by more than eighty percent. The total number of suicides in Vienna declined as well. Research finds an increase in suicide by readers or viewers when:

The number of stories about individual suicides increases.

A particular death is reported at length or in many stories.

The story of an individual death by suicide is placed on the front page or at the beginning of a broadcast.

The headlines about specific suicide deaths are dramatic (a recent example: "Boy, 10, Kills Himself Over Poor Grades").

AFSP recommendations to the media include factual information, questions to ask, and angles for reporters to pursue in the areas of mental illness and suicide, interviewing surviving relatives, language to use in reporting on suicide, and special situations such as celebrity deaths by suicide. For example, information about suicide includes facts such as the following:

Over 90 percent of suicide victims have a significant psychiatric illness at the time of their death. These are often undiagnosed, untreated, or both. Mood disorders and substance abuse are the two most common. When both mood disorders and substance abuse are present, the risk for suicide is much greater, particularly for adolescents and young adults. (AFSP, 2004b)

Suggested questions for media representatives to ask include: "Had the victim ever received treatment for depression or any other mental disorder?" and "Did the victim have a problem with substance abuse?" (AFSP, 2004b).

The AFSP also hopes to ensure a measure of dignity for persons who have completed or attempted suicide and their family and friends. Thus, it is recommended that the deceased be referred to as "having died by suicide" rather than as "a suicide" or as having "committed suicide," because the latter "reduce the person to the mode of death, or connote criminal or sinful behavior." Finally, the AFSP recommends that useful story topics might include suicide myths and warning signs, treatment advances, trends in suicide rates, and "actions individuals can take to prevent suicide by others" (AFSP, 2004b).

In addition to its recommendations to the media, the AFSP is also engaged in universal prevention efforts that specifically target young adults. One such project is a film for college students, *The Truth about Suicide: Real Stories about Depression in College.* The film is expected to be available following piloting during the spring 2004 semester and is intended to encourage students with depression to seek help and to encourage friends in need to seek help (AFSP, 2004c).

Another significant universal preventive intervention is the Air Force Suicide Prevention Program, an ongoing joint project that combines the resources of the U.S. surgeon general, the United States Air Force Medical Service (USAFMS), the Centers for Disease Control, and academic suicidologists. Although the suicide rate for the Air Force is lower than that for the general population, the suicide rate for commissioned and enlisted personnel rose alarmingly between 1990 and 1995, and by 1995 suicide was the second leading cause of death among all Air Force personnel (Office of Public Health and Science, 2004). In 1996 to 1997 the Air Force formed a multidisciplinary committee of civilian and military experts to design a servicewide comprehensive suicide prevention strategy. The program, named LINK, targets both suicide risk reduction and mental and behavioral health promotion. Primary program aspects include coordinating services among agencies, normalizing help-seeking behavior, and increasing protective factors such as effective coping skills, support, and social connectedness (USAFMS, 2000). Further, regular staff development courses have incorporated suicide prevention education for all officers. Finally, the Air Force coordinated its mental health and social services into an integrated delivery system to organize the suicide prevention efforts. After implementing this program, the Air Force saw a significant decrease in suicide rates among its active-duty personnel, from 16.4 per 100,000 to 9.4 per 100,000 ($p < .002$) between 1994 and 1998 (Litts, Moe, Roadman, Janke, & Miller, 2000). In the first half of 1999, the annualized suicide rate was below 3.5 per 100,000, a decline of 80% from the highest rates in the mid-1990s (Office of Public Health and Science, 2004).

The LINK program is unusual insofar as it is a universal preventive intervention for which there is substantial outcome data, making possible a determination of its effectiveness. Some universal programs are implemented without adequate provision for evaluation, and others, by their nature, elude meaningful evaluation. For example, it is probable that educating media reporters and writers helps prevent suicide contagion and that films for students help direct them toward needed intervention services. However, it is unlikely that an accurate and thorough assessment of these efforts' efficiency and effectiveness in preventing suicide will ever be possible.

SELECTIVE PREVENTIVE INTERVENTIONS

Selective interventions to prevent suicide address subsets of the population, focusing on at-risk groups that have a greater probability of becoming suicidal.

Examples include screening programs, gatekeeper training for caregivers, support and skill-building groups for at-risk individuals, and enhanced crisis services and referral services.

An example of an at-risk group of adults is those individuals predisposed to psychiatric disorders, especially depression, substance abuse, and chronic medical illness. Most of these adults will be seen for medical care by primary care physicians; therefore, primary care settings are a critical site for detection of these disorders and prevention of possible suicides. Depression evaluation presents an opportunity for primary care physicians to ask about suicidal ideation. About 6% to 10% of people seen in primary care settings had major depression (Katon & Schulberg, 1992). Seventy-five percent of those seeking help for depression do so through their primary care physician rather than through a mental health professional (Goldman, Nielsen, & Champion, 1999). However, only approximately 30% to 50% of adults with diagnosable depression are accurately diagnosed by primary care physicians (Higgins, 1994; Wells, Katon, Rogers, & Camp, 1994), and only 58% of a random sample of 3,375 primary care physicians directly questioned patients about suicide (Williams et al., 1999). Clearly, efforts toward increased education of primary care physicians are needed.

Treatment of depression in primary care settings was associated with reduced rates of completed suicide in an uncontrolled ecological study on the Swedish island of Gotland (Rutz, von Knorring, & Walinder, 1989, 1992). An educational project for all general practitioners on the island was carried out in 1983 and 1984. The 2-year program consisted of a combination of oral and written information, group work, videotaped and written case reports, and sharing of personal experiences, with a focus on the process of becoming depressed and suicidal, as well as recovery. The training was evaluated prior to the educational intervention and 5 years after the intervention. The general practitioners reported the following results: (1) increased knowledge and capacity to detect patients with depressive conditions, (2) increased willingness to abandon reductionistic psychotherapeutic or biological approaches in favor of a more comprehensive treatment approach, (3) integrating both psychotherapeutic supports and medical interventions, (4) improved capacity for risk assessment concerning suicidality, and (5) improved diagnostic, therapeutic, and monitoring ability to detect and follow up patients with depression in a comprehensive manner. At the time of maximum effect (2 years after the educational intervention) suicides fell dramatically, by 60%, to the lowest suicide rate ever observed on Gotland and in Sweden.

However, by 1988 there was a fading of the previous positive response in Gotland. Suicide increased again to numbers just below the baseline values. Various explanations were offered, including forgetting the information, competition by other educational programs, and a change of focus to other medical problems. However, the main reason described for the change was that 50% of the original group of general practitioners who were present at the time of maximum impact (1986) had left their positions on Gotland (Rutz et al., 1992). In addition, Rihmer and colleagues (Rihmer, Rutz, & Pihlgren, 1998) found that the decrease in suicides was mainly in females and individuals who were in contact with their general practitioners. Male suicides were not affected by the improved abilities of the general practitioners. The influence of gender differences and comorbid substance abuse were cited as important factors to address in the future for suicide prevention education for physicians.

Several American Indian reservation communities have had high suicide rates, and prevention efforts have attempted to address this. Many of these efforts have been geared toward adolescents and young adults. The Jicarilla Apache Tribe of northern New Mexico had a suicide rate exceeding 160 per 100,000 for those age 15 to 24 between 1969 and 1979 (VanWinkle & May, 1986, 1993). A partnership was formed between local councils and health programs, along with the Indian Health Service. These multiple agencies provided public education, risk assessment, counseling, and alcohol abuse prevention initiatives. With these efforts the rate of suicide gestures, attempts, and completions combined were drastically lowered (Serna, May, & Sitaker, 1998). In addition, there was a gradual lowering of the suicide rates as the target population aged (VanWinkle & Williams, 2001).

The College Screening Project, funded by the AFSP, was initiated in 2002 and targets students who may be at risk for suicide (AFSP, 2004c; Painter, 2004). The project began at Emory University in Atlanta, Georgia, where every undergraduate student age 18 and older receives an e-mail once each year asking "Are you depressed?" and offering a link to a brief, anonymous survey. The survey is received and scored at the university's counseling center. If the survey indicates the student is even mildly depressed, she or he receives a reply from a clinical professional suggesting the student come in for help. Some students choose to have only e-mail contact with the counseling center for weeks or months before seeking face-to-face assistance. Once they have seen a professional in the project, students may receive a referral for medication evaluation as well as regular counseling.

In January 2004, the College Screening Project was implemented for seniors at the University of North Carolina-Chapel Hill. On both campuses data are being collected that will become part of larger data-collecting efforts supported by the AFSP. Eventually, the data may help researchers and service providers better understand and prevent suicide among young adults attending college. Meanwhile, an increasing number of universities, for a variety of reasons, are waking up to the need to address depression and the potential for suicide among their students (Painter, 2004).

EFFECTIVE INDICATED PREVENTIVE INTERVENTIONS

Indicated interventions address specific high-risk individuals within a population that have shown early signs of suicide potential. Programs include skill-building support groups, case management, and referral sources for crisis intervention and treatment.

Elderly individuals are especially at risk for suicide. Some of the risk factors in the elderly include aging itself, medical illness, psychiatric illness, substance abuse, and multiple psychosocial factors (Carney, Rich, Burke, & Fowler, 1994). Although elderly suicide victims usually see their primary care physician in the month prior to their death, they face obstacles to receiving appropriate care. Szanto and colleagues (2001) found that elderly suicidal depressed patients can have a favorable outcome, but their treatment response may be more problematic and require continuing use of adjunctive medication to prevent early relapse.

To promote better recognition of and treatment for the problem of suicide in the elderly, NIMH is sponsoring the Prevention of Suicide in the Elderly Project (PROSPECT; Bruce & Pearson, 1999). This study is testing the effectiveness of placing depression care managers in primary care practices to reduce and prevent suicidal ideation and behavior, as well as depressive symptomatology. The PROSPECT study will investigate 1,200 subjects age 60 and older (920 with depressive symptoms and 280 without significant depressive symptomatology). Half of the depressed patients are treated at six primary care practices providing the services of depression care managers. The other half are treated at six comparable practices offering "enhanced care" (information on depression by research team but no care managers). The main tasks of the depression care managers include conveying clinical information to the primary care physician, monitoring the patient's treatment compliance in accordance with the guidelines of the Agency for Health Care Policy and Research, assessing the patient's clinical status, providing counseling when requested, and arranging specialist referrals. The interventions in the PROSPECT study appear to be more effective than current standard medical treatment, according to preliminary data. Although both patient populations had similar base rates, after 12 months, 10% of the patients in the intervention group had suicidal ideation compared to 17% in the standard treatment group (Reynolds et al., 2001). In addition, of those patients in the intervention group who initially had suicidal ideations, 70% were free of them after 8 months, compared to 44% of standard treatment patients (NIMH, 2004). This suggests that a depression care manager can be an effective intervention with the elderly population.

Goldsmith et al. (2002) suggest that psychological, social, biological, and environmental factors all play a significant role in suicide. Our understanding of the impact of these factors individually is uneven, and much less is understood about their combined impact on suicidality. The IOM (Goldsmith et al., 2002), the CDC (2003b), and the surgeon general (U.S. Public Health Service, 1999) have each recognized the limitations of our understanding of suicide and have called for additional research to increase our understanding of and our ability to prevent suicide.

PRACTICE AND POLICY IMPLICATIONS AND FUTURE DIRECTIONS

Implications for practice, policy, and future directions regarding suicide prevention are set forth thoughtfully and in detail both in the *Surgeon General's Call to Action to Prevent Suicide* (U.S. Public Health Service, 1999) and in the IOM study *Preventing Suicide: A National Imperative* (Goldsmith et al., 2002). As we indicated, the recommendations by the surgeon general pertain to his National Strategy for Suicide Prevention, categorized as AIM (awareness, intervention, and methodology). Recommendations regarding awareness and intervention pertain to many of the issues discussed earlier. For example, increasing the public's knowledge about suicide and reducing the stigma associated with mental illness are important aspects of awareness, and enhancing public-private media partnerships are specifically listed among the recommendations for intervention. Increasing primary care physicians' ability to diagnose and treat depression is also recommended by the surgeon general, as is reducing barriers to mental health care. The earlier discussion of universal, selective, and indicated preventive interventions provides one or more examples of each of these recommendations. Future prevention programs should continue these efforts, and providing multiple approaches to preventing suicide is recommended. Because suicidal behavior is multidetermined, communities need to address as many risk factors for suicide as possible and at different levels of intervention.

Goldsmith et al. (2002) propose several improvements to practice and policy in suicide prevention. Their first recommendation pertains to research on suicide and suicidality; given the importance of current, accurate data for developing, targeting, and evaluating interventions, this is not surprising. Funding for prevention, including research in the service of prevention, is never sufficient to meet the need, and governmental budget decisions rarely seem to improve this situation. Therefore, a recommendation that federal funding agencies, including NIMH, CDC, and SAMHSA, encourage the inclusion of measures of suicide and suicidality in each large or longitudinal study is appropriate. This will help address recognized shortcomings in surveillance data, particularly with regard to underreporting. Potter (2001) suggests that mortality data be examined at the state level before sending it on to federal agencies. This would shorten the time lag between the collection of data and their availability to policy makers, practitioners, and researchers. This, in turn, would make it possible to use more current data to develop and implement preventive strategies.

Several changes in public policy might be made to improve the effectiveness of suicide preventive interventions. Reducing easy access to lethal means, especially firearms, has been shown to be an effective intervention (Goldsmith et al., 2002). It is commonly believed that restricting access to firearms, and to handguns in particular, will not affect suicide rates because a suicidal person will simply find another means. However, means replacement is not inevitable, and making access to firearms more difficult can be a useful tool in reducing the number of completed suicides (Goldsmith et al., 2002). Other possibilities for restricting access pertain to barriers on bridges, the content of natural gas used for cooking, and poison control (see Goldsmith et al., 2002).

Another policy change with potential to positively affect suicide prevention pertains to the way government entities address suicide intervention and research. Public-private and interdisciplinary partnerships should be developed at the federal, state, and local levels to work in a concerted fashion, leveraging their resources to develop, evaluate, and expand suicide prevention programs (see Goldsmith et al., 2002; U.S. Public Health Service, 1999).

Finally, public policy must recognize and address differences between the nation's metropolitan and rural areas. Rural areas frequently suffer from shortages of health and mental health care providers. Some risk factors for suicidality appear to differ depending on where people live (Goldsmith et al., 2002), and policies pertaining to funding, implementing, and evaluating suicide prevention efforts should reflect awareness of and sensitivity to these differences.

Much has been learned about suicide in the 40 years since the beginning of systematic suicide prevention and suicidology in this country. In the near future, progress in suicidology is a near certainty as advances are made in areas as diverse as genetic involvement in mental illness and the influence of mass media on behavior. The inclusion of suicidal patients in research studies (Goldsmith et al., 2002), clearer delineation of the role of substance abuse in suicidality (Hawton, 2001), and the study of nearly fatal suicide attempts (Hawton, 2001) are promising steps forward. For the present, prevention efforts at each level of intervention offer significant hope to thousands of people each year.

REFERENCES

American Foundation for Suicide Prevention. (2004a). *History.* Retrieved February 21, 2004, from www.afsp.org.

American Foundation for Suicide Prevention. (2004b). *Reporting on suicide: Recommendations for the media.* Retrieved February 24, 2004, from www.afsp.org.

American Foundation for Suicide Prevention. (2004c). *What's new.* Retrieved February 21, 2004, from www.afsp.org.

Bruce, M., & Pearson, J. (1999). Designing an intervention to prevent suicide: PROSPECT (Prevention of Suicide in Primary Care Elderly: Collaborative Trial). *Dialogues in Clinical Neuroscience, 1*(2), 100–112.

Caplan, G. (1964). *Principles of preventive psychiatry.* New York: Basic Books.

Carney, S., Rich, D., Burke, P., & Fowler, R. (1994). Suicide over 60: The San Diego Study. *Journal of American Geriatric Society, 42,* 174–180.

Centers for Disease Control. (2003a). *Fast stats A to Z: Suicide.* Retrieved January 21, 2004, from www.cdc.gov/nchs/fastats.

Centers for Disease Control. (2003b). *Suicide in the United States.* Retrieved January 6, 2004, from www.cdc.gov.

Day, P. (2003). *A new history of social welfare* (4th ed.). Boston: Allyn & Bacon.

Goldman, L., Nielsen, N., & Champion, H. (1999). Awareness, diagnosis, and treatment of depression. *Journal of General Internal Medicine, 14*(9), 569–580.

Goldsmith, S., Pellmar, T., Kleinment, A., & Bunney, W. (2002). *Reducing suicide: A national imperative.* Washington, DC: National Academy Press.

Hawton, K. (2001). Studying survivors of nearly lethal suicide attempts: An important strategy in suicide research. *Suicide and Life-Threatening Behavior, 32,* 76–84.

Higgins, E. (1994). A review of unrecognized mental illness in primary care: Prevalence, natural history, and efforts to change the course. *Archives of Family Medicine, 3*(10), 908–917.

Katon, W., & Schulberg, H. (1992). Epidemiology of depression in primary care. *General Hospital Psychiatry, 14*(4), 237–247.

Lester, D. (2001). The epidemiology of suicide. In D. Lester (Ed.), *Suicide prevention: Resources for the millennium* (pp. 3–16). Philadelphia: Brunner/Routledge.

Lindemann, E. (1944). Symptomatology and management of acute grief. *American Journal of Psychiatry, 101,* 141–148.

Litts, D., Moe, K., Roadman, C., Janke, R., & Miller, J. (2000). Suicide prevention among active duty Air Force personnel—United States, 1990–1999. *Journal of the American Medical Association, 283*(2), 193–194.

McCarter, A. K., Sowers, K. M., & Dulmus, C. (2004). Adolescent suicide prevention. In L. Rapp-Paglicci, C. Dulmus, & J. Wodarski (Eds.), *Handbook of preventive interventions for children and adolescents* (pp. 85–99). Hoboken, NJ: Wiley.

Muñoz, R., Ying, Y., Perez-Stable, E., & Miranda, J. (1993). *The prevention of depression: Research and practice.* Baltimore: Johns Hopkins University Press.

National Institute of Mental Health. (2004). *Care managers help depressed elderly reduce suicidal thoughts.* Retrieved March 16, 2004, from www.nimh.nih.gov/events.

National Public Radio. (2004, March 8). *Actor Spalding Gray's body found.* Retrieved March 17, 2004, from www.npr.org/features.

Office of Public Health and Science. (2004). *Best practice: Air Force suicide prevention program: A population-based approach.* Retrieved February 24, 2004, from www.osophs.dhhs.gov.

Painter, K. (2004, March 3). Colleges throw lifeline to students. *USA Today,* pp. B1–2.

Potter, L. (2001). Public health and suicide prevention. In D. Lester (Ed.), *Suicide prevention: Resources for the millennium* (pp. 67–72). Philadelphia: Brunner/Routledge.

Rapp-Paglicci, L., Dulmus, C., & Wodarski, J. (Eds.). (2004). *Handbook of preventive interventions for children and adolescents.* Hoboken, NJ: Wiley.

Reynolds, C., Schulberg, H., Bruce, M., Alexopoulous, G., Katz, I., & Mulsant, B. (2001, December 10). *Depression treatment in primary care elderly: Preliminary outcomes of the NIMH PROSPECT Collaborative.* Abstract presented at the annual meeting of the American College of Neuropsychopharmacology in Kona, Hawaii, 2001.

Rihmer, Z., Rutz, W., & Pihlgren, H. (1998). Decreasing tendency of seasonality in suicide may indicate lowering rate of depressive suicides in the population. *Psychiatry Research, 16,* 223–240.

Roy, A. (2001). Psychiatric treatment in suicide. In D. Lester (Ed.), *Suicide prevention: Resources for the millennium* (pp. 103–127). Philadelphia: Brunner/Routledge.

Rutz, W., von Knorring, L., & Walinder, J. (1989). Frequency of suicide on Gotland after systematic postgraduate education of general practitioners. *Acta Psychiatrica Scandinavica, 80*(2), 151–154.

Rutz, W., von Knorring, L., & Walinder, J. (1992). Long-term effects of an educational program for general practitioners given by the Swedish Committee for Prevention and Treatment of Depression. *Acta Psychiatrica Scandinavica, 85*(1), 83–88.

Schneidman, E. S. (1988). Some reflections of a founder. In R. Marris (Ed.), *Understanding and preventing suicide* (pp. 1–12). New York: Guilford Press.

Serna, P., May, P., & Sitaker, M. (1998). Suicide prevention evaluation in a Western Athabaskan American Indian tribe—New Mexico, 1988–1997. *Morbidity and Mortality Weekly Report, 47*(13), 257–261.

Stack, S. (2001). Sociological research into suicide. In D. Lester (Ed.), *Suicide prevention: Resources for the millennium* (pp. 17–29). Philadelphia: Brunner/Routledge.

Substance Abuse and Mental Health Services Administration. (2004a). National strategy for suicide prevention. *National Strategy for Suicide Prevention.* Retrieved January 6, 2004, from www.mentalhealth.samhsa.gov/suicideprevention.

Substance Abuse and Mental Health Services Administration. (2004b). Suicide: Cost to the nation. *National Strategy for Suicide Prevention.* Retrieved January 6, 2004, from www.mentalhealth.samhsa.gov suicideprevention.

Szanto, K., Mulsant, B., Houck, P., Miller, M., Mazumdar, S., & Reynolds, C. (2001). Treatment outcome in suicidal vs. non-suicidal elderly patients. *American Journal of Geriatric Psychiatry, 9*(3), 261–268.

U.S. Air Force Medical Service. (2000). *The Air Force Suicide Prevention Program: A description on program initiatives and outcomes* (USAF Publication No. AFPAM 44-160). Washington, DC: U.S. Air Force.

U.S. Government Printing Office. (2000, February 8). *Suicide awareness and prevention* [Hearing before a Subcommittee of the Committee on Appropriations, United States Senate, 106th Congress; Electronic version]. Washington, DC: Author.

U.S. Public Health Service. (1999). *The Surgeon General's call to action to prevent suicide* [Electronic version]. Washington, DC: U.S. Government Printing Office.

van Praag, H. M. (2001). Suicide and aggression: Are they biologically two sides of the same coin? In D. Lester (Ed.), *Suicide prevention: Resources for the millennium* (pp. 45–64). Philadelphia: Brunner/Routledge.

VanWinkle, N., & May, P. (1986). Native American suicide in New Mexico, 1957–1979: A comparative study. *Human Organization, 45*(4), 296–309.

VanWinkle, N., & May, P. (1993). An update on American Indian suicide in New Mexico, 1980–1987. *Human Organization, 52*(3), 304–315.

VanWinkle, N., & Williams, M. (2001). *Evaluation of the National Model Adolescent Suicide Prevention Project: A comparison of suicide rates among New Mexico American Indian tribes, 1980–1998.* Tulsa: Oklahoma State University, College of Osteopathic Medicine.

Wallace, M. (2001). The origin of suicide prevention in the United States. In D. Lester (Ed.), *Suicide prevention: Resources for the millennium* (pp. 339–354). Philadelphia: Brunner/Routledge.

Wells, K., Katon, W., Rogers, B., & Camp, P. (1994). Use of minor tranquilizers and antidepressant medications by depressed outpatients: Results from the medical outcomes study. *American Journal of Psychiatry, 151*(5), 694–700.

Williams, J. W. J., Rost, K., Dietrich, A. J., Ciotti, M. C., Zyzanski, S. J., & Cornell, J. (1999). Primary care physicians' approach to depressive disorders: Effects of physicians specialty and practice structure. *Archives of Family Medicine, 8,* 58–67.

Chapter 5

UNRESOLVED GRIEF

CAROLYN HILARSKI

Bereaved individuals, who understand their loss as traumatic, are at risk for experiencing severe health and mental health issues (Selby & Prigerson, 2000). The trauma response and its consequences frequently disrupt the mourning process and encourage an unresolved or complicated grief pattern of thinking and behaving (Raphael & Dobson, 2000; Szanto, 2003). Persons struggling with unresolved or complicated grief may report feelings of apathy, weight gain or loss, disturbed sleep, or a need for sleep due to fatigue; they may feel consistently agitated and have trouble concentrating. These individuals may also report intrusive and distressing thoughts and dreams, flashbacks, hypervigilance, concentration difficulties, and feelings of reliving the perceived traumatic event. Indeed, researchers have found a significant number of bereaved individuals meeting the criteria for traumatic stress (Sprang & McNeil, 1995). Further, these symptoms may be present for a year or more after a loss (Szanto & Prigerson, 1997). The consequences of the traumatic response affects not only individuals and families but entire societies (Sherman, 1999; Sprang & McNeil, 1995).

Bereaved persons must modify their identity, roles, and relationships. They are no longer the parent, spouse, sibling, child, coworker, employer, or friend to someone with whom they were close. When the bereaved person is framing the bereavement as traumatic, the "work" of *redefining* the self and the environment can seem overwhelming and unachievable (Hobfoll, Ennis, & Kay, 2000). The outcome of these thoughts and feelings is withdrawing behavior, which can interrupt supportive interpersonal relationships (Lindstrom, 2002). Inefficient social supports and coping skills complicate the mourning process (Carver, 1998).

In summary, unresolved grief finds grievers experiencing the seemingly devastating and complex task of adjusting to a changed external environment, which leads to problems of social maladjustment, ineffective coping skills, and inadequate social supports that may last for years after a loss. The consequences of this may be substance abuse, psychiatric problems, and/or suicide (Knieper, 1999). The elderly are particularly vulnerable to suicide due to the greater likelihood of social isolation and depression (Edelstein, Kalish, Drozdick, & McKee, 1999). Adults over 65 represent 20% of the suicide events each year in the United States, with widowers much more likely to commit suicide than nonwidowers (McIntosh, 1992). It is essential for professionals to be familiar with the factors associated with complicated mourning and the latest empirical universal, selected, and indicated prevention endeavors. This awareness will help to increase the possibility of accurate assessment and prompt and appropriate service delivery for those suffering with the pain of trauma from bereavement.

DEFINITIONS

Bereavement is an objective state of being due to loss (Zeitlin, 2001). Often the circumstance is in the loss of a loved person although it could be the loss of a loved thing (M. Stroebe, Schut, & Finkenauer, 2001).

Mourning is the culturally influenced emotional process of accepting a loss (Foster, 1981). It is the working through or the reframing of a loss with the help of cultural beliefs and traditions (Neimeyer, Prigerson, & Davies, 2002).

Grief is the emotional and psychological reaction to the internal explanation of loss or bereavement (Marwit & Carusa, 1998). This state of being is a subjective response influenced by the nature of the relationship with the loved thing or person; the reactions of others to the loss, in addition to the early childhood attachment experience (Neimeyer et al., 2002). This is a place of "dis-ease" with a path that consists of an initial phase of shock, then, experiences of varied negative thoughts and feelings due to the absence of the attachment figure or thing (Bowlby, 1982; Engel, 1961). Grief is behavior that attempts to maintain the bond to the lost object regardless of the consequences (Bowlby, 1982).

Unresolved grief is a chronic state of grief distinct from anxiety or depressive disorders. However, its presenting symptoms may mirror those categories to some degree (Chen, 1999; Prigerson et al., 1997). The current suggestion is that it is a form of separation anxiety and is associated with health consequences that often require intervention (Selby & Prigerson, 2000).

TRENDS AND INCIDENTS

Approximately 10 million individuals are in a bereaved state each year in the United States (Arias, Anderson, Kung, Murphy, & Kochanek, 2003). A subgroup of this population will perceive their loss as traumatic (Harkness, Shear, Frank, & Silberman, 2002). Bereavement perceived as disturbing, shocking, or overwhelmingly painful is often referred to as atypical, traumatic, pathological, complicated, or unresolved grief (Harkness et al., 2002; Marwit, 1996). These maladaptive responses to bereavement become entrenched if the trauma reaction is not resolved (Bentovim, 1986).

The published prevalence rates for bereaved adult individuals suffering from unresolved grief range from 14% to 64% (Horowitz et al., 1997; Kim & Jacobs, 1991; McDermott et al., 1997; Middleton, Burnett, Raphael, & Martinek, 1996; Prigerson et al., 1997; Zisook & DeVaul, 1984). This wide range of estimates is due to diverse sample selection and a lack of standardized criteria for assessing unresolved grief.

The time line for uncomplicated mourning is believed to be somewhere between 4 and 6 months (Clayton, 1990; Jacobs & Ostfeld, 1980; Parkes, 1972). The presence, for two or more months, of unremitting thoughts of longing, disbelief, shock, wanting to die, life is out of control, in addition to feelings of emptiness, anger, and hopelessness that interfere in daily activities puts the bereaved person in an unresolved grieving pattern (Prigerson & Jacobs, 2001; Selby & Prigerson, 2000). In this pattern, the individual is at increased risk for psychological, physical, and social impairment, as unattended unresolved grief symptoms do not appear to change over time (Prigerson & Jacobs, 2001; Prigerson et al., 1997; Prigerson, Bridge, et al., 1999; Zisook & DeVaul, 1983). The intensity of the unresolved grief response peaks 6 months after a loss and is inclined to remain high for 25 months and beyond (Prigerson, Shear, et al., 1999).

RISK FACTORS FOR UNRESOLVED GRIEF

Age and Gender

Age and gender appear to influence the course of mourning. Specifically, observations of the bereavement response will often differ across age groups (Prigerson, Frank, et al., 1995). This is because individuals face notably diverse stressors across the life stages and coping mechanisms are specific to the developmental level, which is influenced by biology, culture, and life experience (Hayslip, Allen, & McCoy-Roberts, 2001).

Commonly men have greater difficulty expressing emotion following bereavement and self report few coping skills. Moreover, they enter into romantic relationships more rapidly after the death of a partner, experience serious illness and greater social isolation, in addition to demonstrating significant struggles accepting bereavement when compared to women. Men presenting with anxiety in the first 6 months of bereavement are at high risk for suicidal behavior (Chen, 1999).

Women report greater emotional distress (e.g., depressive and anxious type symptoms), feelings of helplessness, and noteworthy changes in identity and social roles (Chen, 1999; Hayslip et al., 2001). Mothers mourning the loss of a child report high levels of grief reactions when compared to their male partners. Denial appeared to be a significant coping response for the males (Zisook & Lyons, 1990). Females presenting with a trauma response within the first 6 months of loss are at risk for cancer and heart disease (Chen, 1999).

Personality

Personality characteristics and preexisting psychological conditions also mediate a persons reaction to bereavement (Meuser & Marwit, 2001). To illustrate, individuals found to be depressed or depressive at the time of bereavement showed a propensity to experience complicated or unresolved grief following a loss (Gilewski, Farberow, Gallagher, & Thompson, 1991).

Early childhood attachment experience may be associated with the bereavement response (Wayment & Vierthaler, 2002). In looking at the attachment style of bereaved persons, it was determined that anxious avoidant persons are at risk for responding to bereavement with depressive and somatic symptoms (Wayment & Vierthaler, 2002).

Social Support

Research finds a relationship between the perception of having close and supportive relationships and uncomplicated mourning in bereaved individuals (Dimond, Lund, & Caserta, 1987). Bereavement self-help groups may encourage supportive interactions for bereaved persons using withdrawal as a coping mechanism. Indeed, bereaved individuals, where the lost object was murdered, reported that self-help groups were exceedingly supportive during the mourning process. The fact that a bereavement group includes a population with similar experiences helps to reduce the bereaved person's thoughts of aloneness and increases the likelihood of interaction both during and outside of the group meetings (Hatton, 2003).

Coping Skills

The lack of effective coping skills further complicates the adjustment process for bereaved individuals (Carver, 1998; Lindstrom, 1997). Studies show that the use of reappraisal, problem-focused decision making, spiritual beliefs and practices, active emotional processing, and drawing positive meaning from stressful events are significant positive coping factors for an individual experiencing bereavement (Folkman, 1997; Lindstrom, 1997).

UNIVERSAL PREVENTIVE INTERVENTIONS

There are no formal universal prevention programs for bereaved individuals. Few persons experiencing loss seek professional help (Parkes, 2002). Avoidance of painful reminders may be one reason. Another may be a concern that the professional helper will reject the problem as insignificant. The U.S. culture demands that individuals handle such a common issue as bereavement. Seeking help is weak behavior. However, the long-term consequences of being strong can be lethal (Chen, 1999). Thus, a universal approach might propose to change the *cultural thinking* about bereavement and how individuals may deal with such a circumstance. The influence of culture on thinking, feeling, and behaving begins early in the life course. Therefore, early prevention endeavors are essential. Schools are an appropriate place to begin such an effort (Charkow, 1998; Findlay, 1999; Milton, 1999a, 1999b). Death education and group sharing is quite appropriate in the health or personal development portion of a school curriculum and most helpful if begun in preschool or kindergarten (Findlay, 1999; Milton, 1999a). It is imperative that parents be included in this prevention effort, as they are the primary influencing factors in the child's response to loss (Charkow, 1998; Cohen, Mannarino, Greenberg, Padlo, & Shipley, 2002; Findlay, 1999; Milton, 1999a). Moreover, *system* prevention is far superior to individual intervention (Black, 1991; Cohen et al., 2002).

Age-appropriate death education in the school curriculum that includes parent participation, helps to inoculate children and their families for future loss exposure (Milton, 1999b). Further, it helps to identify bereaved children and family members that may not be presenting with identifiable symptoms and thwart further escalation of any complicated mourning issues. Additionally, it encourages a dialogue between children—between parents and children—and between parents, children, and *others* regarding this very difficult subject (Cohen et al., 2002). Open communication about death and the accompanying emotions and thoughts is helpful by offering the child the opportunity to ask questions and correct mistaken fantasies about another child, parent, or *other's* feelings concerning loss (Charkow, 1998). Finally, it offers parents the chance to observe helpful age appropriate communication and interaction by other parents, teachers, or group leaders. If honest communication in the family system begins before a loss exposure or anytime during the mourning continuum, reconciliation is more likely (Charkow, 1998).

The parent and child's group needs to feel secure during the school based death education module (Findlay, 1999; Milton, 1999a). To promote group member well-being, the teacher or group leader might share that tears and emotions are normal and natural when talking about loss and death (Milton, 1999a). Questions to explore are: "What is death?" "What happens at a funeral?" "What is it like to lose a pet?" (Milton, 1999a). Some form of group relaxation technique is helpful at termination of the educational and sharing session (Milton, 1999b).

Books are a helpful way for parents and children to explore thoughts and feelings about loss at home (Milton, 1999b). Moreover, books are safe in that the person experiencing the loss and the response to that loss is in the story (Milton, 1999a). Parents need to be encouraged to discuss loss with their children whenever the opportunity presents itself. This reminds and reinforces the parents and informs the child that loss is a normal part of the lived experience.

SELECTED PREVENTIVE INTERVENTIONS

It appears that potential complicated grievers may be distinguished from other bereaved individuals (Bonanno et al., 2002). Thus, assessing for unresolved grief risk factors in persons bereaved or about to be bereaved will enable the appropriate services to be allocated for those identified at risk (Ellifritt, Nelson, & Walsh, 2003). However, Marwit (1996) suggests that bereaved or about to be bereaved individuals need a multiaxial assessment for competent service provision.

Outreach

Individual or family outreach, for a term of 12 months, by a service delivery professional or community layperson to recently (or an anticipated) bereaved person is a way to reduce the possibility of unresolved grief. This vital interaction allows the bereaved (or about to be bereaved) person(s) to recognize that they are not alone. The interface discourages withdrawal behavior and allows the service provider to monitor the mourning path (Berson, 1988; Provini, Everett, & Pfeffer, 2000).

Especially challenging is outreach services for families. Many individuals are not prepared for coping with bereavement (Muller & Thompson, 2003). Parents report difficulty in working through their own mourning process in addition to helping their children. The challenge for parents involves first recognizing the child's presentation of mourning then following through with support. Continuous family member assessment is important toward the prevention effort (Provini et al., 2000), as coping skills may change over time (Muller & Thompson, 2003).

It should be added here that individuals or families might initially reject outreach services. However, gentle reminders, through mailings or drop-in appointments, that services are available may encourage the bereaved person(s) to request assistance when they are ready. Prevention efforts are helpful at any time along the continuum of the mourning process. Moreover, service provision may involve helping the individual or family with everyday tasks such as grocery shopping or with funeral arrangements (Provini et al., 2000).

Family Care

Family members who choose home-based or in-hospital care-giving report a great deal of satisfaction and accomplishment in helping their loved person in the final moments. This behavior encourages the uncomplicated mourning process (Koop & Strang, 2003; Warren, 2002).

Group Therapy

The empirical effectiveness of group therapy interventions for bereaved individuals is in its infancy. Outcome studies are rare. Those that have studied group intervention effectiveness for bereaved persons found that eight weekly 2-hour meetings showed benefits. Interventions employed were: education on the grieving process, relaxation techniques, freedom to vent feelings, and other activities like journalizing, or creating a memorial for the lost object (Morgan, 1994). The intervention components encourage the distressed individual to explore the positive and negative memories and associated feelings related to the lost object. The bereaved individual is then supported in working through the meaning of the loss and the emotions that result from this understanding (Piper, Ogrodniczuk, McCallum, Joyce, & Rosie, 2003).

INDICATED

Complete resolution of a perceived traumatic loss is the exception rather than the rule. An individual presenting with unresolved grief needs trauma symptom assessment, because the presence of perceived trauma from the bereavement is likely and will impede the recovery work (Selby & Prigerson, 2000).

The initial prevention effort will be trauma symptom reduction (van der Kolk, McFarlane, & Weisaeth, 1996). Psychodynamic models are helpful for trauma indicators (Bishop & Lane, 2003; Gerrity & Solomon, 1996), especially in a comorbid circumstance (Bishop & Lane, 2003). Techniques such as exploration of transference and counter transference in addition to counselor empathy and tuning in enable the client to redirect internal energy to more helpful processes (Bishop & Lane, 2003). Cognitive behavioral interventions are effective with intrusive thoughts and recurrent nightmares (Reynolds, 1996). A course of treatment might include learning how to control negative thoughts and feelings through reframing and self-soothing instruction and practice. These new behaviors set the stage for the recounting of disturbing nightmares, daydreams, or the loss event with all their emotional and cognitive content. The telling and retelling of the *story of loss,* in a safe and controlled environment, allows the individual to realize that he or she is able to cope with the negative emotions that may initially be emitted.

Writing or drawing approaches that include the story of loss with the attached responsive emotions and thoughts encourage the perception of the loss to change as new cognitions are integrated with the subjective emotional response (Largo-Marsh & Spates, 2002; Reynolds, 1996). This method relates to exposure therapy where repeated disclosure of the perceived trauma reduces or neutralizes its emotional arousal through habituation. This intervention may be particularly helpful in reducing somatic complaints in individuals suffering with a trauma response (Gramlich, 1968; M. Stroebe, Stroebe, Schut, Zech, & van den Bout, 2002). The writing process entails instructing the bereaved person(s) to first imagine the events surrounding the loss then to write his or her thoughts and feelings regarding the *meaning of these events.* Writing sessions may last 30 minutes or more and occur over several sessions (Range, Kovac, & Marion, 2000). It is important to note that these interventions are for those individuals seeking help for distressing symptoms relating to unresolved grief. Persons experiencing uncomplicated bereavement need to mourn in their own time and manner (W. Stroebe, Stroebe, Abakoumkin, & Schut, 1996) and do not appear to be helped with the aforementioned methods (Schut, Stroebe, van den Bout, & Terheggen, 2001).

Family Prevention

When the majority of family members perceive a loss as traumatic, a family intervention may be useful (Murphy et al., 1998). Specific techniques may include encouraging the family to engage in rituals, reminiscing, and celebratory behaviors to enhance opportunities for collective grief work. To help the family members reduce the sense of aloneness and destructive negative thinking, the helping professional may support the family members in examining their sense of spirituality, for example, a member's perception and relationship with a higher power, in addition to exploring such unhelpful behaviors as blaming (the self or other). An additional issue may be blocked family processes. A common avoidance behavior intended to maintain the lost person within the family is designating a replacement. This allows the family to continue to hold the lost object, however, the burden to the replacement member is staggering and often has long-term detrimental consequences (e.g., substance abuse; Bowser, Word, Stanton, & Coleman, 2003).

Self-Help Group Prevention Effort

Bereaved persons report an overall lack of social supports and this factor relates to a complicated grief response (Carver, 1998). Individuals experiencing the consequences of unresolved grief frequently need assistance, which may include the empathic nature of self-help (Hawton & Simkin, 2003). Support groups are often a valuable supplement to individual and family treatment because they offer members hope for recovery, a level of understanding through shared experiences, tolerant social interactions, normalization, and a safe place to learn and practice new coping skills. Self-help groups are self-governed, self-reliant, conveniently located, and there is no fee to be a member (Lieberman, 1993). Self-help groups do not make up for or take the place of the lost object. They help to fill an empty space and offer new insight (W. Stroebe et al., 1996).

PRACTICE AND POLICY IMPLICATIONS

It is economically and socially profitable for professionals to engage in prevention of unresolved grief (Charkow, 1998; Geis, Whittlesey, McDonald, Smith, & Pfefferbaum, 1998). The consequence of not engaging in such activity is severe health and mental health related disorders (Geis et al., 1998). Therefore, educators and health professionals need to be informed regarding effective assessment and prevention efforts for individuals anticipating or experiencing bereavement, or reporting grief or unresolved grief symptoms (Charkow, 1998; Cohen et al., 2002). Moreover, professionals need to recognize that all individuals require some sort of prevention intervention before a loss, if possible, and certainly during an expected loss or recent loss (Charkow, 1998).

Professionals need to educate and support family members, early in the life stage, to openly share their thoughts and feelings regarding loss. Family members who recognize the importance of open communication and mourning rituals within the developmental constraints of the evolving family are likely to follow an uncomplicated mourning path when exposed to bereavement (Norris-Shortle, Young, & Williams, 1993). Further, professionals and laypersons alike need to be aware of and accept that the individual response to loss is heterogeneous. This awareness decreases the likelihood of disapproving behavior by possible supporters when the bereaved individual displays his or her own unique reaction to loss (Bonanno et al., 2002). Others disapproval of behavior or concern regarding pathology may be internalized by the bereaved individual adding to any distressful bereavement response.

Professionals who modify their intervention techniques to the coping style of their bereaved clients are more effective (Muller & Thompson, 2003). For example, a bereaved client who might fear being overwhelmed by emotions might wish to control the pace of the therapeutic interaction. A person-centered approach might be beneficial for such a client. The helper stands with the client, listening and learning, not leading or advising (Thompson, Rose, Wainwright, Mattar, & Scanlan, 2001). A client who wishes to change a behavior in response to loss may need some type of *reality* technique, while a client who chooses rumination or intellectualization as a coping response, may need a *rational emotive* intervention (e.g., reframing; Muller & Thompson, 2003). As a final point, a Gestalt or empty chair technique might be helpful for a client with unresolved issues relating to the lost object. Journalizing and letter writing is helpful with this type of client (Muller & Thompson, 2003).

Governmental agencies need to comprehensively support unresolved grief prevention efforts. This prevention endeavor needs to focus on families (Dowdney et al., 1999). General screening for unresolved grief symptoms in a group of school age children showed previously unidentified trauma symptoms (March, Amaya-Jackson, Terry, & Costanzo, 1997). Trauma symptoms in youth have long-term academic and health related consequences (Black, 1998). Thus, periodic governmentally funded screening for unresolved grief symptoms is essential. This universal screening will help to identify bereaved children who very likely have bereaved family members in need of help. Early assessment and appropriate intervention is the key to preventing further health related issues in bereaved family members experiencing unresolved grief (Black, 1998; Cohen et al., 2002).

FUTURE DIRECTIONS

There is little empirical evidence supporting the current categories of complicated mourning. If mourning is an individual process relating to the person's age, gender, culture, social supports, and coping skills, is it possible to categorize such possible heterogeneity? Do the grief descriptors pathological, atypical, traumatic, abnormal, or delayed explain the mourning process or the person's perception of the loss? A clear definition for uncomplicated mourning is illusive. Moreover, there is ambiguous acceptance of the associated risk factors that relate to a mourning process that appears complicated. Perhaps, the seeming complicated process is actually the healthy path. Future studies will need to address these concerns.

Finally, outcome studies relating to interventions for individuals struggling with unresolved grief have centered on professional practice. Future studies might include laypersons and the self-help sector to be applicable to current service realities and client needs.

REFERENCES

Arias, E., Anderson, R. N., Kung, H. C., Murphy, S. L., & Kochanek, K. D. (2003). Deaths: Final data for 2001. *National Vital Statistics Reports 52*(3), 1–116. Hyattsville, MD: National Center for Health Statistics.

Bentovim, A. (1986). Bereaved children. *British Medical Journal, 292*(6534), 1482.

Berson, R. J. (1988). A bereavement group for college students. *Journal of American College Health, 37*(3), 101–108.

Bishop, J., & Lane, R. C. (2003). Psychodynamic treatment of a case of grief superimposed on melancholia. *Clinical Case Studies, 2*(1), 3–19.

Black, D. (1991). Family intervention with families bereaved or about to be bereaved. In D. Papadatou & C. Papadatos (Eds.), *Children and death: Series in death education, aging and health* (pp. 135–143). New York: Hemisphere.

Black, D. (1998). Coping with loss: Bereavement in childhood. *British Medical Journal, 316*(7135), 931–933.

Bonanno, G. A., Wortman, C. B., Lehman, D. R., Tweed, R. G., Haring, M., Sonnega, J., et al. (2002). Resilience to loss and chronic grief: A prospective study from preloss to 18-months postloss. *Journal of Personality and Social Psychology, 83*(5), 1150–1164.

Bowlby, J. (1982). Attachment and loss: Retrospect and prospect. *American Journal of Orthopsychiatry, 52*(4), 664–678.

Bowser, B. P., Word, C. O., Stanton, M. D., & Coleman, S. B. (2003). Death in the family and HIV risk-taking among intravenous drug users. *Family Process, 42*(2), 291–304.

Carver, C. S. (1998). Generalization, adverse events, and development of depressive symptoms. *Journal of Personality, 66*(4), 607–619.

Charkow, W. B. (1998). Inviting children to grieve. *Professional School Counseling, 2*(2), 117–123.

Chen, J. H. (1999). Gender differences in the effects of bereavement-related psychological distress in health outcomes. *Psychological Medicine, 29*(2), 367–380.

Clayton, P. J. (1990). Bereavement and depression. *Journal of Clinical Psychiatry, 51*(Suppl.), 34–40.

Cohen, J. A., Mannarino, A. P., Greenberg, T., Padlo, S., & Shipley, C. (2002). Childhood traumatic grief: Concepts and controversies. *Trauma, Violence, and Abuse, 3*(4), 307–327.

Dimond, M., Lund, D. A., & Caserta, M. S. (1987). The role of social support in the first two years of bereavement in an elderly sample. *Gerontologist, 27*(5), 599–604.

Dowdney, L., Wilson, R., Maughan, B., Allerton, M., Schofield, P., & Skuse, D. (1999). Psychological disturbance and service provision in parentally bereaved children: Prospective case-control study. *British Medical Journal, 319*(7206), 354–357.

Edelstein, B., Kalish, K. D., Drozdick, L. W., & McKee, D. R. (1999). Assessment of depression and bereavement in older adults. In P. A. Lichtenberg (Ed.), *Handbook of assessment in clinical gerontology* (pp. 11–58). New York: Wiley.

Ellifritt, J., Nelson, K. A., & Walsh, D. (2003). Complicated bereavement: A national survey of potential risk factors. *American Journal of Hospital and Palliative Care, 20*(2), 114–120.

Engel, G. L. (1961). Is grief a disease? A challenge for medical research. *Psychosomatic Medicine, 23,* 18–22.

Findlay, B. (1999). Using the text "Lucy Bay" to explore loss and grief: Unit overview. *Primary Educator, 5*(3), 17–19.

Folkman, S. (1997). Introduction to the special section: Use of bereavement narratives to predict well-being in gay men whose partners died of AIDS—four theoretical perspectives. *Journal of Personality and Social Psychology, 72*(4), 851–854.

Foster, S. (1981). Explaining death to children. *British Medical Journal, 282*(6263), 540–542.

Geis, H. K., Whittlesey, S. W., McDonald, N. B., Smith, K. L., & Pfefferbaum, B. (1998). Bereavement and loss in childhood. *Child and Adolescent Psychiatric Clinics of North America, 7*(1), viii, 73–85.

Gerrity, E. T., & Solomon, S. D. (1996). The treatment of PTSD and related stress disorders: Current research and clinical knowledge. In A. J. Marsella & M. J. Friedman (Eds.), *Ethnocultural aspects of posttraumatic stress disorder: Issues, research, and clinical applications* (pp. 87–102). Washington, DC: American Psychological Association.

Gilewski, M. J., Farberow, N. L., Gallagher, D. E., & Thompson, L. W. (1991). Interaction of depression and bereavement on mental health in the elderly. *Psychology of Aging, 6*(1), 67–75.

Gramlich, E. P. (1968). Recognition and management of grief in elderly patients. *Geriatrics, 23*(7), 87–92.

Harkness, K. L., Shear, M. K., Frank, E., & Silberman, R. A. (2002). Traumatic grief treatment: Case histories of 4 patients. *Journal of Clinical Psychiatry, 63*(12), 1113–1120.

Hatton, R. (2003). Homicide bereavement counseling: A survey of providers. *Death Studies, 27,* 427–448.

Hawton, K., & Simkin, S. (2003). Helping people bereaved by suicide. *British Medical Journal, 327*(7408), 177–178.

Hayslip, B. J., Allen, S. E., & McCoy-Roberts, L. (2001). The role of gender in a three-year longitudinal study of bereavement: A test of the experienced competence model. In D. A. Lund (Ed.), *Men coping with grief* (pp. 121–146). Amityville, NY: Baywood.

Hobfoll, S. E., Ennis, N., & Kay, J. (2000). Loss, resources, and resiliency in close interpersonal relationships. In J. H. Harvey & E. D. Miller (Eds.), *Loss and trauma: General and close relationship perspectives* (pp. 267–285). New York: Brunner/Routledge.

Horowitz, M. J., Siegel, B., Holen, A., Bonanno, G. A., Milbrath, C., & Stinson, C. H. (1997). Diagnostic criteria for complicated grief disorder. *American Journal of Psychiatry, 154*(7), 904–910.

Jacobs, S., & Ostfeld, A. (1980). The clinical management of grief. *Journal of the American Geriatrics Society, 28*(7), 331–335.

Kim, K., & Jacobs, S. (1991). Pathologic grief and its relationship to their psychiatric disorders. *Journal of Affective Disorders, 21*(4), 257–263.

Knieper, A. J. (1999). The suicide survivor's grief and recovery. *Suicide and Life Threatening Behaviors, 29*(4), 353–345.

Koop, P. M., & Strang, V. R. (2003). The bereavement experience following home-based family caregiving for persons with advanced cancer. *Clinical Nursing Research, 12*(2), 127–144.

Largo-Marsh, L., & Spates, R. C. (2002). The effects of writing therapy in comparison to EMD/R on traumatic stress: The relationship between hypnotizability and client expectancy to outcome. *Professional Psychology, Research and Practice, 33*(6), 581–586.

Lieberman, M. A. (1993). Bereavement, self-help groups: A review of conceptual and methodological issues. In M. S. Stroebe, W. Stroebe, & R. O. Hansson (Eds.), *Handbook of bereavement: Theory, research, and intervention* (pp. 411–426). Cambridge, England: Cambridge University Press.

Lindstrom, T. C. (1997). Immunity and health after bereavement in relation to coping. *Scandinavian Journal of Psychology, 38*(3), 253–259.

Lindstrom, T. C. (2002). "It ain't necessarily so": Challenging mainstream thinking about bereavement. *Family Community Health, 25*(1), 11–21.

March, J. S., Amaya-Jackson, L., Terry, R., & Costanzo, P. (1997). Posttraumatic symptomatology in children and adolescents after an industrial fire. *Journal of American Academy of Child and Adolescent Psychiatry, 36*(8), 1080–1088.

Marwit, S. J. (1996). Reliability of diagnosing complicated grief: A preliminary investigation. *Journal of Consulting and Clinical Psychology, 64*(3), 563–568.

Marwit, S. J., & Carusa, S. S. (1998). Communicated support following loss: Examining the experiences of parental death and parental divorce in adolescence. *Death Studies, 22*(3), 237–255.

McDermott, O. D., Prigerson, H. G., Reynolds, C. F., III, Houck, P. R., Dew, M. A., Hall, M., et al. (1997). Sleep in the wake of complicated grief symptoms: An exploratory study. *Biological Psychiatry, 41*(6), 710–716.

McIntosh, J. L. (1992). Older adults: The next suicide epidemic? *Suicide and Life Threatening Behaviors, 22*(3), 322–332.

Meuser, T. M., & Marwit, S. J. (2001). A comprehensive, stage-sensitive model of grief in dementia caregiving. *Gerontologist, 41*(5), 658–670.

Middleton, W., Burnett, P., Raphael, B., & Martinek, N. (1996). The bereavement response: A cluster analysis. *British Journal of Psychiatry, 169*(2), 167–171.

Milton, J. (1999a). Loss and grief. *Primary Educator, 5*(3), 10–13.

Milton, J. (1999b). Providing anticipatory guidance for our children: Loss and grief education. *Primary Educator, 5*(3), 13–17.

Morgan, J. J. (1994). Bereavement in older adults. *Journal of Mental Health Counseling, 16*(3), 318–327.

Muller, E. D., & Thompson, C. L. (2003). The experience of grief after bereavement: A phenomenological study with implications for mental health counseling. *Journal of Mental Health Counseling, 25*(3), 183–203.

Murphy, S. A., Johnson, C., Cain, K. C., Das Gupta, A., Dimond, M., Lohan, J., et al. (1998). Broad-spectrum group treatment for parents bereaved by the violent deaths of their 12- to 28-year-old children: A randomized controlled trial. *Death Studies, 22*(3), 209–235.

Neimeyer, R. A., Prigerson, H. G., & Davies, B. M. (2002). Mourning and meaning. *American Behavioral Scientist, 46*(2), 235–251.

Norris-Shortle, C., Young, P. A., & Williams, M. A. (1993). Understanding death and grief for children three and younger. *Social Work, 38*(6), 736–742.

Parkes, C. M. (1972). *Bereavement: Studies of grief in adult life.* New York: International Universities Press.

Parkes, C. M. (2002). Grief: Lessons from the past, visions for the future. *Death Studies, 26*(5), 367–386.

Piper, W. E., Ogrodniczuk, J. S., McCallum, M., Joyce, A. S., & Rosie, J. S. (2003). Expression of affect as a mediator of the relationship between quality of object relations and group therapy outcome for patients with complicated grief. *Journal of Consulting and Clinical Psychology, 71*(4), 664–671.

Prigerson, H. G., Bierhals, A. J., Kasl, S. V., Reynolds, C. F., III, Shear, M. K., Day, N., et al. (1997). Traumatic grief as a risk factor for mental and physical morbidity. *American Journal of Psychiatry, 154*(5), 616–623.

Prigerson, H. G., Bridge, J., Maciejewski, P. K., Beery, L. C., Rosenheck, R. A., Jacobs, S. C., et al. (1999). Influence of traumatic grief on suicidal ideation among young adults. *American Journal of Psychiatry, 156*(12), 1994–1995.

Prigerson, H. G., Frank, E., Kasl, S. V., Reynolds, C. F., III, Anderson, B., Zubenko, G. S., et al. (1995). Complicated grief and bereavement-related depression as distinct disorders: Preliminary empirical validation in elderly bereaved spouses. *American Journal of Psychiatry, 152*(1), 22–30.

Prigerson, H. G., & Jacobs, S. C. (Eds.). (2001). *Traumatic grief as a distinct disorder: A rationale, consensus criteria, and a preliminary empirical test.* Washington, DC: American Psychological Association.

Prigerson, H. G., Shear, M. K., Jacobs, S. C., Reynolds, C. F., Maciejewski, P. K., & Davidson, J. R. T. (1999, January). Consensus criteria for traumatic grief: A preliminary empirical test. *British Journal of Psychiatry, 174,* 67–73.

Provini, C., Everett, J. R., & Pfeffer, C. R. (2000, January/February). Adults mourning suicide: Self-reported concerns about bereavement, needs for assistance, and help-seeking behavior. *Death Studies, 24,* 1–19.

Range, L. M., Kovac, S. H., & Marion, M. S. (2000). Does writing about the bereavement lessen grief following sudden, unintentional death? *Death Studies, 24*(2), 115–134.

Raphael, B., & Dobson, M. (2000). Bereavement. In J. H. Harvey & E. D. Miller (Eds.), *Loss and trauma: General and close relationship perspectives* (pp. 45–61). New York: Brunner/Routledge.

Reynolds, F. (1996). Laying mother to rest: Working with grief-related nightmares through exposure therapy and imagery. *Counseling Psychology Quarterly, 9*(3), 229–334.

Schut, H., Stroebe, M., van den Bout, J., & Terheggen, M. (2001). The efficacy of bereavement intervention: Who benefits. In M. S. Stroebe, R. O. Hansson, W. Stroebe, & H. Schut (Eds.), *Handbook of bereavement research: Consequences, coping, and care* (pp. 705–737). Washington, DC: American Psychological Association.

Selby, J., & Prigerson, H. (2000). Psychotherapy of traumatic grief: A review of evidence for psychotherapeutic treatments. *Death Studies, 24*(6), 479–496.

Sherman, J. J. (1999). Effects of psychotherapeutic treatments for PTSD: A meta-analysis of controlled clinical trials. *Clinical Psychology Review, 19*(3), 275–296.

Sprang, G., & McNeil, J. S. (1995). *The many faces of bereavement: The nature and treatment of natural, traumatic, and stigmatized grief.* Philadelphia: Brunner/ Mazel.

Stroebe, M., Schut, H., & Finkenauer, C. (2001). The traumatization of grief? A conceptual framework for understanding the trauma-bereavement interface. *Israel Journal of Psychiatry and Related Sciences, 38*(3/4), 185–201.

Stroebe, M., Stroebe, W., Schut, H., Zech, E., & van den Bout, J. (2002). Does disclosure of emotions facilitate recovery from bereavement? Evidence from two prospective studies. *Journal of Consulting and Clinical Psychology, 70*(1), 169–178.

Stroebe, W., Stroebe, M., Abakoumkin, G., & Schut, H. (1996). The role of loneliness and social support in adjustment to loss: A test of attachment versus stress theory. *Journal of Personality and Social Psychology, 70*(6), 1241–1249.

Szanto, K. (2003). Suicidal behavior in the elderly. *Psychiatric Times, 20*(13), 52–55.

Szanto, K., & Prigerson, H. (1997). Suicidal ideation in elderly bereaved: The role of complicated grief. *Suicide and Life Threatening Behaviors, 27*(2), 194–208.

Thompson, M., Rose, C., Wainwright, W., Mattar, L., & Scanlan, M. (2001). Activities of counsellors in a hospice/palliative care environment. *Journal of Palliative Care, 17*(4), 229–235.

van der Kolk, B. A., McFarlane, A. C., & Weisaeth, L. (1996). *Traumatic stress: The effects of overwhelming experience on mind, body, and society.* New York: Guilford Press.

Warren, N. A. (2002). Critical care family member's satisfaction with bereavement experiences. *Critical Care Nursing Quarterly, 25*(2), 1–7.

Wayment, H. A., & Vierthaler, J. A. (2002). Attachment style and bereavement reactions. *Journal of Loss and Trauma, 7,* 129–149.

Zeitlin, S. V. (2001). Grief and bereavement. *Primary Care, 28*(2), 415–425.

Zisook, S., & DeVaul, R. A. (1983). Grief, unresolved grief, and depression. *Psychosomatics, 24*(3), 247–256.

Zisook, S., & DeVaul, R. A. (1984). Measuring acute grief. *Psychiatric Medicine, 2*(2), 169–176.

Zisook, S., & Lyons, L. E. (1990). Bereavement and unresolved grief in psychiatric outpatients. *Journal of Death and Dying, 20*(4), 307–322.

Chapter 6

SUBSTANCE ABUSE

MATTHEW O. HOWARD, JORGE DELVA, JEFFREY M. JENSON,
TONYA EDMOND, AND MICHAEL G. VAUGHN

Substance use disorders are among the most pernicious, protean, and prevalent of modern human maladies. More than 150,000 U.S. citizens die prematurely each year as a result of alcohol or drug use, at a cost of $300 billion and untold amounts of human suffering (Arias, Anderson, Kung, Murphy, & Kochanek, 2003; Saadat-mand, Stinson, Grant, & Dufour, 1999). Approximately 1.3 million adults annually are discharged with an alcohol-related diagnosis from hospitals participating in the National Hospital Discharge Survey (Whitmore, Chen, & Dufour, 2002). Over the past quarter-century, 30% to 44% of the 39,000 to 51,000 annual traffic crash fatalities were alcohol-related (Yi, Williams, & Dufour, 2002). Substance abuse also often plays a critically important role in homicide and suicide, which together currently claim more than 50,000 lives yearly (Arias et al., 2003). One investigation conservatively estimated that 3.2% of all deaths and 4% of disability-adjusted life years globally were alcohol-related (Rehm et al., 2003).

Few groups escape the damage wrought by substance abuse. Hingson, Heeren, Zakocs, Kopstein, and Wechsler (2002) estimated that 1,400 college students died from alcohol-related injuries in 1998 and that one quarter of the 8 million students in college drove under the influence of alcohol. One study of 283 active-duty Air Force decedents found that 23% had died of alcohol-related causes, resulting in 2,300 years of potential life lost (Stout, Parkinson, & Wolfe, 1993). Surveys of burgeoning jail and prison inmate populations reveal high rates of substance abuse, blood-borne infections acquired through intravenous drug use (IVDU), and substance-motivated or facilitated crime (Abram, Teplin, & McLellan, 2003). IVDU continues to fuel the spread of HIV, hepatitis B (HBV), and hepatitis C (HCV), the last of these now the leading reason for liver transplantation (Seeff & Hoofnagle, 2003). Cities such as Seattle and San Francisco have experienced explosive growth in the incidence of unintentional drug overdose deaths (Davidson et al., 2003; *Morbidity and Mortality Weekly Report,* 2000), and drug-associated deaths currently number close to 1,000 annually in four U.S. cities (Substance Abuse and Mental Health Services Administration [SAMHSA], 2002). Recent findings also indicate that psychiatric disorders and polydrug dependence commonly complicate the clinical presentation of substance abusers who seek or are mandated to treatment (Darke & Ross, 1997; Marsden, Gossop, Stewart, Rolfe, & Farrell, 2000).

Research results bearing on a familiar litany of substance-related social problems—family dysfunction, child and partner abuse, divorce, unemployment, and violence—could easily be adduced to underscore the need for more effective substance abuse prevention practice (National Institute on Alcohol Abuse and Alcoholism [NIAAA], 2000). It may suffice at this juncture, however, simply to note that substance abuse is as damaging to the body politic as it is to the human body. This chapter examines current findings pertaining to the epidemiology of substance use, salient individual, interpersonal, and macrocontexual risk factors for substance use, and promising universal, selective, and indicated substance abuse prevention approaches for adults. Historically, prevention efforts have embodied a range of objectives, including increasing knowledge about alcohol and drugs, delaying or preventing initiation of substance use, reducing levels of current use, and minimizing the harmfulness of any use that does occur (Cuijpers, 2003). Practice and policy implications of substance abuse prevention research and promising future directions for prevention efforts are elucidated.

TRENDS AND INCIDENCE

Ongoing national surveys provide a rich database with which to characterize substance use patterns of U.S. citizens.

Monitoring the Future Survey

The Monitoring the Future survey (MTF) produces reliable estimates of lifetime, annual, and current substance use for high school seniors (Johnston, O'Malley, & Bachman, 2003). Each year since 1975, a nationally representative sample of 9,000 to 17,000 seniors have completed self-report instruments describing their drug use behaviors; thus, MTF data allow for analyses of temporal trends in substance use patterns. Drug use epidemics, such as the spectacular rise in the use of ecstasy between 1998 and 2000, can be identified as they emerge using MTF data.

In 2003, a majority (51.1%) of seniors reported lifetime use of an illicit drug; 58.1% reported one or more episodes of drunkenness. Significant proportions of seniors had used marijuana (46.1%), amphetamines (14.4%), inhalants (11.2%), hallucinogens (10.6%), tranquilizers (10.2%), and ecstasy (8.3%). Overall, substance use rates were lower in 2003 than in recent prior years, and rates of alcohol use and intoxication and tobacco use were at historic lows. Despite these encouraging findings, however, it is apparent that substance use is endemic, if not epidemic, among young adults in the United States.

National Survey on Drug Use and Health

The National Survey on Drug Use and Health (NSDUH) findings provide substance use prevalence data for the noninstitutionalized U.S. population 12 and older (SAMHSA, 2003). In 2002, 68,126 participants completed the study. Results indicated that 19.5 million Americans (8.3%) were current illicit drug users. Of this total, 2 million were current cocaine users, 1.9 million reported current nonmedical use of OxyContin, a synthetic opioid, and 1.2 million were currently using hallucinogens. The highest rate of current illicit drug use (20.2%) was observed among 18- to 25-year-olds. Alcohol abuse and tobacco use were, by any measure, pandemic; approximately 54 million Americans (22.9%) had engaged in binge drinking one or more times in the prior month and 71.5 million (30.4%) reported current tobacco use.

Among pregnant women age 15 to 44, 3.3% reported illicit drug use, 9.1% had used alcohol, and 17.3% had smoked cigarettes in the prior month. Rates of current illicit drug use in unemployed adults were twice the rates of respondents who were employed full time. Approximately 11 million persons (4.7%) drove a car after using an illicit drug in 2002, whereas 33.5 million (14.2%) drove a car under the influence of alcohol. Nearly 10% of the U.S. adult population, a total of 22 million people, met accepted criteria for substance abuse or dependence (American Psychiatric Association, 2000). Approximately 3.2 million people met criteria for alcohol *and* drug dependence. American Indians and Alaska Natives had the highest rates of abuse or dependence (14.1%), Asian Americans the lowest (4.2%), with intermediate rates for Caucasians (9.3%), African Americans (9.5%), and Hispanic Americans (10.4%).

Drug Abuse Warning Network

In 2002, 670,306 substance-related emergency department (ED) visits were reported by the 437 hospitals participating in the Drug Abuse Warning Network (DAWN), a national surveillance system tracking trends in drug-related deaths and hospital ED visits. Between 1994 and 2001, total substance-related ED visits increased 23.1%, compared to an increase of 12.1% in overall ED visits

(SAMHSA, 2003). DAWN data clearly document a growing incidence of substance-related ED visits over the past decade.

Substance-related ED visits were generally motivated by relatively serious medical problems, given that nearly half of all patients admitted to EDs in 2002 for drug-related reasons were hospitalized and 1,618 died. A significant increase in substance-related ED visits for benzodiazepines, narcotic-analgesic combinations, cocaine, and marijuana has been observed in recent years (SAMHSA, 2003).

With regard to mortality, 2001 DAWN medical examiner findings indicate that between 0.3% and 18% of all deaths reviewed in 42 metropolitan areas nationally were substance-related (Drug Abuse Warning Network [DAWN], 2002). In general, heroin, cocaine, and alcohol were the drugs most commonly involved in substance-related deaths.

Arrestee Drug Abuse Monitoring Program

The Arrestee Drug Abuse Monitoring program (ADAM) tracks trends in the nature and extent of substance abuse among booked arrestees in 35 major U.S. urban areas (ADAM, 2003). ADAM findings for 2002 indicate that approximately two-thirds of all adult male arrestees had recently taken cocaine, marijuana, opiates, methamphetamine, or some combination of these drugs. Across ADAM sites, between 25% and 50% of arrestees were deemed to be at high risk for substance dependence, although only 4% to 17% of arrestees had received substance abuse treatment in the prior year. Rates of heavy alcohol consumption ranged from 35% to 70% across sites.

Alcohol-Specific Findings

Rates of per capita alcohol consumption, alcohol-related traffic fatalities, and liver cirrhosis have declined substantially since 1980 (Saadatmand et al., 1999; Yi et al., 2002). However, in absolute terms, the toll taken by alcohol continues to be substantial. Deaths attributable to alcohol exceed 100,000 annually, and alcohol abuse commonly contributes to homicides, suicides, and domestic violence and promotes unsafe sex and other high-risk behaviors (NIAAA, 2000).

Summary

Significant reductions in the prevalence of alcohol and tobacco use have occurred over the past quarter-century. Current rates of illicit drug use are low compared to those observed in the 1970s and 1980s. Concomitant reductions in various adverse substance-related outcomes, including liver cirrhosis rates and alcohol-related traffic fatalities, have also been observed. It is clear, however, that the personal and social costs of substance abuse remain staggeringly high. Moreover, new substance-related problems such as widespread HCV infection among IVD users or "club drug" abuse are continually arising. Effective prevention approaches are needed to reduce the social, economic, and health costs of substance abuse. These efforts should target empirically established risk factors for substance abuse.

RISK FACTORS

Risk factors are characteristics or traits that increase the likelihood of substance abuse. There is a host of individual, interpersonal, social, and macrocontextual factors that place young people and adults at risk for substance abuse (see Belcher & Shinitzky, 1998; J. D. Hawkins, Catalano, & Miller, 1992). Risk factors are summarized and presented by level of effect in the next section. Because evidence about risks for substance abuse is often collected just before initiation of use, our review includes literature assessing factors associated with substance abuse among adolescents *and* adults.

Individual-Level Risk Factors

Individual-level risk factors for substance abuse include biological and psychosocial factors.

Heredity

Evidence from adoption, twin, and half-sibling studies provides support for the genetic transmission of alcoholism (Cadoret, Cain, & Grove, 1980; Clark, Kirisci, & Moss, 1998). Generally, studies investigating genetic links to alcohol use find rates of alcoholism ranging from 20% to 30% for sons of alcoholics, compared to only 5% for males without a biological alcoholic parent (e.g., Cadoret et al., 1980).

Childhood Problem Behaviors and Temperament

Several investigators have found that a sensation-seeking orientation in childhood predicts age of onset and persistent use of alcohol and other drugs (Howard, Kivlahan, & Walker, 1997). Attention Deficit Hyperactivity Disorder, Conduct Disorder, and poor impulse control during childhood and adolescence are associated with later drinking and drug use (Wilens, Biederman, Spencer, & Frances, 1994).

Interpersonal and Social Risk Factors

Interpersonal and social risk factors for substance abuse occur in family, school, employment, marital, and peer contexts.

Family Influences

People whose parents or siblings engage in serious alcohol or illicit substance use are themselves at greater risk for these behaviors during adolescence and adulthood (Anda et al., 2002; Hill, Shen, Lowers, & Locke, 2000). Adolescents who are raised in families with lax supervision, excessively severe or inconsistent disciplinary practices, and little communication between parents and children are also at high risk for substance use disorders in adulthood (Dishion, Capaldi, & Yoerger, 1999). Similarly, parental conflict is related to subsequent alcohol or drug use by young adults (Anda et al., 2002).

School Factors

School failure, low degree of commitment to education, and lack of attachment to school increase the risk of substance abuse during adolescence (Catalano, Oxford, Harachi, Abbott, & Haggerty, 1999). Adolescent drug users are more likely to skip classes, be absent from school, and perform poorly than nondrug users (Gottfredson, Gottfredson, & Hybl, 1993). Predictors of adolescent substance abuse such as school performance and achievement are important because such problems are also associated with criminality and substance abuse during adulthood.

Employment and Marital Factors

Employment status and marital problems during adulthood pose significant risks for substance abuse. Marital conflict and divorce are associated with alcohol and other types of substance abuse (Anda et al., 2002). Job loss and unemployment also increase risk for substance abuse (Friedmann, Lemon, Anderson, & Stein, 2003).

Peer Influence

Associating with friends who use drugs is among the strongest predictors of adolescent substance abuse (Fergusson & Horwood, 1999; Jenson & Howard, 1999). Spending time with drug-using peers or partners is also a strong predictor of substance abuse during adulthood (Tuten & Jones, 2003); the influence of drug-using peers on substance use is particularly strong among IVD users (W. E. Hawkins, Latkin, Mandel, & Oziemkowska, 1999).

Some researchers have suggested that the peer rejection experienced by some young people in elementary school leads to the creation of antisocial peer networks that extend into adolescence and adulthood (Coie, 1990). These investigators hypothesize that rejected children form friendships with other rejected children and that such groups become more heavily involved in delinquent and substance abusing behaviors as they progress through adolescence and into adulthood (Patterson, Dishion, & Chamberlain, 1993).

Macrocontexual Risk Factors

Risk factors at the macrocontexual level of effect include laws and norms about substance abuse, poverty, child abuse, community disorganization, and residential mobility.

Laws and Norms

Community laws and norms that favor substance use, such as comparatively low legal drinking age and low taxes on alcoholic beverages, increase the risk of substance abuse (Joksch, 1988). Laws and norms that express intolerance for alcohol and illicit drug use are associated with a lower prevalence of substance use (Johnston, 1991).

Poverty

The relationship between poverty and problems such as delinquency, criminality, and violence are well-known (Farrington, Gallagher, Morley, St. Leger, & West, 1988). Being raised in adverse economic conditions is also related to substance abuse among adolescents and adults. Several longitudinal studies have found a direct effect between family economic hardship and substance use among adult substance abusers (e.g., Kost & Smyth, 2002).

Poverty may also have indirect effects on substance use. Family income is associated with many other risk factors for substance use (e.g., parenting practices); low family income may affect substance use indirectly through such risk factors.

Child Abuse

Men and women who experience physical or sexual abuse as children are at elevated risk for substance abuse during adulthood. Galaif, Stein, Newcomb, and Bernstein (2001) found that adults who were physically or sexually abused as children had significantly more alcohol-related problems than men and women who had not been abused. Childhood abuse is also associated with an increased risk for opiate use during adulthood (Heffernan et al., 2000).

Community Disorganization and Residential Mobility

Individuals residing in communities with high rates of unemployment, school dropout, crime, low neighborhood attachment, and other measures of neighborhood disorganization are at elevated risk for substance abuse. Neighborhoods with high population density and high rates of adult crime also have high rates of drug use (Simcha-Fagan & Schwartz, 1986). Neighborhood disorganization may also indirectly affect risk for substance abuse by eroding the ability of parents to supervise their children. High rates of residential mobility are positively associated with substance abuse (Smith & Jarjoura, 1988).

Most of what is known about risk and protective factors for substance abuse has been drawn from studies of male and Caucasian adolescents and adults residing in middle-class neighborhoods. Prevention and treatment programs often assume that risk and protective factors related to substance abuse are the same for different populations. However, age, gender, and ethnic minority status are central issues in the development of young adults and warrant additional research attention.

Age

Practitioners need to be aware that different risk factors are salient at different developmental stages during adolescence and adulthood (J. D. Hawkins et al., 1992). For example, aggressiveness in children as young as 5 predicts later substance use (Kellam, Rebok, Ialongo, & Mayer, 1994), and association with deviant peers is strongly related to use in adolescence and early adulthood (Dishion, 1990). Poor parenting and family management practices are related to substance use during childhood and adolescence (Kendziora & O'Leary, 1993). Lack of community supports and of extended family members are associated with substance abuse in older adolescents and adults (Werner, 1994).

Gender

The few investigations that have studied the relationship between gender and risk factors have identified surprisingly few differences between males and females (e.g., Fishbein & Perez, 2000; Khoury, 1998). Girls and young women evidence higher rates of prior abuse and victimization than males, two risk factors that are significantly related to substance abuse (Boyd, 2000). There is also evidence suggesting that girls and young women are at greater risk for mental health disorders than boys and young men (Timmons-Mitchell et al., 1997); mental health problems may in turn increase the likelihood of substance abuse (Loeber, Farrington, Stouthamer-Loeber, & Van Kammen, 1998). Investigators have also speculated that different patterns of development between boys and girls, including pubertal changes, gender role characteristics, and self-esteem, are related to substance use and delinquency (Khoury, 1998).

Race and Ethnicity

Adolescents and adults in the United States receive differential exposure to risk based on racial/ethnic characteristics. Persons of color are overrepresented among the persistently poor and are more likely to be incarcerated, victims of violent crime, and raised in single-parent households than Caucasians (D. F. Hawkins, Laub, & Lauritsen, 1998). Differential exposure to predisposing factors because of race/ethnicity may increase risk for substance abuse among adolescents and adults.

Summary

Current knowledge of risk factors for substance abuse is only correlational in nature; that is, the presence of risk factors only increases the likelihood that an adolescent or adult may develop problem alcohol or drug use. The interaction of risk factors is poorly understood (Blum, 1997; J. D. Hawkins et al., 1992), and some investigators even argue that such factors may be consequences of substance abuse rather than characteristics that increase risk for use. Despite these limitations, several conclusions about risk factors for substance abuse can be drawn.

First, risk factors have been shown to be stable over the past 25 years. The factors summarized earlier consistently predict substance use even though social norms about the acceptability of drinking and other drug use changed several times during this period. Second, research indicates that the more risk factors that are present, the greater the risk a person will have for alcohol or drug problems (Bry, McKeon, & Pandina, 1982; Pollard, Hawkins, & Arthur, 1999). These findings suggest that prevention and treatment programs should, at a minimum, target risk factors at all levels of effect. Third, theorists increasingly agree that effective prevention programs should target risk factors at multiple levels of influence, including personal, interpersonal, and contextual (Hanlon, Bateman, Simon, O'Grady, & Carswell, 2002).

EFFECTIVE UNIVERSAL PREVENTIVE INTERVENTIONS

For more than a century, individuals and citizen groups in the United States have sought ways to prevent youth and adults from using substances, help those who have already commenced use to discontinue their use before it becomes more frequent and harmful, and assist those who already use substances problematically to reduce or cease their use (Musto, 1999). In this section, we review a selection of recently implemented universal substance abuse preventive interventions and examine evidence pertaining to their effectiveness in successfully preventing or reducing substance use.

By universal interventions, we mean interventions that target the public or whole populations rather than specific groups identified as at risk for substance abuse. Examples of broad-based population interventions include the passage of laws to increase the legal drinking age to 21 and driving under the influence (DUI) laws that lower the blood alcohol concentration (BAC) threshold for legal intoxication. These policy interventions target the entire population of drivers rather than high-risk subgroups. Interventions aimed at specific high-risk sub-populations, such as mandated use of ignition interlocking devices with repeat DUI offenders, are discussed later in this chapter. Several recently implemented universal preventive interventions for alcohol abuse, illicit drug abuse, and tobacco dependence are highlighted next.

Alcohol Use

Ever since the failure of the federal government to successfully regulate the manufacture, distribution, and sale of alcohol during the 1920s and early 1930s through national prohibition of alcohol, broad-based universal interventions have become more specific. Universal preventive interventions are intended to minimize the harm to the user and society at large rather than prevent individuals from consuming alcohol. A recent report lists over a dozen universal interventions that have been found to reduce alcohol consumption and alcohol-related harm. These interventions include raising the minimum legal drinking age, zero tolerance laws that make it illegal for individuals under 21 to drive after consuming alcohol, lowering the legal limits for BAC-defined legal intoxication, passing laws to allow police officers to confiscate the license of drivers whose BAC exceeds the state's legal limit (i.e., administrative license revocation), comprehensive community programs, increased taxation on alcoholic beverages, reducing alcohol sales outlet density, and programs promoting the use of designated drivers (NIAAA, 2000). Each of these intervention approaches has produced effects ranging from small to large with regard to preventing alcohol-related harm.

A number of interventions have attempted to curb alcohol consumption among the general population of college students. The Task Force of the National Advisory Council on Alcohol Abuse and Alcoholism (2002) recently conducted an extensive review of interventions aimed at reducing alcohol consumption and related problems among college students, concluding that only multidimensional interventions will lead to changes in alcohol consumption in this population. Promising interventions for this population include brief motivational enhancement, which provides students with feedback about their drinking behavior and its consequences using a social norms approach, interventions that target members of sororities and fraternities and athletes, and interventions that do not rely solely on alcohol or drug education. The report also recommends that colleges and universities become involved in joint college-community interventions, build community coalitions, and work with local businesses to monitor alcohol marketing, sales, and consumption practices.

Illicit Drug Use

In the United States, illicit drug use prevention efforts span more than a century (Musto, 1999). The apex of the fight against drug use came in 1971, when President Nixon declared the War on Drugs, whereby the Office of National Drug Control Policy (ONDCP) was created. ONDCP is charged with coordinating all state and nationwide efforts aimed at reducing the supply of drugs in the country through such measures as interdiction efforts, crop eradication, and crop substitution and with demand reduction efforts founded on substance abuse prevention programs.

One of ONDCP's most controversial recent campaigns is the National Youth Anti-Drug Media Campaign authorized by the Drug-Free Media Campaign Act of 1998. The campaign's focus is to convince participants to avoid use of illegal drugs through exposure to repeated advertisements in a manner similar to contemporary antitobacco media campaigns. The campaign's advertisements are produced by the Partnership for a Drug Free America. Eddy (2003) reported that data presented at a hearing on the media campaign held by the House Government Reform Subcommittee on Criminal Justice, Drug Policy, and Human Resources on March 27, 2003, indicated that the campaign has had no general positive results. However, recent findings suggest that media campaigns based on expectancy and health persuasion theoretical models, which employ interactive media and appropriate pretesting methods, can be an important component of multilevel universal substance abuse preventive interventions (Crano & Burgoo, 2002).

Another intervention approach promoted by the executive branch through ONDCP is drug testing. However, one recent study showed that drug testing is not associated with decreased marijuana and other illicit drug use (Yamaguchi, Johnston, & O'Malley, 2003).

Despite the general lack of effectiveness of the War on Drugs, there has been a slight decline in the use of marijuana, ecstasy, LSD, amphetamines, tranquilizers, and sedatives among high school youths in recent years (Johnston et al., 2003). However, the extent to which these minimal decrements might be attributed to any antidrug campaign is unclear. Furthermore, the same study indicated that there has been a significant increase in the use of inhalants, OxyContin, and Vicodin and no significant changes in the use of drugs such as Rohypnol, Ketamine, hallucinogens other than LSD, power cocaine, crack cocaine, and heroin. Thus, optimism regarding the slight decrease observed in the use of some drugs among some age groups is tempered by the observed increase in the use of other substances by the same age group or the same substances by other age groups.

Another program that has received considerable funding from federal and state governments is the Drug Abuse Resistance Education (DARE) program. This program can be considered a universal preventive intervention because it is implemented in most school systems in the country and has the objective of preventing all participants from initiating drug use. Despite its popularity, a recent General Accounting Office (2003) review of DARE evaluations concluded that it has largely been ineffective in preventing drug involvement and changing participants' attitudes about drug use. Furthermore, the report suggested that those studies that show a positive effect also show that the benefits are short-lived.

Evaluating the effectiveness of universal preventive interventions is extremely difficult because too many potentially relevant factors cannot be ruled out as causes of changes in drug use rates. During the past two decades there have been a number of fluctuations in drug use among adults (SAMHSA, 2003), but the extent to which these fluctuations can be attributed to universal interventions remains unclear for at least three reasons.

First, changes in drug use patterns cannot unequivocally be attributed to governmental policies, as it appears that most policies reflect population norms, values, and beliefs at a particular time, which in turn affect society's tolerance of drug-using behaviors (Musto, 1999). The obverse scenario, that broad-based drug prevention policies influence drug involvement, is less plausible.

Second, despite the recent declining trend in the use of some illicit drugs, there have been substantial increases in the use of inhalants and synthetic narcotics such as Vicodin and OxyContin, as well as stable levels of use of several drugs mentioned earlier. The nature of this phenomenon is not well understood, but it appears that when the use of one drug declines, the use of other drugs often increases or new drugs of abuse emerge in patterns of local, regional, or national epidemics.

Third, careful examination of drug use trends since the 1980s shows peaks and valleys in the prevalence of use of several illicit drugs that do not correspond to the constantly increasing budget used by the federal government to fight illicit drug use during the same period. As a result of this disconnect, and serious unanticipated consequences of the War on Drugs (e.g., incarceration of a greater proportion of African Americans when in fact the greatest prevalence of illicit drug use is among non-Hispanic Whites), public health advocates, libertarians, and citizens concerned about the lack of effectiveness of these programs argue that universal drug use preventive interventions should be based on entirely different models than the one currently in place. A review of the philosophical underpinnings of these models is beyond the scope of this chapter (see MacCoun & Reuter, 2001; Piper, Briggs, Huffman, & Lubot-Conke, 2003, for detailed discussions).

Tobacco Use

A number of universal interventions have been implemented in recent years to prevent or decrease tobacco use among adults that may inform efforts to prevent psychoactive substance abuse. These efforts include taxation, advertising regulations, smoking regulations, litigation, antitobacco media campaigns, and community-based interventions. Comprehensive reviews of these interventions and their effectiveness are provided by Fiore, Bailey, and Cohen (2000) and the American Public Health Association (2003). A recent systematic review of the effectiveness of community-based interventions to reduce smoking concluded that there is limited evidence that these interventions lead to significant reductions in the prevalence of cigarette smoking, although the authors also concluded that community-based programs in conjunction with mass media campaigns were the most effective approach to reducing the prevalence of smoking—but again, the effects were small (Secker-Walker, Gnich, Platt, & Lancaster, 2003).

One recently evaluated program is the American Stop Smoking Intervention Study (ASSIST; Stillman et al., 2003). Funded by the National Cancer Institute and the American Cancer Society in the 1990s, the ASSIST program involved the establishment of state tobacco control programs to support smoke-free environments, increase tobacco taxes, and reduce opportunities for youth to acquire tobacco products. Seventeen participating states created statewide prevention programs. When participating and nonparticipating states were compared, the effects of ASSIST in reducing the prevalence of tobacco use among adults were, at best, modest. The authors pointed out that program effects might have been underestimated because many of the states that did not participate in the ASSIST program had implemented their own antitobacco programs during the same period. Further, the tobacco industry spent billions of dollars advertising their products during the period ASSIST was under way.

Stillman and colleagues (2003) estimated that ASSIST could have resulted in approximately 278,700 fewer smokers if it had been implemented nationwide. Thus, even with relatively small effects, population-based interventions can produce large net benefits. Although the effects associated with universal antitobacco prevention campaigns are much weaker than those associated with smaller, intensive, individually tailored interventions, the overall *impact* of population-based interventions is significantly greater than that of smaller programs (Fiore et al., 2000). Even when universal smoking interventions achieve only a 5% quit rate, this percentage often translates into thousands of individuals who will lead healthier lives and significant reductions in health care costs to the individual and society at large (Friend & Levy, 2002; Siegel, 2002).

EFFECTIVE SELECTIVE PREVENTIVE INTERVENTIONS

Selective preventive interventions target adults who are deemed, by virtue of empirical findings or theoretical considerations, to be at high risk for substance abuse (Gordon, 1983). Indicated prevention approaches are also directed to high-risk persons, but they focus on individuals who already demonstrate some signs and symptoms of substance use disorders. In practice, prevention programs commonly include heterogeneous groups of high-risk individuals, including participants with and without established signs and symptoms of substance abuse. Promising selective prevention efforts targeting high-risk subpopulations are discussed next.

College Students

Current binge drinking rates among college students nationally exceed 40%; thus, college students are increasingly considered to be at high risk for adverse alcohol-related events (Perkins, 2003). However, the authors of a recent report based on a survey of 365 colleges concluded that most schools "have not yet installed the basic infrastructure required for developing, implementing, and evaluating environmental management strategies" (DeJong & Langford, 2002, p. 140).

Evaluations of social norms-based preventive interventions at Western Washington University (Fabiano, 2003), Northern Illinois University (Haines & Barker, 2003), and the Hobart and William Smith Colleges (Perkins & Craig, 2003), designed to correct students' misperceptions about the extent and acceptability of student drinking, suggest that such interventions produced immediate and ongoing reductions in student binge and heavy drinking and their consequences. Normative reeducation interventions employed print media campaigns, cocurricular activities, electronic media, and other strategies to effectively change norms regarding drinking across these campuses.

Attempts have also been made to evaluate promising cognitive preventive interventions that aim to change college students' positive outcome expectancies regarding the effects of alcohol, examine the utility of social mentoring by upper-class students, and examine factors that predict greater use of designated drivers by students who continue to use substances in off-campus settings (Hubner, 2002; Musher-Eizenman & Kulick, 2003).

Pregnant Women

Substance abuse by pregnant women can have devastating and enduring consequences to the developing fetus. Farber and Olney (2003) noted that alcohol, PCP, ketamine, and benzodiazepines can cause millions of neurons to die in neonates, resulting in reduced brain size and severely impaired function later in life. Psychiatric impairments attributable to maternal alcohol use, including Attention Deficit Hyperactivity Disorder, learning disorders, cerebral palsy, and epilepsy, are relatively common among persons with prenatal alcohol exposure (Burd, Cotsonas-Hassler, Martsolf, & Kerbeshian, 2003).

As a leading cause of preventable birth defects in the United States, fetal alcohol syndrome (FAS), a disorder marked by a characteristic set of facial deformities and profound growth and intellectual impairments, affects between 0.5% and 2% of every 1,000 live births in the United States (May & Gossage, 2001). Surprisingly, few evaluations of FAS prevention efforts with high-risk women have been conducted. Recent developments supporting selective FAS preventive interventions include efforts to validate substance use screening instruments specifically designed for women, such as the T-ACE and TWEAK, along with practice guidelines facilitating greater detection of at-risk pregnant drinkers in primary care settings (NIAAA, 2000). Risk factors for FAS births have been identified, which should enhance future efforts to target preventive interventions to women at high risk for FAS birth outcomes (NIAAA, 2000).

Among the promising FAS preventive interventions are those that employ brief motivational interventions (Chang, Goetz, Wilkins-Haug, & Berman, 2000) and enhanced blood screening methods to identify drinking mothers (Stoler et al., 1998) and incorporate prevention efforts into public health programs in urban and rural settings for women with FAS risk factors (Walsh, Henderson, & Magraw, 2003).

The Elderly

Substance abuse among the elderly plays a role in disease susceptibility and aging. Neuropsychological studies indicate that alcohol abuse is associated with premature aging of the brain (NIAAA, 1997). Research has also established heavy drinking as a risk factor for depression, suicide, and serious functional impairment in older persons (Whelan, 2003). Few selective preventive interventions have been evaluated with elderly participants, although a recent evaluation of an intervention for health professionals indicated that a statewide alcohol dependence screening and prevention training intervention in Virginia produced effects that persisted for 7 years (Coogle & Parham, 2001). Program participants were more likely to seek further training related to substance abuse in the elderly, detect substance abuse in elderly patients, and provide preventive interventions to high-risk older persons. Fleming (2002) reviewed a number of promising motivational interventions and pharmacologic treatments that have been used with older substance users. Brief educational interventions with elderly women are effective in increasing awareness of substance-related issues, but their efficacy in reducing risk for subsequent substance use problems is unclear (e.g., Eliason & Skinstad, 2001).

Health Care Professionals

Health care professionals may be at elevated risk for substance misuse due to their access to potent psychoactive medications. Although substance abuse by health care workers can have disastrous professional consequences, evaluations of selective preventive interventions with members of this subgroup are uncommon. One exception was Lapham et al.'s (2003a, 2003b) evaluation of a binge-drinking preventive intervention for managed care professionals. Intervention components included educational videos addressing binge drinking, depression, and stress-reduction techniques, instruction in health risk self-appraisal, and substance misuse training for managers. Intervention efforts at one site were compared to those at nonintervention sites while controlling for potentially confounding factors. Results indicated that binge-drinking health professionals at the intervention site were significantly more likely to report a desire to cut down on their alcohol use than were their control group counterparts. In addition, following the intervention, employee assistance program referrals increased significantly and there was a slight decline in the monthly rate of nonsubstance-related outpatient health care use.

Emergency Department, Trauma Unit, and Primary Care Patients

One in three ED patients are intoxicated at the time they seek treatment and high proportions of patients also arrive intoxicated at hospital trauma units (Blondell, Looney, Hottman, & Boaz, 2002). A recent evaluation of patients with traumatic brain injuries found that "a vast majority of victims test positive for alcohol or illicit drugs at the time of hospital admission" (Soderstrom et al., 2001). Substance abuse and dependency were prevalent among study patients, supporting the need for selective and indicated prevention approaches with this group.

Substance abusers suffer a host of medical ailments; thus, selective and indicated preventive interventions delivered in health care settings by primary practitioners hold great potential for reducing the toll taken by substance abuse. Kristenson, Oesterline, Nilsson, and Lindgaerde (2002) randomly assigned one group of middle-aged drinkers to a control condition and another group to a brief physician-delivered preventive intervention. Both groups were identified on the basis of elevations in serum gamma-glutamyltransferase and current excessive drinking. Subjects were followed for 13 years, during which time 12.7% died— nearly half from alcohol-related causes. Death rates for the intervention and control groups were 10% and 14%, respectively, suggesting that treatment may have been weakly efficacious in terms of reducing mortality. Earlier and more intense efforts might produce significantly better outcomes. Unfortunately, physicians inquire about alcohol intake far less often than they do about other health care conditions (Arndt, Schultz, Turvey, & Petersen, 2002). Promising methods to increase the likelihood that hospital inpatients being treated for medical illness will enter outpatient substance abuse treatment when needed have been reported (O'Toole, Strain, Wand, McCaul, & Barnhart, 2002).

Employees

The U.S. Department of Labor (2004) estimated that 74.6% of the country's 16.6 million illegal drug users work full or part time. Substance abusers are more often absent from work or tardy, have more accidents and lower productivity, and evidence higher rates of health care utilization than nonabusers (Lipscomb, Dement, & Li, 2003). Thus, a number of workplace selective and indicated preventive interventions have been implemented in recent years to increase the detection and improve the outcomes of employees who are at risk for, or are currently engaged in, substance abuse. Roman and Blum (1996) reviewed 24 evaluations of worksite alcohol preventive interventions published between 1970 and 1995, concluding that employee assistance programs are effective in rehabilitating employees with alcohol problems and in changing the attitudes of employees and supervisors.

New approaches to workplace substance abuse prevention have been implemented in recent years as it has become clear that drug testing alone does not identify alcohol abuse, fails to address factors motivating substance abuse, and does not address contextual issues that foster and maintain substance use. Current approaches to substance abuse prevention with employees include peer intervention programs, workplace coping skills interventions that help employees cope more effectively with work and family stressors, programs based on social-cognitive theory that integrate substance abuse prevention into larger health promotion programs, interactive and participatory team-oriented approaches for workplace substance abuse training, and a Department of Labor web site (www.dol.gov/dol/workingpartners.htm) designed to help employers set up drug-free programs for their workplaces (Bennett & Lehman, 2003).

Gay, Lesbian, Bisexual, and Transgendered Persons

Gay, lesbian, bisexual, and transgendered (GLBT) persons may be at high risk for substance abuse (e.g., Cochran, Keenan, Schober, & Mays, 2000), although evidence supporting this contention is not conclusive (Gorman, 2003). Evaluations of prevention efforts with these populations are sorely needed, especially those that might reduce substance-related sexual risk-taking behavior.

Victims and Perpetrators of Violence

Etiological, clinical, and policy issues relevant to the drugs-violence nexus have long been the focus of energetic debate (Wekerle & Wall, 2003). Substance abuse is commonly identified in individuals who commit homicide, suicide, and domestic and other interpersonal violence, and in those who abuse and neglect children (NIAAA, 2000). On a broader level, neighborhoods and communities evincing high rates of substance use also tend to have more severe problems with violence. An ecological study in New Mexico, for example, found rates of suicide and alcohol-related car crashes and crash fatalities to be significantly positively associated with liquor sales outlet density across counties (Escobedo & Ortiz, 2002).

Substance abuse prevention efforts directed to victims and perpetrators of violent crime might reduce rates of substance abuse and associated violence. Project Towards No Drug Abuse was a high school-based drug prevention program targeting youth 14 to 19 years of age who were followed for 1 year (Simon, Sussman, Dahlberg, & Dent, 2002). Males who received the intervention were significantly less likely to report having been victimized in the year following the preventive intervention than were their control condition counterparts. The authors concluded that substance abuse prevention reduced the likelihood of violent victimization among program participants. A noteworthy prevention initiative in Stockholm combined community mobilization efforts, alcohol server training, and stricter enforcement of extant alcohol laws in an effort to prevent alcohol-related violence (Wallin, Norstroem, & Andreasson, 2003). Findings indicated that violent crimes declined by 29% over a 7-year period for the intervention area, a substantial improvement over the reduction in control areas.

The Mentally Ill

National studies reveal high rates of comorbid substance use and psychiatric disorders in clinical and human service populations (Crawford, Crome, & Clancy, 2003). Experimental findings support the need for prevention approaches specifically targeting individuals with mental disorders. For example, Sinha (2001) reviewed clinical findings suggesting that high levels of stress increase the likelihood of substance abuse, which in turn alters stress responses and coping in a manner that further increases the probability of substance abuse. In a related vein, Dehaas (2003) found that a self-reported measure of anxiety sensitivity was significantly positively related to substance abuse in negative situations among a sample of substance users.

Studies of psychiatrically disordered opioid abusers in outpatient settings (King, Kidorf, Stoller, & Brooner, 2000), homeless mentally ill substance users (Linn et al., 2003), and dually diagnosed prison inmates (e.g., Edens, Peters, & Hills, 1997) suggest that early intervention with mentally ill substance abusers may prevent a variety of adverse outcomes.

Ethnic Minorities

Although they are characterized by large within- and between-group differences, ethnic minorities can be considered at risk for substance abuse by virtue of the acculturation stresses, intergenerational trauma, and poverty to which many have been subjected (Orozco & Lukas, 2000). Research has elucidated cross-ethnicity differences in conceptions of addiction, patterns of substance use, and responses to substance abuse preventive interventions (Castillo & Henderson, 2002). However, despite calls for more culturally relevant prevention approaches, including approaches targeted to stages of acculturation (Castillo & Henderson, 2002), and the actual implementation of prevention programs targeted to American Indian (Ellis, 2003), Hispanic/Latino (Cervantes, Kappos, Duenas, & Arellano, 2003), Asian American (Lew & Tanjasiri, 2003), and African American (Spoth, Guyll, Chao, & Molgaard, 2003) adults, formal evaluations of prevention program effectiveness with different ethnic minority groups are needed.

EFFECTIVE INDICATED PREVENTIVE INTERVENTIONS

Indicated prevention approaches target high-risk persons who have detectable signs and symptoms of substance use disorders but do not meet full criteria for substance dependence. Promising indicated prevention approaches for different client populations are identified next.

Intravenous Drug Users

IVD users are at high risk for HIV, HCV, and HBV infection, leading causes of morbidity and mortality in the United States (Bailey, Huo, Garfein, & Ouellet, 2003). Research supports the need for substantially more HCV/HBV prevention programming in outpatient drug-free and methadone maintenance treatment programs nationally (Strauss, Astone, Vassilev, Des Jarlais, & Hagan, 2003). Jail and prison inmates are a particularly important subset of clients vis-à-vis HIV risk, given their comparatively high rates of IVDU and other risk factors for HIV (Farabee & Leukefeld, 2002). Although HIV-infected inmates are twice as likely to report an IVDU-acquired infection than their general population counterparts are, jail and prison authorities have been slow in implementing substance use prevention and treatment programs (Leukefeld & Tims, 2002).

Various approaches to reducing risk for blood-borne infections among IVD users have been evaluated recently. Needle exchange programs have demonstrated significant positive effects in a number of studies. Jenkins, Rahman, Saidel, Jana, and Hussain (2001) reported significantly lower HIV risk behaviors, including reductions in the average proportion of needles shared and in the proportion of male addicts never sharing needles, in a large population of IVD users. Efforts to change laws so that syringes can be purchased and possessed legally by IVD users have also been undertaken, although support for syringe prescription programs appears to be stronger. Rich, Macaline, McKenzie, Taylor, and Burris (2001) evaluated the efficacy of a novel program involving physician prescription of syringes for 267 IVD users in Rhode Island, concluding that syringe prescription programs promote important connections between health care providers that can prevent acquisition of infections and other adverse IVDU-related outcomes.

Some evidence is available supporting the utility of HIV counseling and testing in reducing risk for HIV and other blood-borne infections among substance users. Methadone maintenance treatment also prevents acquisition of blood-borne infections among IVD users (De Castro & Sabate, 2003).

Substance abuse prevention programs for HIV/HCV/HBV-infected clients are clearly needed for prevention personnel. Copenhaver, Avants, Warburton, and Margolin (2003) noted that many HIV positive substance users enter treatment with significant cognitive impairment that limits their ability to learn, retain, and execute HIV preventive interventions. Findings from Project EXPLORE, an individually tailored HIV prevention program targeting men who have sex with men, found that alcoholism and non-IVDU were important risk factors for high-risk sexual behavior and that the EXPLORE intervention was effective in reducing sexual risk-taking behavior (Chesney et al., 2003). Additional preventive interventions designed to reduce the risk of overdose, such as naloxone prescription (Coffin et al., 2003) and monitored injection (Darke & Hall, 2003), have also been implemented effectively in select sites.

Individuals with Subclinical Substance Use Disorders

Various pharmacotherapeutic agents have proven effective in treating substance abusers. Naltrexone and Acamprosate appear to reduce the likelihood and severity of relapse in abstinent alcohol abusers (Stromberg, Mackler, Volpicelli, & O'Brien, 2001). A recent meta-analysis of controlled trials found that naltrexone-treated abstinent alcohol abusers had significantly lower rates of relapse and higher rates of abstinence compared to alcohol abusers treated with a placebo (Streeton & Whelan, 2001).

Pharmacologic agents such as Buprenorphine and naltrexone have proven useful in treating some populations of opioid abusers. Naltrexone blocks the psychoactive effects of illicit opioids, thereby discouraging their use; however, compliance with the medication has been a major factor limiting intervention efficacy. Buprenorphine appears to be effective in office-based opioid detoxification treatment (Welsh & Liberto, 2001).

Preventive interventions for substance abusers that combine pharmacologic treatments with case management and psychosocial interventions have only recently been developed. For example, the BRENDA approach combines naltrexone and case management interventions and may well be effective with substance users of many types, although formal evaluations have not been published (Volpicelli, Pettinati, McLellan, & O'Brien, 2001).

PRACTICE AND POLICY IMPLICATIONS

Per capital alcohol consumption and tobacco use and rates of many substance-related social and health problems have declined significantly over the past quarter-century. Greater awareness of the damage wrought by substance abuse along with individual, social, and policy changes supportive of healthier lifestyles are undoubtedly among the many factors accounting for these positive developments. However, substance abuse remains one of the most important causes of morbidity, mortality, and social dysfunction in the United States and many other countries.

Although clinicians and policy practitioners have long recognized the potential cost-effectiveness of prevention, research evaluating varied prevention approaches has not been vigorously undertaken until very recently. The findings reviewed here suggest many promising avenues for future research and indicate that prevention can reduce substance abuse problems, especially when programs target empirically established risk factors for abuse.

Comprehensive, integrated community-based prevention programs addressing individual and social risk factors can reduce community substance abuse problems. Universal prevention programs of even modest effectiveness can save many lives. Promising selective and indicated prevention efforts are under way in a variety of areas, including efforts to reduce substance abuse problems in college students, pregnant women, the elderly, the mentally ill, patients utilizing primary, ED, or trauma unit care, and individuals at risk for blood-borne infections such as HIV. Dramatically more research in these areas and new efforts to evaluate prevention programs designed specifically for women, the GLBT community, ethnic minority populations, and victims and perpetrators of violence are sorely needed.

FUTURE DIRECTIONS

Policy analysts and clinical practitioners in the substance abuse field strongly support prevention initiatives, provided they employ interventions of established effectiveness (Saunders & Brady, 2002). Proponents of "prevention science," a relatively new movement, contend that prevention programs should explicitly target empirically identified risk factors for substance abuse and its consequences (J. D. Hawkins, Catalano, & Arthur, 2002). It is increasingly clear that effective prevention programming requires an understanding of etiological factors pertinent to substance abuse and research designs, statistical methodologies, and conceptual models specific to the prevention practice area itself (Hogan, Gabrielsen, Luna, & Grothaus, 2003).

Recent developments in prevention science include more sophisticated approaches to accounting for missing data in longitudinal studies, more widespread use of meta-analysis and other efforts to evaluate the comparative effectiveness of promising prevention approaches, and more commonplace reporting of effect sizes, confidence intervals, and statistical power estimates. Multilevel modeling, latent-growth-curve analysis, and structural equation modeling have also contributed significantly to the rigor of substance abuse prevention research in the past decade (MacKinnon & Lockwood, 2003).

Perhaps the most important theoretical development relevant to substance abuse prevention has been the growing acceptance of harm reduction as a conceptual model supporting prevention efforts. Recently implemented harm reduction interventions include needle exchange programs, monitored injection, and syringe prescription. Each of these initiatives shares the aim of reducing drug users' risk for a variety of adverse outcomes, even when substance abuse itself cannot be entirely curtailed. Harm reduction approaches to prevention and treatment in active alcohol abusers evince levels of efficacy at least equivalent to those of abstinence-only approaches and may engender less resistance on the part of substance abusers, who are often reluctant to enter formal treatment or prevention programs (Marlatt & Witkiewitz, 2002).

Future prevention research must also address the issue of technology transfer. Greater elucidation and evaluation of the methods by which interventions of established experimental effectiveness can be successfully adapted to diverse community contexts is needed (Sloboda & Schildhaus, 2002). Rogers (2002) offered five strategies for increasing the rapidity with which effective new prevention approaches are adopted, noting the slow diffusion of prevention innovations that has historically characterized the substance abuse area.

Other areas for future exploration include the need for additional efforts to evaluate the cultural appropriateness of preventive intervention strategies and the need for more interaction between substance abuse prevention practitioners and researchers and their counterparts working in crime, suicide, and allied areas (Spooner & Hall, 2002).

REFERENCES

Abram, K. M., Teplin, L. A., & McLellan, G. M. (2003). Comorbidity or severe psychiatric disorders and substance use disorders among women in jail. *American Journal of Psychiatry, 160,* 1007–1010.

American Psychiatric Association. (2000). *Diagnostic and statistical manual of mental disorders* (4th ed., text rev.). Washington, DC: Author.

American Public Health Association. (2003). *Tobacco and public health: Selections from the American Journal of Public Health.* Washington, DC: Author.

Anda, R. F., Whitfield, C. L., Felitti, V. J., Chapman, D., Edwards, V. J., Dube, S. R., et al. (2002). Adverse childhood experiences, alcoholic parents, and later risk of alcoholism and depression. *Psychiatric Services, 53,* 1001–1009.

Arias, E., Anderson, R. N., Kung, H., Murphy, S. L., & Kochanek, M. A. (2003). *Deaths: Final data for 2001* (National Vital Statistics Reports No. 50). Hyattsville, MD: National Center for Health Statistics.

Arndt, S., Schultz, S. K., Turvey, C., & Petersen, A. (2002). Screening for alcoholism in the primary care setting: Are we talking to the right people? *Journal of Family Practice, 51,* 41–46.

Arrestee Drug Abuse Monitoring Program. (2003). *Annual report, Arrestee Drug Abuse Monitoring Program.* Washington, DC: U.S. Department of Justice, Office of Justice Programs.

Bailey, S. L., Huo, D., Garfein, R. S., & Ouellet, L. J. (2003). The use of needle exchange by young injection users. *Journal of the Acquired Immune Deficiency Syndrome, 34,* 67–70.

Belcher, H. M., & Shinitzky, H. E. (1998). Substance abuse in children: Prediction, protection, and prevention. *Archives of Pediatrics and Adolescent Medicine, 152,* 952–960.

Bennett, J. B., & Lehman, W. E. K. (2003). *Preventing workplace substance abuse: Beyond drug testing to wellness.* Washington, DC: American Psychological Association.

Blondell, R. D., Looney, S. W., Hottman, L. M., & Boaz, P. W. (2002). Characteristics of intoxicated trauma patients. *Journal of Addictive Diseases, 2,* 1–12.

Blum, R. W. (1997). Adolescent substance use and abuse. *Archives of Pediatric Adolescent Medicine, 151,* 805–808.

Boyd, M. R. (2000). Predicting substance abuse and comorbidity in rural women. *Archives of Psychiatric Nursing, 14,* 64–72.

Bry, B. H., McKeon, P., & Pandina, R. J. (1982). Extent of drug use as a function of number of risk factors. *Journal of Abnormal Psychology, 91,* 273–279.

Burd, L., Cotsonas-Hassler, T. M., Martsolf, J. T., & Kerbeshian, J. (2003). Recognition and management of fetal alcohol syndrome. *Neurotoxicology and Teratology, 25,* 681–688.

Cadoret, R. J., Cain, C. A., & Grove, W. M. (1980). Development of alcoholism in adoptees raised apart from alcoholic biologic relatives. *Archives of General Psychiatry, 37,* 561–563.

Castillo, M., & Henderson, G. (2002). Hispanic substance abusers in the United States. In G. X. Ma & G. Henderson (Eds.), *Ethnicity and substance abuse: Prevention and intervention* (pp. 1–22). Springfield, IL: Charles C. Thomas.

Catalano, R. F., Oxford, M., Harachi, T. W., Abbott, R. D., & Haggerty, K. P. (1999). A test of the social development model to predict problem behavior during the elementary school period. *Criminal Behaviour and Mental Health, 9,* 39–56.

Cervantes, R. C., Kappos, B., Duenas, N., & Arellano, D. (2003). Culturally focused HIV prevention and substance abuse treatment for Hispanic women. *Addictive Disorders and Their Treatment, 2,* 69–77.

Chang, G., Goetz, M. A., Wilkins-Haug, L., & Berman, S. (2000). A brief intervention for prenatal alcohol use: An in-depth look. *Journal of Substance Abuse Treatment, 18,* 365–369.

Chesney, M. A., Kobline, B. A., Barresi, P. J., Husnik, M. J., Celum, C. L., Colfax, G., et al. (2003). An individually-tailored intervention for HIV prevention: Baseline data from the EXPLORE study. *American Journal of Public Health, 93,* 933–938.

Clark, D. B., Kirisci, L., & Moss, H. B. (1998). Early adolescent gateway drug use in sons of fathers with substance use disorders. *Addictive Behaviors, 23,* 561–566.

Cochran, S. D., Keenan, C., Schober, C., & Mays, V. M. (2000). Estimates of alcohol use and clinical treatment needs among homosexually active men and women in the U.S. population. *Journal of Consulting and Clinical Psychology, 68,* 1062–1071.

Coffin, P. O., Fuller, C., Vadnai, L., Blaney, S., Galea, S., & Vlahov, D. (2003). Preliminary evidence of health care provider support for naloxone prescription as overdose fatality prevention strategy in New York City. *Journal of Urban Health, 80,* 288–289.

Coie, J. D. (1990). Towards a theory of peer rejection. In S. R. Asher & J. D. Coie (Eds.), *Peer rejection in childhood* (pp. 365–398). New York: Cambridge University Press.

Coogle, C. L., & Parham, I. A. (2001). Addictions services: Follow-up to the statewide model detection and prevention program for geriatric alcoholism and alcohol abuse. *Community Mental Health Journal, 37,* 381–391.

Copenhaver, M., Avants, S. K., Warburton, L. A., & Margolin, A. (2003). Intervening effectively with drug abusers infected with HIV: Taking into account the potential for cognitive impairment. *Journal of Psychoactive Drugs, 35,* 209–218.

Crano, W. D., & Burgoo, M. (2002). *Mass media and drug prevention: Classic and contemporary theories and research.* Claremont Symposium on Applied Social Psychology, Claremont Graduate School, Claremont, CA.

Crawford, V., Crome, I. B., & Clancy, C. (2003). Co-existing problems of mental health and substance misuse (dual diagnosis): A literature review. *Drugs: Education, Prevention, and Policy,* S1–S74.

Cuijpers, P. (2003). Three decades of drug prevention research. *Drugs: Education, Prevention, and Policy, 10,* 7–20.

Darke, S., & Hall, W. (2003). Heroin overdose: Research and evidence-based intervention. *Journal of Urban Health, 80,* 189–200.

Darke, S., & Ross, J. (1997). Polydrug dependence and psychiatric comorbidity among heroin injectors. *Drug and Alcohol Dependence, 48,* 135–141.

Davidson, P. J., McLean, R. L., Kral, A. H., Gleghorn, A. A., Edlin, B. R., & Moss, A. R. (2003). Fatal heroin-related overdose in San Francisco, 1997–2000: A case for targeted intervention. *Journal of Urban Health, 80,* 261–273.

De Castro, S., & Sabate, E. (2003). Adherence to heroin dependence therapies and human immunodeficiency virus/acquired immunodeficiency syndrome infection rates among drug abusers. *Clinical and Infectious Diseases, 15,* S464–S467.

Dehaas, R. A. B. (2003). Anxiety sensitivity and substance use situations: A comparison of clinical substance abusing populations. *Dissertation Abstracts International, 63*(8-B), 3909.

DeJong, W., & Langford, L. M. (2002). A typology for campus-based alcohol prevention: Moving toward environmental management strategies. *Journal of Studies on Alcohol, 14,* 140–147.

Dishion, T. J. (1990). The peer context of troublesome behavior in children and adolescents. In P. Leone (Ed.), *Understanding troubled and troublesome youth* (pp. 128–153). Beverly Hills, CA: Sage.

Dishion, T. J., Capaldi, D. M., & Yoerger, K. (1999). Middle childhood antecedents to progressions in male adolescent substance use: An ecological analysis of risk and protective factors. *Journal of Adolescent Research, 14,* 175–205.

Drug Abuse Warning Network. (2002). Medical examiner findings. Department of Health and Human Services, Washington, DC.

Eddy, M. (2003, April). *War on drugs: The national youth anti-drug media campaign. Congressional Research Service Library of Congress. Report for Congress* [Electronic version]. Retrieved December 31, 2003, from www.drugpolicy.org/docUploads /RS21490.pdf.

Edens, J. F., Peters, R. H., & Hills, H. A. (1997). Treating prison inmates with co-occurring disorders: An integrative review of existing programs. *Behavior Science and the Law, 15,* 439–457.

Eliason, M. J., & Skinstad, A. H. (2001). Drug and alcohol intervention for older women: A pilot study. *Journal of Gerontological Nursing, 27,* 18–24.

Ellis, B. H. (2003). Mobilizing communities to reduce substance abuse in Indian country. *Journal of Psychoactive Drugs, 35,* 89–96.

Escobedo, L. G., & Ortiz, M. (2002). The relationship between liquor outlet density and violence in New Mexico. *Accident Analysis and Prevention, 34,* 689–694.

Fabiano, P. M. (2003). Applying the social norms model to universal and indicated alcohol interventions at Western Washington University. In H. W. Perkins (Ed.), *The social norms approach to preventing school and college age substance abuse: A handbook for educators, counselors, and clinicians* (pp. 3–17). San Francisco: Jossey-Bass.

Farabee, D., & Leukefeld, C. G. (2002). HIV and AIDS prevention strategies. In C. G. Leukefeld & F. Tims (Eds.), *Treatment of drug offenders: Policies and issues* (pp. 12–47). New York: Springer.

Farber, N. B., & Olney, J. W. (2003). Drugs of abuse that cause developing neurons to commit suicide. *Brain Research and Developmental Brain Research, 147,* 37–45.

Farrington, D. P., Gallagher, B., Morley, L., St. Leger, R., & West, D. (1988). Are there any successful men from criminogenic backgrounds? *Psychiatry, 51,* 116–130.

Fergusson, D. M., & Horwood, L. J. (1999). Prospective childhood predictors of deviant peer affiliations in adolescence. *Journal of Child Psychology and Psychiatry and Allied Disciplines, 40,* 581–592.

Fiore, M. C., Bailey, W. C., & Cohen, S. J. (2000). *Treating tobacco use and dependence: Clinical practice guideline.* Rockville, MD: U.S. Department of Health and Human Services, Public Health Service.

Fishbein, D. H., & Perez, D. M. (2000). A regional study of risk factors for drug abuse and delinquency: Sex and racial differences. *Journal of Child and Family Studies, 9,* 461–479.

Fleming, M. F. (2002). Identification and treatment of alcohol use disorders in older adults. In A. M. Gurnack, R. Atkinson, & N. J. Osgood (Eds.), *Treating alcohol and drug abuse in the elderly* (pp. 85–108). New York: Springer.

Friedmann, P. D., Lemon, S. C., Anderson, B. J., & Stein, M. D. (2003). Predictors of follow-up health status in the Drug Abuse Treatment Outcome Study (DATOS). *Drug and Alcohol Dependence, 69,* 243–251.

Friend, K., & Levy, D. (2002). Reductions in smoking prevalence and cigarette consumption associated with mass-media campaigns. *Health Education Research, 17,* 85–98.

Galaif, E. R., Stein, J. A., Newcomb, M. D., & Bernstein, D. P. (2001). Gender differences in the prediction of problem alcohol use in adulthood: Exploring the influence of family factors and childhood maltreatment. *Journal of Studies on Alcohol, 62,* 486–493.

General Accounting Office. (2003). *Youth illicit drug use prevention: DARE long-term evaluations and federal efforts to identify effective programs.* (Report No. GAO-03-172R). Washington, DC: Author.

Gordon, R. (1983). An operational classification of disease prevention. *Public Health Reports, 98,* 107–109.

Gorman, E. M. (2003). Research with gay drug users and the interface with HIV: Current methodological issues for social work research. *Journal of Gay and Lesbian Social Services: Issues in Practice, Policy, and Research, 15,* 79–94.

Gottfredson, D. C., Gottfredson, G. D., & Hybl, L. G. (1993). Managing adolescent behavior: A multiyear, multischool study. *American Educational Research Journal, 30,* 179–215.

Haines, M. P., & Barker, G. P. (2003). The Northern IL University experiment: A longitudinal case study of the social norms approach. In H. W. Perkins (Ed.), *The social norms approach to preventing school and college age substance abuse: A handbook for educators, counselors, and clinicians* (pp. 83–99). San Francisco: Jossey-Bass.

Hanlon, T. E., Bateman, R. W., Simon, B. D., O'Grady, K. E., & Carswell, S. B. (2002). An early community-based intervention for the prevention of substance abuse and other delinquent behavior. *Journal of Youth and Adolescence, 31,* 459–471.

Hawkins, D. F., Laub, J. H., & Lauritsen, J. L. (1998). Race, ethnicity, and serious juvenile offending. In R. Loeber & D. P. Farrington (Eds.), *Serious and violent juvenile offenders: Risk factors and successful interventions* (pp. 30–46). Thousand Oaks, CA: Sage.

Hawkins, J. D., Catalano, R. F., & Arthur, M. W. (2002). Promoting science-based prevention in communities. *Addictive Behaviors, 27,* 951–976.

Hawkins, J. D., Catalano, R. F., & Miller, J. Y. (1992). Risk and protective factors for alcohol and other drug problems in adolescence and early adulthood: Implications for substance abuse prevention. *Psychological Bulletin, 112,* 64–105.

Hawkins, W. E., Latkin, C., Mandel, W., & Oziemkowska, M. (1999). Do actions speak louder than words? Perceived peer influence on needle sharing and cleaning in a sample of injection drug users. *AIDS Education and Prevention, 11,* 122–131.

Heffernan, K., Cloitre, M., Tardiff, K., Marzuk, P. M., Portera, L., & Leon, A. C. (2000). Childhood trauma as a correlate of lifetime opiate use in psychiatric patients. *Addictive Behaviors, 25,* 797–803.

Hill, S. Y., Shen, S., Lowers, L., & Locke, J. (2000). Factors predicting the onset of adolescent drinking in families at high risk for developing alcoholism. *Biological Psychiatry, 48,* 265–275.

Hingson, R. W., Heeren, T., Zakocs, R. C., Kopstein, A., & Wechsler, H. (2002). Magnitude of alcohol-related mortality and morbidity among U.S. college students ages 18–24. *Journal of Studies on Alcohol, 63,* 136–144.

Hogan, J. A., Gabrielsen, K. R., Luna, N., & Grothaus, D. (2003). *Substance abuse prevention: The intersection of science and practice.* Needham Heights, MA: Allyn & Bacon.

Howard, M. O., Kivlahan, D., & Walker, R. D. (1997). Cloninger's tridimensional theory of personality and psychopathology: Applications to substance use disorders. *Journal of Studies on Alcohol, 58,* 48–66.

Hubner, L. S. (2002). Social mentoring as an alcohol prevention program for undergraduate college freshmen on a commuter campus. *Dissertation Abstracts International, 62-B,* 3849.

Jenkins, C., Rahman, H., Saidel, T. S., Jana, S., & Hussain, A. M. Z. (2001). Measuring the impact of needle exchange programs among injecting drug users through the National Behavioural Surveillance in Bangladesh. *AIDS Education and Prevention, 13,* 452–461.

Jenson, J. M., & Howard, M. O. (1999). Hallucinogen use among juvenile probationers: Prevalence and characteristics. *Criminal Justice and Behavior, 26,* 357–372.

Johnston, L. D. (1991). Toward a theory of drug epidemics. In L. Donohew, H. E. Sypher, & W. J. Bukoski (Eds.), *Pervasive communication and drug abuse prevention* (pp. 93–131). Hillsdale, NJ: Erlbaum.

Johnston, L. D., O'Malley, P. M., & Bachman, J. G. (2003). *Monitoring the Future national survey results on drug use, 1975–2002: Vol. I. Secondary school students* (NIH Publication No. 03-5375). Bethesda, MD: National Institute on Drug Abuse.

Joksch, H. C. (1988). *The impact of severe penalties on drinking and driving.* Washington, DC: AAA Foundation for Traffic Safety.

Kellam, S. G., Rebok, G. W., Ialongo, N., & Mayer, L. S. (1994). The course and malleability of aggressive behavior from early first grade into middle school: Results of a developmental epidemiologically based preventive trial. *Journal of Child Psychology and Psychiatry, 35,* 259–281.

Kendziora, K. T., & O'Leary, S. G. (1993). Dysfunctional parenting as a focus for prevention and treatment of child behavior problems. In T. H. Ollendick & R. J. Prinz (Eds.), *Advances in clinical child psychology* (Vol. 15, pp. 19–26). New York: Plenum Press.

Khoury, E. L. (1998). Are girls different? A developmental perspective on gender differences in risk factors for substance use among adolescents. In W. A. Vega, A. G. Gil, & Associates (Eds.), *Drug use and ethnicity in early adolescence* (pp. 42–80). New York: Plenum Press.

King, V. L., Kidorf, M. S., Stoller, K. B., & Brooner, R. K. (2000). Influence of psychiatric comorbidity on HIV risk behaviors: Changes during drug abuse treatment. *Journal of Addictive Diseases, 19,* 65–83.

Kost, K. A., & Smyth, N. J. (2002). Two strikes against them? Exploring the influence of a history of poverty and growing up in an alcoholic family on alcohol problems and income. *Journal of Social Service Research, 28,* 23–52.

Kristenson, H., Oesterline, A., Nilsson, J., & Lindgaerde, F. (2002). Prevention of alcohol-related deaths in middle-aged heavy drinkers. *Alcoholism: Clinical and Experimental Research, 26,* 478–484.

Lapham, S. C., Gregory, C., & McMillan, G. (2003a). Impact of an alcohol misuse intervention for health care workers: 1. Frequency of binge drinking and desire to reduce alcohol use. *Alcohol and Alcoholism, 38,* 176–182.

Lapham, S. C., Gregory, C., & McMillan, G. (2003b). Impact of an alcohol misuse intervention for health care workers: 2. Employee assistance programme utilization, on-the-job injuries, job loss and health services utilization. *Alcohol and Alcoholism, 38,* 182–188.

Leukefeld, C. G., & Tims, F. (Eds.). (2002). *Treatment of drug offenders: Policies and issues.* New York: Springer.

Lew, R., & Tanjasiri, S. P. (2003). Slowing the epidemic of tobacco use among Asian Americans and Pacific Islanders. *American Journal of Public Health, 93,* 764–768.

Linn, J. G., Neff, J. A., Theriot, R., Harris, J. L., Interrante, J., & Graham, M. E. (2003). Reaching impaired populations with HIV prevention programs: A clinical trial for homeless mentally ill African-American men. *Cell and Molecular Biology, 49,* 1167–1175.

Lipscomb, H. J., Dement, J. M., & Li, L. (2003). Health care utilization of carpenters with substance abuse-related diagnoses. *American Journal of Independent Medicine, 43,* 120–131.

Loeber, R., Farrington, D. P., Stouthamer-Loeber, M., & Van Kammen, W. B. (1998). Multiple risk factors for multiproblem boys: Co-occurrence of delinquency, substance use, attention deficit, conduct problems, physical aggression, covert behavior, depressed mood, and shy/withdrawn behavior. In R. Jessor (Ed.), *New perspectives on adolescent risk behavior* (pp. 91–149). New York: Cambridge University Press.

MacCoun, R. J., & Reuter, P. (2001). *Drug war heresies.* Cambridge, MA: Cambridge University Press.

MacKinnon, D. P., & Lockwood, C. M. (2003). Advances in statistical methods for substance abuse prevention. *Prevention Sciences, 4,* 155–171.

Marlatt, G. A., & Witkiewitz, K. (2002). Harm reduction approaches to alcohol use: Health promotion, prevention, and treatment. *Addictive Behaviors, 27,* 867–886.

Marsden, J., Gossop, M., Stewart, D., Rolfe, A., & Farrell, M. (2000). Psychiatric symptoms among clients seeking treatment for drug dependence. Intake data from the National Treatment Outcome Research Study. *British Journal of Psychiatry, 176,* 285–289.

May, P. A., & Gossage, J. P. (2001). Estimating the prevalence of fetal alcohol syndrome. A summary. *Alcohol Research and Health, 25,* 159–167.

Morbidity and Mortality Weekly Report. (2000). *Unintentional opiate overdose deaths—King County, Washington, 1990–1999.* Atlanta, GA: Centers for Disease Control and Prevention.

Musher-Eizenman, D. R., & Kulick, A. D. (2003). An alcohol expectancy-challenge prevention program for at risk college women. *Psychology of Addictive Behaviors, 17,* 163–166.

Musto, D. F. (1999). *The American disease, Origins of narcotic control* (3rd ed.). New York: Oxford University Press.

National Institute on Alcohol Abuse and Alcoholism. (1997). *Alcohol and health.* Health and Human Services, Washington, DC.

National Institute on Alcohol Abuse and Alcoholism. (2000). *Tenth special report to congress on alcohol and health.* Bethesda, MD: U.S. Department of Health and Human Services.

Orozco, S., & Lukas, S. (2000). Gender differences in acculturation and aggression as predictors of drug use. *Drug and Alcohol Dependence, 59,* 165–172.

O'Toole, T. P., Strain, E. C., Wand, G., McCaul, M. E., & Barnhart, M. (2002). Outpatient treatment entry and health care utilization after a combined medical/substance abuse intervention for hospitalized medical patients. *Journal of General Internal Medicine, 17,* 334–340.

Patterson, G. R., Dishion, T. J., & Chamberlain, P. (1993). Outcomes and methodological issues relating to treatment of antisocial children. In T. R. Giles (Ed.), *Effective psychotherapy: A handbook of comparative research* (pp. 43–88). New York: Plenum Press.

Perkins, H. W. (2003). The emergence and evolution of the social norms approach to substance abuse prevention. In H. W. Perkins (Ed.), *The social norms approach to preventing school and college age substance abuse: A handbook for educators, counselors, and clinicians* (pp. 3–17). San Francisco: Jossey-Bass.

Perkins, H. W., & Craig, D. W. (2003). The Hobart and William Smith Colleges experiment: A synergistic social norms approach using print, electronic media, and curriculum infusion to reduce collegiate problem drinking. In H. W. Perkins (Ed.), *The social norms to preventing school and college age substance abuse: A handbook for educators, counselors, and clinicians* (pp. 35–64). San Francisco: Jossey-Bass.

Piper, B., Briggs, M., Huffman, K., & Lubot-Conke, R. (2003, September). *State of the states, drug policy reforms: 1996–2002, a report by the drug policy alliance* [Electronic version]. New York: Drug Policy Alliance. Retrieved December 14, 2003, from www.drugpolicy.org/docUploads/sos_report2003.pdf.

Pollard, J. A., Hawkins, J. D., & Arthur, M. W. (1999). Risk and protection: Are both necessary to understand diverse behavioral outcomes in adolescence? *Social Work Research, 23,* 145–158.

Rehm, J., Room, R., Monteiro, M., Gmel, G., Graham, K., Rehn, N., et al. (2003). Alcohol as a risk factor for global burden of disease. *European Journal of Addiction Research, 9,* 157–164.

Rich, J. D., Macaline, G. E., McKenzie, M., Taylor, L. E., & Burris, S. (2001). Syringe prescription to prevent HIV infection in Rhode Island: A case study. *American Journal of Public Health, 91,* 699–700.

Rogers, E. M. (2002). Diffusion of preventive interventions. *Addictive Behaviors, 27,* 989–993.

Roman, P. M., & Blum, T. C. (1996). Alcohol: A review of the impact of worksite interventions on health and behavioral outcomes. *American Journal of Health Promotion, 11,* 136–149.

Saadatmand, F., Stinson, F. S., Grant, B. F., & Dufour, M. C. (1999). *Liver mortality in the United States, 1970–96* (Surveillance report No. 52). Rockville, MD: National Institute on Alcohol Abuse and Alcoholism.

Saunders, J. B., & Brady, K. T. (2002). The scientific basis for the prevention and treatment of substance misuse. *Current Opinion in Psychiatry, 15,* 231–234.

Secker-Walker, R. H., Gnich, W., Platt, S., & Lancaster, T. (2003). Community interventions for reducing smoking among adults (Cochrane Review). *Cochrane Library* (Vol. 4). Chichester, England: Wiley.

Seeff, L. B., & Hoofnagle, J. H. (2003). Appendix: The National Institutes of Health Consensus Development Conference Management of Hepatitis C, 2002. *Clinical Liver Diseases, 7,* 261–287.

Siegel, M. (2002). The effectiveness of state-level tobacco control interventions: A review of program implementation and behavioral outcomes. *Annual Review of Public Health, 23,* 45–71.

Simcha-Fagan, O., & Schwartz, J. E. (1986). Neighborhood and delinquency: An assessment of contextual effects. *Criminology, 24,* 667–703.

Simon, T. R., Sussman, S., Dahlberg, L. L., & Dent, C. W. (2002). Influence of a substance-abuse-prevention curriculum on violence-related behavior. *American Journal of Health Behavior, 26,* 103–110.

Sinha, R. (2001). How does stress increase risk of drug abuse and relapse? *Psychopharmacology, 158,* 343–359.

Sloboda, Z., & Schildhaus, S. (2002). A discussion of the concept of technology transfer of research-based drug "abuse" prevention and treatment interventions. *Substance Use and Misuse, 37,* 1079–1087.

Smith, D. R., & Jarjoura, G. R. (1988). Social structure and criminal victimization. *Journal of Research on Crime and Delinquency, 25,* 27–52.

Soderstrom, C. A., Ballesteros, M. F., Dischinger, P. C., Kerns, T. J., Flint, R. D., & Smith, G. S. (2001). Alcohol/drug abuse, driving convictions, and risk-taking dispositions among trauma center patients. *Accident Analysis and Prevention, 33,* 771–782.

Spooner, C., & Hall, W. (2002). Public policy and the prevention of substance-use disorders. *Current Opinion in Psychiatry, 15,* 235–239.

Spoth, R., Guyll, M., Chao, W., & Molgaard, V. (2003). Exploratory study of a preventive intervention with general population African-American families. *Journal of Early Adolescence, 23,* 435–468.

Stillman, F. A., Hartman, A. M., Graubard, B. I., Gilpin, E. A., Murray, D. M., & Gibson, J. T. (2003). Evaluation of the American Stop Smoking Intervention Study (ASSIST): A report of outcomes. *Journal of the National Cancer Institute, 95,* 1681–1691.

Stoler, J. M., Huntington, K. S., Peterson, C. M., Peterson, K. P., Daniel, P., Aboagye, K. K., et al. (1998). The prenatal detection of significant alcohol exposure with maternal blood markers. *Journal of Pediatrics, 133,* 346–352.

Stout, R. W., Parkinson, M. D., & Wolfe, W. H. (1993). Alcohol-related mortality in the U.S. Air Force, 1990. *American Journal of Preventive Medicine, 9,* 220–223.

Strauss, S. M., Astone, J., Vassilev, Z., Des Jarlais, D. C., & Hagan, H. (2003). Gaps in the drug-free and methadone treatment program response to Hepatitis C. *Journal of Substance Abuse Treatment, 24,* 291–297.

Streeton, C., & Whelan, G. (2001). Naltrexone, a relapse prevention maintenance treatment of alcohol dependence: A meta-analysis of randomized controlled trials. *Alcohol and Alcoholism, 36,* 544–552.

Stromberg, M. F., Mackler, S. A., Volpicelli, J. R., & O'Brien, C. P. (2001). Effect of acamprosate and naltrexone, alone or in combination, on ethanol consumption. *Alcohol, 23,* 109–116.

Substance Abuse and Mental Health Services Administration. (2002). *Mortality data from the Drug Abuse Warning Network, 2000* [Press release announced March 1, 2002]. Available from www.samhas.gov/news/newsreleases.

Substance Abuse and Mental Health Services Administration. (2003). *Results from the 2002 National Survey on Drug Use and Health: National findings* (Office of Applied Studies, NHSDA Series H-22, DHHS Publication No. SMA 03-3836). Rockville, MD: Author.

Task Force of the National Advisory Council on Alcohol Abuse and Alcoholism. (2002). *How to reduce high-risk college drinking: Use proven strategies, fill research Gaps: Final report of the panel on prevention and treatment.* Bethesda, MD: U.S. Department of Health and Human Services.

Timmons-Mitchell, J., Brown, C., Schulz, S. C., Webster, S. E., Underwood, L. A., & Semple, W. E. (1997). Comparing the mental health needs of female and male incarcerated juvenile delinquents. *Behavioral Sciences and the Law, 15,* 195–202.

Tuten, M., & Jones, H. E. (2003). A partner's drug-using status impacts women's drug treatment outcome. *Drug and Alcohol Dependence, 70,* 327–330.

U.S. Department of Labor. (2004). Available from www.dol.gov/dol/workingpartners .htm.

Volpicelli, J. R., Pettinati, H. M., McLellan, A. T., & O'Brien, C. P. (2001). *Combining medications and psychosocial treatments for addictions.* New York: Guilford Press.

Wallin, E., Norstroem, T., & Andreasson, S. (2003). Alcohol prevention targeting licensed premises: A study of effects on violence. *Journal of Studies on Alcohol, 64,* 270–277.

Walsh, D. J. A., Henderson, D., & Magraw, M. (2003). A public health program for preventing fetal alcohol syndrome among women at risk in Montana. *Neurotoxicology and Teratology, 25,* 757–761.

Wekerle, C., & Wall, A. M. (2003). The violence and addiction equation: Theoretical and clinical issues in substance abuse and relationship violence. *Adolescence, 38,* 203.

Welsh, C. J., & Liberto, J. (2001). The use of medication for relapse prevention in substance dependence disorders. *Journal of Psychiatric Practice, 7,* 15–31.

Werner, E. E. (1994). Overcoming the odds. *Developmental and Behavioral Pediatrics, 15,* 131–136.

Whelan, G. (2003). Alcohol: A much neglected risk factor in elderly mental disorders. *Current Opinion in Psychiatry, 16,* 609–614.

Whitmore, C. C., Yi, H., Chen, C. M., & Dufour, M. C. (2002). *Trends in alcohol-related morbidity among short-stay community hospital discharges, United States, 1979–1999* (Surveillance report No. 58, revised). Rockville, MD: National Institute on Alcohol Abuse and Alcoholism.

Wilens, T. E., Biederman, J., Spencer, T. J., & Frances, R. J. (1994). Comorbidity of attention deficit hyperactivity and psychoactive substance use disorders. *Hospital and Community Psychiatry, 45,* 421–423.

Yamaguchi, R., Johnston, L. D., & O'Malley, P. M. (2003). The relationship between student illicit drug use and school drug-testing policies. *Journal of School Health, 73,* 159–164.

Yi, H., Williams, G. D., & Dufour, M. C. (2002). *Trends in alcohol-related fatal traffic crashes, United States, 1977–2000* (Surveillance report No. 61). Rockville, MD: National Institute on Alcohol Abuse and Alcoholism.

Chapter 7

SEXUAL DYSFUNCTION

KAREN M. SOWERS, WILLIAM S. ROWE, AND ANDREA K. McCARTER

What type of therapy works with what type of patient experiencing what type of dysfunction (McCarthy, 1995)? After more than 30 years of attention on this topic, this question still awaits an answer. Sexual dysfunction affects numerous men and women and yet is underdiagnosed and underinvestigated as a medical problem (Lechtenberger & Ohl, 1994). Based on the high numbers of occurrence, there is a need for continued research and discussion of treatment interventions in this area.

This chapter first examines pertinent definitions and history for a beginning understanding of sexual dysfunction. Next, the authors review the risk factors identified in the professional literature. In the third section, trends, incidence, and prevalence rates are addressed. The fourth section reviews research studies, treatment methods, and assessment techniques over the past 30 years. Finally, the authors provide suggestions for practice and policy implications within the social work field as well as future directions for research.

DEFINITIONS AND HISTORY

Although sexual dysfunction has probably existed since the beginning of humankind, the scientific study of human sexuality is a relatively recent phenomenon (Rowe & Savage, 1987). There is still lack of knowledge regarding the development of sexuality (Dziegielewski, Resnick, Nelson-Gardell, & Harrison, 1998). The first major attempts to understand human sexuality from a viewpoint of psychological normalcy came at the turn of the twentieth century. At the forefront of this movement were Sigmund Freud and Havelock Ellis. Both recognized the reality of childhood sexuality and normal stages of psychosexual development (Rowe & Savage, 1987). The first significant attempt to gather information about the actual sexual practices and beliefs of people was made by Alfred Kinsey. Much of the treatment for sexual dysfunction began from research conducted and published by Masters and Johnson (1970). As the recognition of sexual problems has grown, there has been an increase in sophistication of technologies for treating such dysfunctions (H. R. Conte, 1986). An example of this, discussed in detail later, is the movement over time from a psychological focus with counseling-type therapy to a focus on physical aspects of dysfunction and treatment with drug therapy. Yet, despite the increase in attention to the topic, there still remains a need to develop a universal definition of sexual dysfunction and a universal method of assessment (Conte, 1986).

The professional literature attempts to address the difference between a sexual problem and a sexual dysfunction related primarily to females (Bancroft, 2002). Bancroft attempts to differentiate the two by referring to a sexual problem as an "inhibition of sexual responsiveness in the presence of stress, depression, or marked tiredness, or the continuing presence of negative or threatening patterns of behavior in the partner" (p. 454). Sexual dysfunction is diagnosed in those with an "undue propensity for inhibition, [that] may maladaptively inhibit response, or for whom an unusually low propensity for excitation may make sexual response unlikely" (p. 455).

The *DSM-IV* (American Psychological Association, 1994) defines sexual dysfunction as a "disturbance in the processes that characterize the sexual response cycle or by pain associated with sexual intercourse" (p. 493). Within this broad definition of sexual dysfunction are five more specific categories: sexual desire disorders, sexual arousal disorders, orgasmic disorders, sexual pain disorders, and sexual dysfunction due to a general medical condition (American Psychological Association, 1994; Dziegielewski et al., 1998).

The sexual response cycle has been defined and discussed by a number of authors. It consists of a desire phase, often represented by fantasies; an excitement phase, in which physiological changes occur; an orgasm phase, witnessed by muscle tensions and contractions; and finally, a resolution phase or relaxation (Dziegielewski et al., 1998).

There are several categories of specific dysfunctions under the broad umbrella term *sexual dysfunction*. Females suffering from sexual dysfunction may experience primary orgasmic dysfunction (never experiencing orgasm), secondary orgasmic dysfunction (experiencing orgasm at some point), or vaginismus (inability to have intercourse due to extreme physical pain; LoPiccolo & Stock, 1986). Males experiencing some form of sexual dysfunction may suffer from erectile dysfunction, premature ejaculation, or inhibited ejaculation (LoPiccolo & Stock, 1986).

With the wide range of dysfunctions that a person can suffer sexually, there needs to be careful consideration of the treatment interventions that are available.

It has been "three decades since the advent of sex therapy" (Weiderman, 1998, p. 88), with numerous changes occurring in the treatment practices. In the late 1960s, sexual dysfunctions were seen as part of a greater psychopathology and were therefore treated within a psychoanalytic framework (E. Rosen & Weinstein, 1988). In the 1970s, treatment moved to a more behavioral approach, beginning with Masters and Johnson's (1970) development of brief, problem-focused, directive, behavioral techniques. During this time, there was also a noticeable increase in the attention paid to sexual dysfunction by the mass media (Leiblum & Rosen, 1995). Due to the increased amount of educational information available in the media, there was a decrease in the use of sex therapists in the 1980s (LoPiccolo, 1994). This led to a decrease in success rates of sex therapy because the only people seeking assistance were those with severe problems who presented more of a challenge to therapists (Wiederman, 1998).

In addition to the increase in sex therapy treatments available and in use, there has been a small increase in research on sexual dysfunction and interventions, although a number of authors have reported a paucity of evidence for the use of one intervention over another (Dziegielewski et al., 1998; Fisher, Swingen, & O'Donohue, 1997; Kinder & Blakeney, 1977). Another issue is the definition of effective treatment and the application of this term to treatment interventions in use by clinicians. Heiman (2002a, 2002b) discusses two categories of treatment proposed by the 1995 American Psychological Task Force on the Promotion and Dissemination of Psychological Procedures that are well-established treatments and probably efficacious treatments. According to Heiman (2002a, 2002b), some well-established treatments have been studied by a number of researchers and are shown to be superior to other treatments. However, a probably efficacious treatment may also be used which is a treatment method shown to be more effective "than [using] a waiting list control group" (Heiman, 2002a, p. 446). She asserts that "a number of sexual dysfunctions have treatment data that meet the probably efficacious criteria [while] few meet the well-established criteria" (2002b, p. 74). With the great number of risk factors and high prevalence rates, discussed in the following sections, it is imperative that research be conducted to determine the most effective treatment interventions.

RISK FACTORS

Sexual dysfunction has roots in two major areas of a person's life. The dysfunction may be caused by physical factors such as illness, use of drugs and medications, or injury. However, little is known about the physiological aspect of sexual response (Barlow, 1986). Psychological and psychosocial factors, such as rape, incest, depression, religious beliefs, and marital problems, may also play a role in sexual dysfunction.

Studying anxiety and sexual dysfunction, Barlow (1986) cites five areas of difference between sexually functional and sexually dysfunctional individuals:

1. Affect during sexual stimulation
2. Differences of sexual arousal
3. Perceptions of control over arousal
4. Distractibility during sexual stimulation
5. Sexual response while anxious

Different levels of anxiety could cause these differences. Anxiety, both performance anxiety and fear of failure, is a contributing factor to sexual dysfunction (Barlow, 1986).

Several recent studies have looked at the possibility of child sexual abuse as a cause or risk factor of sexual dysfunction in later adult life. Most of the studies do not show a direct correlation between child sexual abuse and sexual dysfunction, but rather a link between the two by another risk factor. Beitchman and associates (1992), however, did find that victims of child sexual abuse show greater levels of adult sexual dysfunction. Similarly, Sarwar, Crawford, and Durlak (1997) assert that child sexual abuse does have long-lasting effects on sexual functioning, but more so for women than men. A number of authors have indicated that childhood abuse leads to more general than specifically sexual problems (Finklehor, 1979; Fromuth, 1986; D. Russell, 1986). The general life problems may then lead to or cause a sexual dysfunction. Bendixen, Muus, and Schei (1994) and Kinzl and Biebl (1992) show that child sexual abuse often leads to health problems, which also can have effects on sexual functioning. Finally, Finklehor, Hotaling, Lewis, and Smith (1990) demonstrate that more children who are raised in dysfunctional families experience sexual abuse and that people raised in dysfunctional families are more susceptible to sexual dysfunction in adulthood. There is not a direct link, however, between sexual abuse and adult sexual dysfunction.

Masters and Johnson (1970) provide numerous case studies from their research showing the potential for a sexually restrictive and religiously orthodox upbringing to be a risk factor for adult sexual dysfunction. Some studies have looked at sexual dysfunction as a medical problem. Lechtenberger and Ohl (1994) indicate that risk factors are not only psychological, but also can be urological, gynecological, and neurological. Social, cultural, and psychiatric factors also play a role in the patterns of sexual behavior (Lechtenberger & Ohl, 1994). The National Health and Social Life Survey (NHSLS, 1992) identified a number of potential risk factors for sexual dysfunction. Demographic factors such as age, education, and race/ethnicity were considered (Heiman, 2002b). Stress and emotional problems were examined as health and lifestyle variables. Other variables were social status, income level, and sexual experience history.

A review of the literature from 1966 to 1990 by Ussher (1993) showed risk factors of sexual dysfunction stemming from a number of areas in a person's life: sexual abuse, psychological factors, cognitions, menopause, physical aspects, social aspects, contraceptive anxiety, sociobiology, marital problems, alcohol use, and hormones. Although some of these factors are gender-specific, this literature review indicates that there are many areas of a person's life that must be considered in assessing and treating sexual dysfunction. More recently, it has been reiterated that one should consider physiological factors, mental health, use of medications, substance abuse, and life stress in treating sexual dysfunction (Dziegielewski et al., 1998).

TRENDS, INCIDENCE, PREVALENCE RATES

There have been a number of studies conducted to determine the prevalence rates of sexual dysfunction. Although rates differ among the studies, their ranges are similar: from 10% to 52% for men and 25% to 63% for women (H. A. Feldman, Goldstein, Hatzichristou, Krane, & McKinlay, 1994; Spector & Carey, 1990). Laumann and associates (Laumann, Paik, & Rosen, 1999) found that 43% of women and 31% of men surveyed, who had been sexually active in the previous 12 months, had experienced some type of dysfunction. In 1986, Conte found that 50% to 60% of all couples surveyed experience difficulties. These results indicate that sexual dysfunction is a very common issue among both men and women that take on a variety of forms.

In addition to the studies providing general statistics for sexual dysfunction, there are also studies that discuss the statistics of specific dysfunctions. Spector and Carey (1990) found that the most common dysfunction among males is premature ejaculation, with a prevalence rate of 36% to 38%. Men also experience erectile disorder at a rate of 4% to 9%. Inhibited orgasm occurs in both males (4% to 10%) and females (5% to 10%). Palace (1995) researched the sexual experiences of females in the United States and discovered that 30% or 23.5 million females experience orgasmic difficulties. Another 20%, or 15 million females, experience sexual desire disorders.

There are several categories of sexual dysfunction occurrence. Nadelson (2001) divides the broad category into people who have had a dysfunction present since puberty, or *lifelong,* people who have *acquired* a dysfunction at some point due to an incident or change in life that caused it, people who have a *situational* dysfunction in which they experience problems only in certain situations, and people who have *generalized* dysfunction and experience problems regardless of the situation. There are no studies available to indicate how many people or what percentage of people with sexual dysfunction fit into each of the categories.

LITERATURE REVIEW

The literature contains articles defining and explaining sexual dysfunction. There is literature available on the types of assessment that have been and should be used with patients with sexual dysfunction. Then there are research studies on the prevalence rates of specific dysfunctions, treatments and their success rates, and occurrence of sexual dysfunction based on specific risk factors.

Assessment

Authors are consistent on the methods that should be used in assessing and diagnosing sexual dysfunction. Almost all of the articles describe the use of person-to-person interviews, physical examinations, and self-report instruments that are available.

Conte (1986) conducted a review of the assessment techniques that have been used to evaluate females, males, and couples. Most of the assessment tools discussed are self-report because other methods of assessing sexual dysfunction are intrusive. Self-report methods include interviews, questionnaires, and behavioral records. An objective structure for the assessment interview was created in the 1960s and published by Masters and Johnson (1970). Several questionnaires have been created for use in assessing different aspects of sexual dysfunction, including the Sexual Orientation Method (M. P. Feldman, MacCulloch, Mellor, & Pinschot, 1966), the Sexual Interest Questionnaire (Harbison, Graham, Quinn, MacAllister, & Woodward, 1974), the Sexual Interaction Inventory (LoPiccolo & Steger, 1974), the Self-Evaluation of Sexual Behavior and Gratification (Lief, 1981), and the Sexual Arousability Index (Hoon, Hoon, & Wincze, 1976). Other methods of assessing sexual dysfunction rely on self-report behavioral records comparing successful and unsuccessful experiences, evaluation of erection during sleep, and physiological assessments (Conte, 1986).

Lechtenberger and Ohl (1994) agree with earlier literature that a person's sexual history is an important factor in treating her or him. They recommend using a person-to-person interview to obtain the history because then the researcher/clinician is able to clarify questions, tailor language to different patients' needs, and obtain clearer information from the patient about the problem.

Also important in assessment is a physical exam, including general, neurological, vascular, and endocrinological testing. The authors indicate, however, that only tests that will produce results that will directly affect the treatment interventions should be performed.

R. C. Rosen (2002) presents four categories of outcome measures that can be used in researching sexual dysfunction and treating patients that present with such problems. Self-administered measures that have been shown to be reliable and valid include questionnaires and event logs or daily diaries, in which a patient records episodes of sexual activity and satisfaction. Both of these measurements are subject to the patient's responses and opinions. Interviews for in-depth assessment conducted by a practitioner and physiological measures performed by a medical doctor are also reliable and valid measures of sexual dysfunction. These are the most common methods currently being used to assess patients for treatment.

Before deciding on a route of treatment for sexual dysfunction, therapists must consider the psychological, behavioral, and physiological domains of the individual's life.

Research Studies and Treatment Methods

The Gordon Model (Gordon, 1983, 1987) divides preventive interventions into three categories: universal, selective, and indicated. Although there is still a stigma attached to having a sexual dysfunction, healthy sexuality contributes to a person's overall well-being, and so treatment for such dysfunctions should be taken as seriously as treatment for any other health problem. Treatment for sexual dysfunction can be viewed as a continuum ranging from education for people of all ages to focusing education on specific populations who are prone to develop problems to treatment of the dysfunction once it has developed.

Universal Preventive Interventions

Universal preventive interventions are those created for the general population. In terms of sexual dysfunction, the only universal intervention is education about risk factors and symptoms. Education on sexual dysfunction should begin as early as sex education in general begins, with adolescents. This would provide the information to people as they begin to become sexually active and potentially prevent problems from occurring. Such early education may also help eliminate the stigma of seeking treatment.

Selective Preventive Interventions

Selective preventive interventions are focused on individuals who are at high risk for developing a problem. There are no selective interventions noted in the sexual dysfunction literature. One population that has been examined minimally in the literature in terms of sexual dysfunction is the aging. As one ages, one's general health changes (e.g., menopause), which can be a cause of decreasing sexual appetite or increasing dysfunction (Kingsberg, 2002). Although this population has been identified as a possible high-risk population, there has not been any intervention for treatment tested to date. Sexual dysfunction needs to be assessed by social workers, physicians, and other caregivers working with this population in an attempt to provide the highest quality of life possible.

Indicated Preventive Interventions

Indicated preventive interventions are those targeted to individuals who have detectable signs or symptoms of a disorder. Interventions and treatment programs discussed earlier fit the category of indicated treatment interventions.

As in any area of treatment intervention, theory guides which treatments are used. Weiderman (1998) examines some of the theories behind sex therapy. One of the most popular is systems theory, in which the therapist works to understand the couple or family as a whole (Maddock, 1983, 1990). The couple is viewed as the unit of treatment and the changes that occur must be initiated by both individuals (Wiederman, 1998). Other theories include the psychogenic perspective, which indicates that the past plays a role in one's current state, and the biogenic perspective, which states that physical health and disease have a role in one's current state. A medical model proposes the individual as the unit of treatment rather than the couple or the individual with her or his partner.

The first notable published research on sexual dysfunction appeared in 1956, with an article about the treatment of premature ejaculation (Semans, 1956). The article describes and discusses the success rates of the use of manual stimulation in the male population suffering this dysfunction. A 100% success rate is reported.

In 1970, Masters and Johnson published *Human Sexual Inadequacy.* The book elaborated on the results of their study on different dysfunctions and follow-up relapse results. Individuals (both male and female) participated in a 2-week intensive treatment session. The authors defined success as a reversal of basic symptomatology. Results are broken down by dysfunction: primary impotence (54.4% success; 0% relapse), secondary impotence (73.3% success; 11.1% relapse), premature ejaculation (97.8% success; 1.5% relapse), ejaculatory incompetence (82.4% success; 0% relapse), vaginismus (100% success; relapse not reported), primary inorgasmic (83.4% success; 2.6% relapse), and situational inorgasmic (77.2% success; 5% relapse). The total success rate of their study was 81.1%, with a total relapse rate of 5.1%. This book adds greatly to our knowledge of the authors' development and use of the "pinch and squeeze" method of treatment for males, sexual history assessment tools, and case study examples.

In the 1970s, numerous authors studied and reported on different types of dysfunctions and treatments (Kinder & Blakeney, 1977). Zilbergeld (1975) used the Semans (1956) manual stimulation approach to treatment with the addition of group discussions and information sessions with males experiencing sexual dysfunction but currently without a partner. A 66% success rate was reported. In 1974, Barbach reported a 91.6% success rate after working with preorgasmic females using group discussion and homework consisting of Kegel exercises and masturbation as a treatment program. Kohlenberg combined individual therapy and masturbation as treatment methods and reported a 100% success rate in 1974. Other treatment approaches that have been described are couples therapy (Kaplan, Kohl, Pomeroy, Offit, & Hogan, 1974), weekly therapy sessions in addition to the Masters and Johnson (1970) "pinch and squeeze" treatment (Lansky & Davenport, 1975; Meyer, Schmidt, Lucan, & Smith, 1975), and the Masters and Johnson approach in addition to a workshop (Powell, Blakeney, Croft, & Pulliam, 1974).

LoPiccolo and Stock (1986) discuss treatment interventions for specific sexual dysfunctions. They indicate that primary orgasmic dysfunction is best treated with masturbation training, and relaxation training is an effective way to treat vaginismus. A number of treatments can be used with secondary orgasmic disorder, such as directed masturbation, communication training, sexual techniques training, and individual therapy (Andersen, 1983; Kilmann, 1988; LoPiccolo & Stock, 1986). Also included in this review are treatment options for male sexual dysfunctions such as the use of cognitive-behavioral therapy for treatment of low sexual desire; hormonal treatment or surgery for erectile dysfunction; and physical stimulation, use of vibrators, and participation in role-play (LoPiccolo, 1977) for treatment of premature and inhibited ejaculation.

Studies conducted in the 1990s elaborated on a variety of commonly used interventions in treating sexual dysfunction. Crooks and Baur (1990) designate sex education, communication training, sexual technique training, and systematic desensitization as interventions for treating sexual desire disorders and sexual arousal disorders. Hyposexual desire disorder can be treated with hormonal therapy, sex therapy, and treatment of depression (Trudel, 1991). In relation to this, there may be an increase in the success rates of the female with hyposexual desire disorder with an increase in motivation for success by the male (Hawton, Catalan, & Fagg, 1991). A cognitive approach using self-disclosure is an intervention that has been used with couples (either partner having the problem; L. Russell, 1990). Hulbert (1993) compared groups of people who received a standard intervention of marital and sex therapy with those who received the standard intervention plus orgasm consistency training. Hulbert found that the experimental group experienced more positive results.

In *Sexual Dysfunction,* Lechtenberger and Ohl (1994) discuss such interventions as drug therapy, hormonal therapy, penile implants, intrapenile injections, communication, masturbation and relaxation therapy, hypnotherapy, sex education, and cognitive restructuring.

More recently, pharmacotherapy has been used in the treatment of sexual dysfunction. Rowland and Burnett (2000) report that oral, intraurethral, and intravenous forms of drug therapy are the most successful in the treatment of erectile dysfunction, at rates of 40% to 82%. Premature ejaculation, another common form of dysfunction for males, has been treated effectively with oral, topical, and alpha-blocker medications (50% to 100% success; Rowland & Burnett, 2000). "The current 'gold standard' for clinical trials in male and female sexual dysfunction is the randomized, double-blind, placebo-controlled, parallel group design, with one or more dosages of the specific drug being investigated" (R. C. Rosen, 2002, p. 440). With this in mind, there have been few studies on the use of "vasoactive drugs for the treatment of female sexual dysfunction" (Rosen, 2002, p. 441), thus supporting the notion that the "sexuality of some women [has] been largely ignored" (Bancroft, 2002b; Sanders, Graham, Bass, & Bancroft, 2001).

Treatment has ranged from various therapies to surgeries to, most recently, drug and hormone interventions. Yet, even with the increased availability of medical treatment for sexual dysfunction, there needs to be continued research and advancement of psychological treatments (Heiman, 2002a) to allow for patient choice in interventions. There is a need for "treatments that compare and combine psychological and pharmacological approaches to dysfunctions" (Heiman, 2002b, p. 77). After 30 years of research and treatment of sexual dysfunction, there are still no definite answers regarding the effectiveness of interventions.

FUTURE DIRECTIONS

There are a number of directions in which the research could progress in the area of sexual dysfunction prevention. One is toward greater understanding of the theories most influencing sex therapy (Wiederman, 1998). Another need is continued research on the relationship between child sexual abuse and adult sexual dysfunction (Kinzl, Mangweth, Trawger, & Biebl, 1996; Sarwar et al., 1997). There is also a need for increased education in the general society to eliminate the stigma that prevents many people from seeking treatment. A number of years ago, Kinder and Blakeney (1977) provided a list of research needs that are still pertinent. There is a need for more accurate pretreatment assessment and reporting, data on the process of treatment, more accurate and definitive posttherapy evaluations, a more objective, measurable database, and statistical success rates for specific diagnoses. Research to date indicates mixed results for treatment methods and there is a lack of specificity regarding treatment techniques with the general population that needs to be resolved if we are to be effective in treating people with sexual dysfunctions.

CONCLUSION

"Sexual problems and dysfunctions have been notably under-researched, particularly from the perspective of consequences to individual mental health, relationships, and family functioning" (Heiman, 2002b, p. 73). Considering the number of people experiencing these problems, this is a tragedy in the field of social work, where people expect to find help with their problems. As seen in this review of the literature, McCarthy's question posed in the introduction is still relevant.

REFERENCES

American Psychological Association. (1994). *Diagnostic and statistical manual of mental disorders* (4th ed.). Washington, DC: Author.

American Psychological Association. (1995). Training in and dissemination of empirically-validated psychological treatments: Report and recommendations. *Clinical Psychologist, 48,* 3–24.

Andersen, B. L. (1983). Primary orgasmic dysfunction. *Psychological Bulletin, 43,* 105–136.

Bancroft, J. (2002). The medicalization of female sexual dysfunction: The need for caution. *Archives of Sexual Behavior, 31*(5), 451–455.

Barbach, L. G. (1974). Group treatment of "preorgasmic" women. *Journal of Sex and Marital Therapy, 1,* 139–145.

Barlow, D. H. (1986). Causes of sexual dysfunction: The role of anxiety and cognitive interference. *Journal of Consulting and Clinical Psychology, 54*(2), 140–148.

Beitchman, J. H., Zucker, K. J., Hood, J. E., DaCosta, G. A., Akman, D., & Cassavia, E. (1992). A review of the long term effects of child sexual abuse. *Child Abuse and Neglect, 16,* 101–118.

Bendixen, M., Muus, K. M., & Schei, B. (1994). The impact of child sexual abuse: A study of a random sample of Norwegian students. *Child Abuse and Neglect, 18,* 837–847.

Conte, H. R. (1986). Multivariate assessment of sexual dysfunction. *Journal of Consulting and Clinical Psychology, 42*(2), 149–157.

Crooks, R., & Baur, K. (1990). *Our sexuality* (4th ed.). Redwood City, CA: Benjamin-Cummings.

Dziegielewski, S. F., Resnick, C., Nelson-Gardell, D., & Harrison, D. F. (1998). Treatment of sexual dysfunction: What social workers need to know. *Research on Social Work Practice, 8*(6), 685–697.

Feldman, H. A., Goldstein, I., Hatzichristou, D. G., Krane, R. J., & McKinlay, J. B. (1994). Impotence and its medical and psychosocial correlates: Results of the Massachusetts male aging study. *Journal of Urology, 151,* 54–61.

Feldman, M. P., MacCulloch, M. J., Mellor, V., & Pinschot, J. M. (1966). The application of anticipatory avoidance learning to the treatment of homosexuality: The sexual orientation method. *Behavior Research and Therapy, 4,* 289–299.

Finklehor, D. (1979). *Sexually victimized children.* New York: Free Press.

Finklehor, D., Hotaling, G., Lewis, J. A., & Smith, C. H. (1990). Sexual abuse in a national survey of adult men and women: Prevalence, characteristics, and risk factors. *Child Abuse and Neglect, 14,* 19–28.

Fisher, J. E., Swingen, D. N., & O'Donohue, W. (1997). Behavior interventions of sexual dysfunction in the elderly. *Behavior Therapy, 28*(1), 65–82.

Fromuth, M. E. (1986). The relationship of childhood sexual abuse with later psychological and sexual adjustment in a sample of college women. *Child Abuse and Neglect, 10,* 5–15.

Gordon, R. (1983). An operational classification of disease prevention. *Public Health Reports, 98,* 107–109.

Gordon, R. (1987). An operational classification of disease prevention. In J. A. Steinberg & M. M. Silverman (Eds.), *Preventing mental disorders* (pp. 20–26). Rockville, MD: U.S. Department of Health and Human Services.

Harbison, J. J. M., Graham, P. J., Quinn, J. T., MacAllister, H., & Woodward, R. (1974). A questionnaire measure of sexual interest. *Archives of Sexual Behavior, 3,* 357–366.

Hawton, K., Catalan, J., & Fagg, J. (1991). Low sexual desire: Sex therapy results and prognostic factors. *Behavior Research and Therapy, 29,* 217–224.

Heiman, J. R. (2002a). Psychologic treatments for female sexual dysfunction: Are they effective and do we need them? *Archives of Sexual Behavior, 31*(5), 445–450.

Heiman, J. R. (2002b). Sexual dysfunction: Overview of prevalence, etiological factors, and treatments. *Journal of Sex Research, 39*(1), 73–78.

Hoon, E. F., Hoon, P. W., & Wincze, J. (1976). An inventory of the measurement of female sexual arousability: The SAI. *Archives of Sexual Behavior, 5,* 291–300.

Hulbert, D. F. (1993). A comparative study using orgasm consistency training in the treatment of females reporting hypoactive sexual desire. *Journal of Sex and Marital Therapy, 19,* 41–55.

Kaplan, H. S., Kohl, R. N., Pomeroy, W. B., Offit, A. K., & Hogan, B. (1974). Group treatment of premature ejaculation. *Archives of Sexual Behavior, 3,* 443–452.

Kilmann, P. R. (1988). The treatment of primary and secondary orgasmic dysfunction: A methodological review of the literature since 1970. *Journal of Sex and Marital Therapy, 4,* 155.

Kinder, B. N., & Blakeney, P. (1977). Treatment of sexual dysfunction: A review of outcome studies. *Journal of Clinical Psychology, 33*(2), 523–530.

Kingsberg, S. A. (2002). The impact of aging on sexual function in women and their partners. *Archives of Sexual Behavior, 31*(5), 431–437.

Kinzl, J. F., & Biebl, W. (1992). Long-term effects of incest: Life events triggering mental disorders in female patients with sexual abuse in childhood. *Child Abuse and Neglect, 16,* 567–573.

Kinzl, J. R., Mangweth, B., Trawger, C., & Biebl, W. (1996). Sexual dysfunction in males: Significance of adverse childhood experiences. *Child Abuse and Neglect, 20*(8), 759–766.

Kohlenberg, R. J. (1974). Directed masturbation and the treatment of primary orgasmic dysfunction. *Archives of Sexual Behavior, 3,* 349–356.

Lansky, M. R., & Davenport, A. E. (1975). Difficulties in brief conjoint treatment of sexual dysfunction. *American Journal of Psychiatry, 132,* 177–179.

Laumann, E. O., Paik, A., & Rosen, R. C. (1999). Sexual dysfunction in the United States: Prevalence and predictors. *Journal of the American Medical Association, 281,* 537–544.

Lechtenberger, R., & Ohl, D. A. (1994). *Sexual dysfunction.* Philadelphia: Lea & Febiger.

Leiblum, S. R., & Rosen, R. C. (1995). The changing focus of sex therapy. In R. C. Rosen & S. C. Leiblum (Eds.), *Case studies in sex therapy* (pp. 3–17). New York: Guilford Press.

Lief, H. I. (1981). Self-evaluation of sexual behavior and gratification. In H. I. Lief (Ed.), *Sexual problems in medical practice* (pp. 389–399). Monroe, WI: American Medical Association.

LoPiccolo, J. (1977). Direct treatment of sexual dysfunction in the couple. In J. Money & H. Musaph (Eds.), *Handbook of sexology* (pp. 1214–1227). New York: Elsevier.

LoPiccolo, J. (1994). The evolution of sex therapy. *Journal of Sex and Marital Therapy, 9,* 5–7.

LoPiccolo, J., & Steger, J. (1974). The sexual interaction inventory: A new instrument for assessment of sexual dysfunction. *Archives of Sexual Behavior, 3,* 585–595.

LoPiccolo, J., & Stock, W. E. (1986). Treatment of sexual dysfunction. *Journal of Consulting and Clinical Psychology, 54*(2), 158–167.

Maddock, J. W. (1983). Sex in the family system. *Marriage and Family Review, 6*(3–4), 9–20.

Maddock, J. W. (1990). Promoting healthy family sexuality. *Journal of Family Psychotherapy, 1,* 49–63.

Masters, W. H., & Johnson, V. E. (1970). *Human sexual inadequacy.* Boston: Little, Brown.

McCarthy, B. W. (1995). Learning from unsuccessful sex therapy patients. *Journal of Sex and Marital Therapy, 21,* 31–38.

Meyer, J. K., Schmidt, C. W., Lucan, M. J., & Smith, E. (1975). Short term treatment of sexual problems: Interim report. *American Journal of Psychiatry, 132,* 172–176.

Nadelson, C. C. (2001). *Sexual disorders.* Philadelphia: Chelsea House.

Palace, E. (1995). Modification of dysfunctional patterns of sexual response through automatic arousal and false physiological feedback. *Journal of Consulting and Clinical Psychology, 63,* 604–615.

Powell, L. C., Blakeney, P., Croft, H., & Pulliam, G. P. (1974). Rapid treatment approach to human sexual inadequacy. *American Journal of Obstetrics and Gynecology, 119,* 89–97.

Rosen, E., & Weinstein, E. (1988). Introduction: Sexuality counseling. In E. Weinstein & E. Rosen (Eds.), *Sexuality counseling: Issues and complications* (pp. 1–15). Pacific Grove, CA: Brooks/Cole.

Rosen, R. C. (2002). Sexual function assessment and the role of vasoactive drugs in female sexual dysfunction. *Archives of Sexual Behavior, 31*(50), 439–443.

Rowe, W. S., & Savage, S. (1987). *Sexuality and the developmentally handicapped: A guidebook for health care professionals.* Queenston, Ontario, Canada: Edwin Mellen Press.

Rowland, D. L., & Burnett, A. L. (2000). Pharmacotherapy in the treatment of male sexual dysfunction. *Journal of Sex Research, 37*(3), 226–243.

Russell, D. (1986). *The secret trauma: Incest in the lives of girls and women.* New York: Basic Books.

Russell, L. (1990). Sex and couple therapy: A method of treatment to enhance physical and emotional intimacy. *Journal of Sex and Marital Therapy, 16,* 111–120.

Sanders, S. A., Graham, C. M., Bass, J., & Bancroft, J. (2001). A prospective study of the effects of oral contraceptives on sexuality and well being and their relationship to discontinuation. *Contraception, 64,* 51–58.

Sarwar, D. B., Crawford, L., & Durlak, J. A. (1997). The relationship between childhood sexual abuse and adult male sexual dysfunction. *Child Abuse and Neglect, 21*(7), 649–655.

Semans, J. H. (1956). Premature ejaculation: A new approach. *Southern Medical Journal, 49,* 353–358.

Spector, L., & Carey, M. (1990). Incidence and prevalence of sexual dysfunction: A critical review of the literature. *Archives of Sexual Behavior, 19,* 389–408.

Trudel, G. (1991). Review of psychological factors in low sexual desire. *Sexual and Marital Therapy, 6,* 261–272.

Ussher, J. M. (1993). The construction of female sexual problems: Regulating sex, regulating women. In J. M. Ussher & C. D. Baker (Eds.), *Psychological perspectives in sexual problems: New direction in theory and practice* (pp. 9–40). London: Routledge.

Wiederman, M. W. (1998). The state of theory in sex therapy. *Journal of Sex Research, 35*(1), 88–99.

Zilbergeld, B. (1975). Group treatment of sexual dysfunction in men without partners. *Journal of Sex and Marital Therapy, 1,* 204–214.

PART III

Preventive Interventions for Adult Health Problems

Chapter 8

HYPERTENSION

THOMAS M. VOGT

Although there are many causes of hypertension, some of them still obscure, the effects of high blood pressure on health and illness have been studied extensively in epidemiologic studies and clinical trials with great consistency in results. This research has two clear messages: (1) prevention works and (2) treatment works.

Hypertension is the direct cause of major cardiovascular morbidities. Except in extreme cases, it is painless and silent until it induces congestive heart failure, stroke, kidney failure, or other manifestations of vascular disease. Its negative effects are enhanced in the presence of other major cardiovascular risk factors, such as smoking and hyperlipidemia. Consequently, both the prevention *and* the treatment of high blood pressure can be viewed as preventive measures aimed at reducing vascular morbidity. It is beyond the scope of this chapter to discuss the details of the treatment of hypertension, rather, we address the importance of treatment as a preventive intervention. Details on treatment recommendations can be obtained from the *Seventh Report of the Joint National Committee on Prevention, Detection, Evaluation, and Treatment of High Blood Pressure* (National High Blood Pressure Education Program [NHBPEP], 2003) or on the World Wide Web at http://www.nhlbi.nih.gov/guidelines/hypertension/jncintro.htm.

Blood pressure is measured as the height of a column of mercury (mm Hg) that can be supported by the pressure inside a major artery. The systolic pressure (upper number) is the pressure during the contraction of the heart. The diastolic pressure (lower number) is the pressure during the relaxation phase of the heart. In younger persons, the arteries are elastic and their expansion during heart contraction keeps the systolic pressure lower. As people age, their arteries become calcified and unable to expand as readily. This results in higher systolic blood pressures. The condition of systolic hypertension occurs when the systolic pressure is elevated and the diastolic pressure is normal. Because it results from arterial rigidity, it is increasingly prevalent with advancing age.

High blood pressure is present when pressures are above "normal," usually considered to be > 140/90 mm Hg. Because everyone has periods of high blood pressure (e.g., during exercise or severe emotional distress), hypertension is diagnosed only when high blood pressure is detected on several successive occasions and with proper blood pressure measurement techniques (see the discussion that follows). *Essential hypertension* refers to elevations in both systolic and diastolic pressure that arise from uncertain causes. *Secondary hypertension* refers to elevated blood pressures arising from identified causes such as a pheochromocytoma (a tumor that produces hormones that raise blood pressure) or a blockage of the renal artery.

Before the late 1960s, the term *hypertension* referred only to very high blood pressure levels that conferred a risk of imminent morbidity or death. The notion that asymptomatic levels of blood pressure might be treated arose from epidemiologic studies that showed a linear association between blood pressure and risk of vascular events. The first large, well-designed randomized trial of hypertension therapy for nonemergent blood pressure levels, the Veterans Administration Cooperative Study on Antihypertensive Agents (VA Cooperative Study, 1967, 1970) defined "moderate" hypertension as a diastolic blood pressure of 115 to 129 mm Hg—a pressure that might now be considered a medical emergency. The 1967 trial surprised its investigators by demonstrating reduced mortality within 2 years among those with initial diastolic blood pressures of 115 to 129 mm Hg. Many subsequent trials were aimed at clarifying the levels of blood pressure that required treatment, the parameters for treatment, and the potential for prevention through lifestyle modification. These studies included the Hypertension Detection and Follow-Up Program (HDFP, 1979), the Medical Research Council Trial of Treatment of Mild Hypertension (MRC, 1985), the European Working Party on High Blood Pressure in the Elderly Trial (Amery et al., 1985), and the Systolic Hypertension in the Elderly Program (SHEP, 1991). The HDFP and the MRC showed the effectiveness of therapy on diastolic blood pressures of 90 to 114, and the European Working Party and the SHEP demonstrated the effectiveness of therapy among older persons with isolated systolic hypertension.

In recent years, systolic pressure has been recognized as a better predictor of risk than diastolic pressure, and more recent studies and consensus reports have tended to shift the emphasis from diastolic to systolic pressure, although both are important (e.g., NHBPEP, 2003) and should be treated until goal blood pressures are achieved.

Generally, the higher the blood pressure, the higher the risk, and the more blood pressure is lowered, the lower the morbidity and mortality rates. But there are exceptions to this generalization that have created confusion about the proper goal levels for blood pressure. The Multiple Risk Factor Intervention Trial (MRFIT, 1985) found that patients with electrocardiographic (ECG) abnormalities at entry had an increased risk of death if they were placed on hydrochlorothiazide, at a dose of 100 mg per day. This effect was not present, however, among those with no evidence of myocardial ischemia or among persons who were treated with chlorthalidone or lower doses of hydrochlorothiazide, Warram, Laffel, Valsania, Christlieb, and Krolewski (1991) found that diabetic patients had increased mortality risk when treated with diuretics. The hydrochlorothiazide maximum dose was reduced by half in the 1980s as a consequence of the MRFIT experience, although these findings were not confirmed in randomized trials with a priori hypotheses relating to the negative effects of lower blood pressures. Other studies suggested that, although calcium channel blockers lower blood pressure, they may not produce the health benefits seen with other antihypertensive medications (Held, Usuf, & Furberg, 1989), and, indeed, may be harmful to some patients (Chobanian, 1996). Despite their high cost and concerns about safety, calcium channel blockers still retain a disturbingly large share of the market for first-line antihypertensive therapy.

THE J-CURVE—HOW LOW SHOULD BLOOD PRESSURE GO?

Because the relation of high blood pressure to heart failure and stroke is nearly linear, we probably understand the value of prevention and treatment of high blood pressure better than for any other disease. Antihypertensive therapy is associated with reductions in congestive heart failure of 50%, in stroke of 35% to 40%, and in myocardial infarction of 20% to 25% (Neal, MacMahon, & Chapman, 2000). However, the linear relationship between cardiovascular morbidity and diastolic blood pressure may be attenuated or even reversed at lower levels of diastolic pressure. This phenomenon is termed the "J-curve," and, until recently, its cause was not well understood, but it is an important consideration when deciding how aggressively to treat hypertension. One review of 13 studies concluded that the J-curve was consistently present, but that its shape and the blood pressure level at which it appeared was not consistent (Farnett, Mulrow, Linn, Lucey, & Tuley, 1991). Overall, it appeared that diastolic pressures below 85 mm Hg were associated with higher morbidity rates. This cut-off is considerably higher than most clinicians would apply as a standard of therapy, and some even recommend initiating nonpharmacologic treatment at this level. A study of women in Holland (Witteman et al., 1994) found that 19% of them showed increased calcification of the abdominal aorta over an 8-year follow-up. Among that group, those persons whose diastolic blood pressure declined the most (10 mm Hg or more) had significantly more morbid events than those whose pressure declined less. However, those who had little or no increase in calcifications and also the greatest declines in blood pressure had the fewest morbid events. The authors concluded that the J-curve may result from mixing two different populations. The first is a group in which advancing vessel wall stiffening leads to a mechanical decline in diastolic pressure because the artery loses its elasticity. This is a sign of arterial disease and is associated with increased morbidity. For those with normal elasticity, however, lower diastolic pressure is a positive sign and is associated with fewer events. The prospective, randomized Hypertension Optimal Treatment (HOT) study has confirmed this view (Cruickshank, 2003). The J-curve relationship between blood pressure and cardiovascular/noncardiovascular events is due to reverse causality, where underlying disease (e.g., poor left ventricular function, poor general health, poorly compliant/stiff arteries) is the cause of both the low blood pressure and the increased risk of both cardiovascular and noncardiovascular events. The negative effects of low blood pressure in patients with stiff arteries (wide pulse pressure) may be exacerbated by treatment. For nonischemic hypertensive subjects, the therapeutic lowering of diastolic blood pressure (DBP) to the low 80s mm Hg is beneficial, but it is safe (though unproductive) to go lower. However, in the presence of coronary artery disease (limited coronary flow reserve), there is a J-curve relationship between treated DBP and myocardial infarction, but not for stroke. In such high-risk (for myocardial infarction) cases, it would be prudent to avoid lowering DBP to below the low 80s mm Hg. These findings may explain the anomalous results of the MRFIT (1985) and Warram et al. (1991) studies described earlier.

There are less precise data relating to the effects of changes in diet, weight, and physical activity on blood pressure. However, it is clear that: (1) changes in lifestyle can produce substantial reductions in blood pressure without medication and (2) the changes that benefit blood pressure also reduce risk of diabetes and its complications, atherosclerosis, osteoporosis, cancer, and other diseases.

JOINT NATIONAL COMMITTEE REPORTS

The National Institutes of Health has convened seven sequential expert panels called the Joint National Committee (JNC) on Prevention, Detection, Evaluation, and Treatment of High Blood Pressure. Each panel has produced an updated report and recommendations summarizing the current state of knowledge about high blood pressure. The report of the seventh panel was issued in 2003 (NHBPEP, 2003). It contains current recommendations on prevention, assessment, and treatment.

TRENDS AND INCIDENCE

Between 1960 and 1980, improved understanding about the relationship of high blood pressure to morbid events and the effectiveness of treatment led to changes in the definition of hypertension. Because the definition of hypertension became broader and more inclusive, the shift from *International Classification of Diseases, (ICD-8)* to *ICD-9* created an artificial three- to fourfold rise in the "prevalence" of hypertension (Rothenberg & Aubert, 1990). This rise was based on disease definition and not on any real change. This highlights the problem of examining secular trends in prevalence or incidence of diseases when their very definition evolves over time. Despite this problem, it seems clear that the prevalence of hypertension in the United States declined modestly between the 1960s and 1991. More recent National Health and Nutrition Examination Surveys (NHANES) suggest that the rate has been rising since that time. The 1999 to 2000 survey showed a 3.7% rise in hypertension prevalence compared to 1988 to 1991. Nearly 29% of Americans reported that they had been diagnosed with hypertension (Hajjar & Kotchen, 2003). Hypertension prevalence varies from 14.0% for Arizona to 31.6% for residents of Alabama (MMWR, 2002). From 1991 to 1999, significant increases in self-reported prevalence of hypertension on the Behavioral Risk Factor Surveillance System (BRFSS) survey occurred in 17 states, while only three states showed declines (MMWR, 2002). Selected BRFSS survey results are summarized in Table 8.1. There were declines in the proportion of screened persons 20 to 44 and 45 to 64 years of age, and increases over age 65. Screening declined among non-Hispanic Whites and persons with high school or less education. Self-reported hypertension prevalence is highest among African Americans compared to other ethnic groups, and is higher among men than women and among those with less education.

Blood pressure screening rates are high, but treatment and control leaves something to be desired. Currently, about two-thirds of Americans with hypertension are aware that they have it; but only 58% of those with hypertension are under active treatment (Natarajan & Nietert, 2003), and only 31% of persons with hypertension are appropriately controlled (Hajjar & Kotchen, 2003). These data are little improved from 30 years ago, despite the rising prevalence of the condition, the relatively high rates of screening, and the proliferation of effective drug therapies.

Blood pressure is measured in our health care system with an intensity that borders on obsession. The sixth report of the Joint National Committee (NHBPEP, 1997) recommended screening every 2 years for persons with SBP and DBP below 130 mm Hg and 85 mm Hg, respectively, and more frequent for screening those with blood pressure at higher levels. In one study, however, the

Table 8.1   BRFSS Survey Results on High Blood Pressure (1991–1999)

	Blood Pressure Checked				Told of High Blood Pressure			
Characteristic	1991 (%)	1999 (%)	Percent Change	(95% CI)	1991 (%)	1999 (%)	Percent Change	(95% CI)
Age group (years)								
20–44	94.3	93.0	−1.3	(+0.5)	11.7	12.2	0.5	(+0.6)
45–64	95.7	95.1	−0.6	(+0.5)	30.8	32.7	2.0	(+1.2)
>65	97.2	97.8	0.6	(+0.5)	41.8	48.5	6.7	(+1.5)
Race/ethnicity								
Non-Hispanic White	95.4	94.8	−0.6	(+0.3)	22.2	23.9	1.7	(+0.6)
Non-Hispanic Black	97.0	96.8	−0.2	(+0.8)	31.2	23.9	4.7	(+2.0)
Hispanic	93.2	91.6	−1.6	(+1.7)	21.6	23.1	1.9	(+2.7)
Other	92.6	93.1	0.5	(+1.9)	19.4	23.8	4.4	(+3.6)
Sex								
Male	93.6	92.5	−1.1	(+0.5)	22.2	25.1	2.9	(+0.8)
Female	96.9	96.5	−0.4	(+0.3)	23.2	24.7	1.5	(+0.7)
Education								
<High school	93.0	90.1	−2.9	(+1.3)	27.4	30.4	3.0	(+1.7)
High school/GED	95.0	93.8	−1.1	(+0.6)	23.4	26.1	2.7	(+1.0)
Some college	95.8	95.5	−0.4	(+0.5)	22.3	24.7	2.4	(+1.1)
College graduate	96.1	95.9	−0.2	(+0.5)	19.5	21.5	1.9	(+1.1)

Source: Adapted from "State-Specific Trends in Self-Reported Blood Pressure Screening and High Blood Pressure," 2002, *Morbidity and Mortality Weekly Reports, 51*(21), pp. 456–460; adjusted to U.S. 2000 Standard population.

average adult HMO member with no history of hypertension or cardiovascular disease, had 13 medical office blood pressure determinations over a 5-year period, or 2.6 pressures per year (Vogt & Stevens, 2003). This number does not include screening blood pressures taken elsewhere (e.g., dentist's office, blood bank). Given the plethora of blood pressures taken, why are adequate treatment and control achieved so infrequently? Except in extreme cases, hypertension produces no symptoms. Consequently, it does not provide much motivation for prescribing or for accepting treatment.

RISK FACTORS

Hypertension is a disease of modern society. Hunter-gatherer tribes rarely exhibit hypertension. Contrary to popular assumption, the "stress" of modern life is not the primary cause of hypertension. The role of stress in causing hypertension remains unclear, despite a large number of often contradictory studies on the subject (e.g., Beilin, Puddey, & Burke, 1999; Patel et al., 1985; Whelton, He, et al., 1997). But the roles of obesity, sedentary lifestyle, and poor diet are clear and important. Prevention and treatment of hypertension absolutely requires attention to lifestyle. Despite common, often annoying, side effects, the many effective drugs available to lower blood pressure have tended to deemphasize the potential for the individual with elevated blood pressure to manage the condition by modifying lifestyle. Mild hypertension can be effectively managed with lifestyle changes, and management of moderate to severe hypertension is enhanced by lifestyle change. Further, the lifestyle changes that control blood pressure also benefit general health and many other disease risks. Table 8.2 summarizes the JNC7 recommendations for preventive measures.

Weight/BMI

There is a direct relationship between body mass index (BMI) and blood pressure, even within the normal range (Hardy, Kuh, Langenberg, & Wadsworth, 2003; He, Whelton, Appel, Charleston, & Klag, 2000; Trials of Hypertension Prevention [TOHP], 1997). The heavier the individual, the higher the blood

Table 8.2   Preventing the Consequences of Hypertension

Modification	Recommendations	Approximate SBP Reduction (Range)
Weight reduction	Maintain BMI 18.5–24.9 kg/m^2 weight loss	5–20 mm Hg per 10 kg weight loss
DASH diet	Diet rich in fruits, vegetables, lowfat dairy products, and reduced saturated and total fat	8–14 mm Hg
Dietary sodium reduction	Limit sodium to 100 mmol per day (2.4g sodium or 6g salt)	2–8 mm Hg
Physical activity	Regular aerobic physical activity (e.g., brisk walking) at least 30 minutes per day, most days	4–9 mm Hg
Moderation of alcohol use	Limit to two drinks (1 oz. ethanol, 24 oz. beer, 10 oz. wine, 3 oz. 80-proof liquor) per day, less in small persons	2–4 mm Hg

Source: Adapted from Table 5 of "The Seventh Report of the Joint National Committee on Prevention, Detection, Evaluation, and Treatment of High Blood Pressure," by National High Blood Pressure Education Program, 2003, Rockville, MD: U.S. Department of Health and Human Services.

pressure. Nevertheless, some thin people have hypertension, while some obese people have normal blood pressures. Regardless of the initial blood pressure and weight, however, weight loss will lead to a blood pressure decline that is proportional to the amount of weight loss.

Diet

The role of diet in determining blood pressure has been extensively studied. Vegetarians have lower blood pressures than nonvegetarians (Anholm, 1974; Armstrong et al., 1979; Armstrong, Van Merwyk, & Coates, 1977; Haines, Chakabarti, Fisher, & Meade, 1980; Rouse, Beilin, Armstrong, & Vandongen, 1983; Sacks, Rosner, & Kass, 1974). Randomized trials have confirmed that this relationship is causal (Margetts, Beilin, Vandongen, & Armstrong, 1986; Rouse et al., 1983), but have not defined the responsible nutrients.

Many micronutrients are involved with blood pressure regulation and are associated in epidemiologic studies with lower blood pressure. These include calcium, magnesium, and potassium (Allender et al., 1996; Cappuccio & MacGregor, 1991; Simpson, 1985; Whelton, Kumanyika, et al., 1997). Macronutrients may also affect blood pressure, including omega three fatty acids (Knapp & FitzGerald, 1989), other forms of dietary fat (Iacono, Dougherty, & Puska, 1990), and protein (Elliott, 2003). Many studies have examined the effects of giving supplements of macro- and micronutrients on blood pressure and the results have been mixed at best (Aro et al., 1998; Plum-Wirell, Stegmayr, & Wester, 1994; Simpson, 1985; Whelton, Kumanyika, et al., 1997; Yamamoto et al., 1995). The cited studies are a small representation of many that were consistent only in their inconsistency. The Trials of Hypertension Prevention (TOHP), Phase I (Whelton, Kumanyika, et al., 1997) was designed to settle these contradictions by comparing the effects on blood pressure of weight loss, sodium reduction, stress management, and supplements of potassium, calcium, magnesium, and fish oil using an identical randomized study design for each intervention (Whelton, Kumanyika, et al., 1997). Weight reduction produced the most blood pressure decline; sodium restriction produced a lesser amount, and the others had no significant effects. The stress management arm of TOHP, however, tested a very brief and limited form of stress management training that was much less intensive than the successful yoga approach of Patel et al. (1985). Additional well-designed areas in stress management are needed to determine if these approaches can be reliably used to reduce blood pressure.

The TOHP's failure to show any impact from micronutrient supplements is more difficult to explain in light of the physiological evidence that these nutrients are involved in blood pressure regulations and the epidemiological evidence that consumption of diets rich in fish oil, magnesium, potassium, and calcium is associated with lower blood pressures. However, nutrients interact with one another, and single supplements may not provide a fair test of their effects on blood pressure (Beilin, 1994; McCarron, 1987). The TOHP study found no effects of supplements of potassium, magnesium, calcium, or omega-3 fatty acid on blood pressure using a common study design that did show effects for weight reduction and sodium reduction. These results led directly to the design of a study that used the epidemiological and physiological data to design what appeared to be an optimal diet. There was considerable resistance to combining multiple nutrients into a single diet on the grounds that, if the study worked, it would not be possible to tell which nutrients were responsible. On the other hand, single supplement studies had produced inconsistent results, and it is just possible that all of them, in combination, are necessary. The Dietary Approaches to Stop Hypertension (DASH) study developed a diet with many of the characteristics of vegetarian diets, but it included meat, allowed alcohol in limited quantities, and was designed to be palatable and acceptable to the general public (Appel et al., 1997; Vogt et al., 1999). The DASH diet emphasized high consumption (8 to 10 servings per day) of fruits and vegetables (high in potassium, magnesium, and related, but unspecified, nutrients), high consumption of nonfat dairy products (for calcium and protein), and a low-fat intake. This diet was about as effective as a first line antihypertensive monotherapy in reducing blood pressure. A follow-up study, DASH 2, combined the DASH diet with sodium restriction and achieved greater blood pressure reduction (Sacks et al., 2001). The DASH diet also nearly doubled the blood pressure reduction from losartan therapy in a related study (Conlin et al., 2003), and the effect was greater for African Americans than for Whites.

In the DASH study, subjects were provided all of their food. The question remained as to whether people could follow the diet successfully on their own. The Premier trial (Premier, 2003) confirmed that the DASH diet could enhance the affect of aggressive intervention aimed at weight, activity, sodium, and alcohol, but only modestly. The impact of weight reduction is more dramatic than that of all other lifestyle approaches.

The TOHP and DASH studies helped to define the ideal diet for hypertension, but this diet is also perfectly congruent with recommendations for prevention of heart disease, cancer, and osteoporosis. In other words, it appears to be optimal for human nutrition.

Alcohol Intake

Alcohol intake is consistently related to blood pressure (Fortmann, Haskell, Vranizan, Brown, & Farquhar, 1983; Henriksson et al., 2003; Klatsky, Friedman, Siegelaub, & Gerard, 1977; Saunders, 1987) and to hemorrhagic stroke

(Diaz, Cumsille, & Bevilacqua, 2003). This relationship appears to be relatively linear and, at high levels of consumption, alcohol is an important cause of hypertension and its consequent morbidities. Hypertensive patients should be asked about their alcohol intake and advised to reduce it to one drink per day or less (Saunders, 1987).

Dietary Sodium Intake

There is an enormous literature on sodium intake and blood pressure. Sodium restriction was first suggested in Chinese medicine around 2300 BC (Veith, 1966). Extreme sodium restriction was the first therapy available for life-threatening malignant hypertension. The salt hypothesis asserts that salt is a necessary, but insufficient, etiologic factor for essential hypertension (Joossens & Geboers, 1983). There is so much literature on this topic, and so much controversy associated with that literature, that it is difficult to summarize, although many articles have attempted to provide an overview of that literature (Cutler et al., 1997; Grobbee & Hoffman, 1986; Joossens & Geboers, 1983; Midgley et al., 1996; Pickering, 2002; Weinsier, 1976). Inconsistencies in study findings led to the hypothesis that some persons are "salt-sensitive" while others are much less so (Fujita et al., 1980; Kurtz et al., 1987). The salt industry has strongly argued against the salt hypothesis and the controversy has, at times, become very heated (Taubes, 1998). The National Heart, Lung and Blood Institute has argued strongly and consistently in favor of reducing the nation's salt intake (Cutler et al., 1997). Well-designed studies suggest that dietary sodium reduction can lower blood pressure (Sacks et al., 2001; TOHP, 1997), although the effect is modest and is not limited to a subset of "salt responders" (Obarzanek et al., 2003). The Trials of Hypertension Prevention I (Whelton, Kumanyika, et al., 1997; Yamamoto et al., 1995) clarified the relative impact of seven nonpharmacologic interventions on blood pressure among persons with high normal blood pressure. Weight reduction was most effective; sodium reduction was modestly effective; the other five interventions were not effective.

Physical Activity

Regular aerobic exercise can produce mean reductions in blood pressure of 4 to 9 mm Hg. A meta-analysis of 54 randomized trials confirmed that this effect is independent of body mass or whether or not the individual is hypertensive (Whelton et al., 2002). Another meta-analysis of progressive resistance exercise also showed consistent blood pressure reductions (Kelley & Kelley, 2000). Although physical activity appears to have a direct benefit on blood pressure, its primary value in sustaining lower pressure is that physical activity appears to be essential to maintaining achieved weight loss (Ewbank, Darga, & Lucas, 1995; Glasgow et al., 1997; Stevens et al., 2001; Vogt & Stevens, 2003). Because it has both direct and indirect effects on blood pressure, physical activity is an essential feature of lifestyle programs aimed at preventing hypertension. Clinically significant declines in blood pressure occur with relatively modest increases in physical activity above sedentary levels (Ishikawa-Takata, 2003).

The risk factors discussed (weight/BMI, diet, alcohol intake, sodium intake, physical activity) relate to personal behaviors. The health care system also exhibits behaviors that are associated with failures to diagnose and/or treat hypertension adequately. These system behaviors are analogous to personal lifestyle behaviors in that they represent enculturated ways of operating that produce enhanced disease risk. Changing organizational behaviors is at least as difficult as changing personal ones. The very fact that discussions of risk factors rarely address institutional behaviors illustrates the fact the where a problem is not recognized, it is unlikely to be corrected.

Poor Blood Pressure Assessment

There is a major contrast between the attention clinical laboratories give to reducing measurement error of blood tests and the almost complete lack of attention in clinical settings to proper blood pressure assessment. Blood pressure changes as conditions change. Generally, people have higher blood pressures during the day when they are active than at night when they are sleeping. Because blood pressure is affected by emotional state and by way it is measured, it is sometimes difficult to determine the true "normal" blood pressure for an individual. Some people are nervous in the doctor's office and have higher blood pressure there than when they are at home ("white coat" hypertension). Medical office blood pressures, often taken in haste, can result in pressures that are higher or lower than the true level and may lead to unnecessary treatment or to failure to prescribe needed treatment. The JNC reports (e.g., NHBPEP, 2003) describe careful procedures for taking an accurate blood pressure—procedures that are rarely used in real clinical settings. Yet, those same settings have defined poorly taken blood pressures as a "vital sign," assuming that a large quantity of bad data are more valuable than a lesser amount of good information. The JNC recommends blood pressure screening once every 2 years (NHBPEP, 1997). In one study of a large HMO, the average adult health plan member (excluding those with hypertension or other conditions requiring blood pressure monitoring) received 13 blood pressures screenings over a 5-year period, or one every 4.65 months (Vogt & Stevens, 2003). This is more than five times the recommended frequency. In addition to the poor treatment decisions that sloppy blood pressure measurements produce, frequent measurements can be costly. If blood pressure screening on healthy people was done biennially as recommended by the JNC6 report, not only would the quality of care improve, but it has been estimated that the costs of care would be reduced by approximately $7.66 (1996 dollars) per person per year (Vogt & Aickin, 2001). Nationally, the savings could approach two billion dollars per year. Why is this important? The most common argument for not using JNC standards is that health systems lack the resources to do it. Improper assessment of blood pressure is a risk factor for preventing the consequences of hypertension because it leads to incorrect diagnoses and treatments, and also because it wastes resources that could be used to improve screening, diagnosis, and treatment.

Correct diagnosis of hypertension requires multiple measurements taken after a brief resting period in a quiet location while *slowly* deflating the blood pressure cuff. These pressures should be taken on at least three different occasions to be certain that sustained high blood pressure is present. If hypertension is present, treatment is important and will clearly reduce risk of premature death and disability.

Self-Measurement

Many people now have their own blood pressure devices and take their pressure at home. This practice can improve blood pressure control among persons with hypertension and reduce their frequency of outpatient visits *if* the pressures are taken correctly and are reported regularly to the clinician (Soghikian et al., 1992). This requires both training of the individual in proper blood pressure procedures and a system for reporting the results back to the clinician. Neither of these is present in most settings.

Lifestyle Advice and Counseling

More than 60 randomized trials have shown that physician assessment and counseling substantially raises long-term smoking cessation rates among patients (Hollis, Lichtenstein, Mount, Vogt, & Stevens, 1993; Kottke, Battista, DeFriese, & Brekke, 1988; Smoking Cessation Clinical Practice Guideline Panel & Staff, 1996). Although many fewer studies have been conducted in other areas of lifestyle interventions, studies suggest that advice and counseling from physicians also has strong impact when it addresses diet (Neil et al., 1995; Ockene et al., 1995) and exercise (Calfas et al., 1997; Long et al., 1996; Marcus, Bock, & Pinto, 1997; Weisemann, Metz, Nuessel, Scheidt, & Scheuermann, 1997). Most behavioral interventions are characterized by a short-term period of success followed by relapse (e.g., Beresford et al., 1997; Kottke et al., 1988). Most programs that support lifestyle changes are short term and focus on the initial period of change. Long-term maintenance of changes, however, is the real challenge. There is a growing body of evidence that chronic disease management models improve the long-term success of lifestyle change (Bodenheimer, Wagner, & Grumback, 2002; Perri et al., 1983; Vogt & Stevens, 2003).

Table 8.3 summarizes the reasons that counseling on lifestyle fails in the medical care system. If we did surgery with the same level of interest, funding, and quality control that we apply to lifestyle counseling in medicine, we would not do it aseptically even though the medical journals were filled with data on the benefits of the germ-free operating room. Office-based tobacco interventions are more cost effective in saving life than any activity that can occur in the medical care office except immunization (Vogt et al., 1998). Despite a literature supporting the effectiveness of medical office behavioral counseling, despite overwhelming evidence that the leading causes of death and disability are diseases that are preventable with lifestyle change, health care systems regard intervention programs that address lifestyle issues largely as public relations programs rather than medical care. Health systems are not accountable for applying state-of-the-art methods; they often do not use trained and dedicated staff; quality of outcomes is not assessed and corrected when it declines; accreditation does not require such programs; failure to offer them confers no legal liability; and funding is often woefully inadequate.

Since the prevention of hypertension (and many other diseases) requires lifestyle change, the failure of health care systems to treat lifestyle interventions

Table 8.3   Health System Actions for Preventing the Consequences of Hypertension

Blood pressure assessment	Use JNC7 methods; 5 minutes quiet sitting in chair, feet on floor, arm at heart level, proper cuff size; minute two measures, SBP = 1st Kortokoof sound, DBP = 5th Korotkoff sound
Accurate devices	Conduct periodic checks of blood pressure device accuracy; correct inaccurate devices
Screen at proper intervals	Once every 2 years for general public; more often for those with hypertension, elevated BP, or high cardiovascular risk
Lifestyle risk assessment and counseling	Assess, counsel, and follow-up on weight, diet, physical activity, and alcohol intake as they relate to controlling blood pressure; provide state-of-the-art interventions
Treat hypertension	Prescribe therapy, including lifestyle interventions, and appropriate medication to assure blood pressure remains below 140/90 mm Hg

as "real" medicine, is an important barrier to the prevention of hypertension and its consequences. The public depends on advice from experts on how to stay well. When the advice is inadequate, at least some of the responsibility for the consequences falls on the advisors.

EFFECTIVE UNIVERSAL PREVENTIVE INTERVENTIONS

General preventive measures for hypertension that individuals can apply are summarized in Tables 8.2 and 8.3. These measures are straightforward. Individuals should maintain a reasonable weight, be physically active, eat a diet rich in fruits and vegetables, low in fat, and high in calcium (the DASH diet), and they should avoid excessive alcohol consumption. Healthy adults should have their blood pressure assessed every 2 years. The good news is that these measures will also provide protection against heart disease, diabetes, osteoporosis, and other conditions. The bad news is that lifestyle change isn't easy.

Because most health care systems don't support these measures very effectively, Table 8.3 also suggests the practices that health systems should adopt in order to improve the prevention of hypertension and reduce the consequences of sustained high blood pressure. Medical offices should adopt JNC7 standards for blood pressure assessment and abandon the senseless standard practice of frequent hasty and inaccurate blood pressure assessment. Sphygmomanometers are not always accurate. They need occasional quality control adjustments. Standard procedures for quality control checks should be implemented in all health care settings. Health systems should also integrate the tasks of lifestyle assessment and counseling into their standards of care. This means that, like other medical practices, the services should meet the standards of medical guidelines, the personnel should be appropriately trained, and the programs are accountable for their results.

EFFECTIVE, SELECTIVE, AND INDICATED PREVENTIVE INTERVENTIONS

High Risk Individuals

People with the high risk conditions shown in Table 8.4 have an increased risk for developing hypertension and/or for suffering morbid events as a result of their blood pressure. For example, cigarette smoking does not appear to cause hypertension, but persons with hypertension who smoke are more likely to suffer vascular events for other reasons. Consequently, smoking is a factor in

**Table 8.4   Risk Factors for Complications of Hypertension:
Indications for Increased Screening Frequency**

Hypertension
Cigarette smoking
Obesity (BMI $\geq$ 30 kg/m^2)
Physical inactivity
Dyslipidemia
Diabetes
Microalbuminuria or estimated GFR <60 mL/min
Age: males >55; females >65
Family history of early cardiovascular disease (male <55; female <65)
Existing target organ damage:
    Left ventricular hypertrophy
    Angina or prior myocardial infarction
    Prior coronary revascularization
    Heart failure
    Stroke or transient ischemic attack
    Chronic kidney disease
    Peripheral arterial disease
    Retinopathy

Source: Adapted from Express Report, Table 3, p. 6; "The Seventh Report of the Joint National Committee on Prevention, Detection, Evaluation, and Treatment of High Blood Pressure," by National High Blood Pressure Education Program, 2003, Rockville, MD: U.S. Department of Health and Human Services.

identifying high risk groups. Persons with high risk conditions should have more frequent blood pressure screening, although the JNC7 report does specify intervals. The appropriate interval depends on the mix of blood pressure and risk factors in each individual, but certainly screening in these groups should be at least annual. And, when elevated pressures are found, it is even more important to respond with aggressive interventions to normalize pressure.

Borderline High Blood Pressure

Persons with borderline high blood pressure (130 to 139 mm Hg/80 to 89 mm Hg) should be monitored more frequently and also receive lifestyle counseling to delay or prevent the onset of hypertension.

Hypertension

Persons with Stage 1 hypertension (140 to 159 mm Hg/90 to 99 mm Hg) should receive lifestyle interventions plus medication (primarily diuretics, beta blockers, or ace inhibitors) if blood pressure is not controlled within a few months on lifestyle management alone. Stage 2 hypertension (> 160 mm Hg ≠ > 100 mm Hg) should receive two-dose drug combinations. Other persons may have compelling indications for other therapies as described in JNC7 (NHBPEP, 2003). Active and aggressive efforts are needed to achieve and sustain goal blood pressures.

PRACTICE AND POLICY IMPLICATIONS

Blood pressure assessment is rampant. Quality control of blood pressure assessment is rare. Blood pressure control among those with hypertension is often inadequate. State-of-the-art lifestyle counseling in health care systems is uncommon and is not a standard of care. These few sentences define the practice and policy changes needed to improve blood pressure control. Screening rates are as high as they can be, and exhortations to screen more cannot address the causes of our failure to adequately prevent the consequences of high blood pressure. The major actions needed relate, rather, to changes, not only in process, but in culture of health care systems.

Blood Pressure Assessment

The U.S. medical culture views blood pressure as a *vital sign* (that is, we need to take it every time we encounter a patient), but the accuracy of the blood pressure is regarded as irrelevant, and there is a wide-spread perspective that clinical personnel don't have the time to do it properly. Although proper blood pressure assessment techniques were developed for clinical trials more than 30 years ago, health providers have never been held accountable for applying these standards, and clinical blood pressure techniques have hardly changed in 50 years. We have digital devices and ambulatory devices, but, like mercury sphygmomanometers, they are rarely checked for accuracy, incorrect cuff sizes are frequently used, and the technique is nearly always hasty and inaccurate.

Lifestyle Interventions

Health systems must become accountable for delivering lifestyle interventions that address diet, smoking, and physical activity according to standard guidelines. The Diabetes Prevention Study (Tuomilehto et al., 2001) and the Diabetes Prevention Program (Knowler et al., 2002) have clearly demonstrated that lifestyle interventions are effective—indeed, more effective than medication—in reducing the incidence of diabetes among those at high risk. The DASH study (Appel et al., 1997) has demonstrated the same thing for hypertension. These are only three examples of a rich and growing literature. Well-designed lifestyle interventions based in the medical setting and using state-of-the-art methods do lead to behavior change (Vogt & Stevens, 2003; Vogt et al., 1998). Effective prevention of the consequences of hypertension and many other conditions requires a fundamental cultural change so that advice and counseling about lifestyle are viewed as legitimate, integral components of medical care that are accountable both in delivery and outcomes.

FUTURE DIRECTIONS

We already have a plethora of effective medications for treating hypertension, most of them generic and inexpensive. However, we lack effective preventive interventions that are integrated into routine clinical care. Hypertension is largely a preventable disease as are the strokes, myocardial infarctions, and heart and renal failures that result from it. The provision of effective preventive services requires that the quality of those services becomes a subject of attention to a much greater degree than it has been up to this time. The proliferation of computerized medical records systems will permit the assessment of the frequency and content of lifestyle interventions without expensive chart reviews and will also provide the capacity for reminding the clinician about services required by the patient (Vogt et al., 2003). Research is currently underway on ways to use these computerized medical records to improve the quality of preventive care and of treatment. More research and more clinical attention are needed to improve compliance to treatment regimens. We need systematic attention to defining and ameliorating the barriers to acceptance and adherence to therapy.

Ultimately, the changes that are needed are primarily cultural rather than technological. Hypertension is easy to detect and responds readily to prevention and to treatment. The problems relate to sloppy assessment and low compliance, which, in turn, require different approaches to care. Until health care systems become accountable for the delivery of preventive care in the same way that they are accountable for the delivery of medical treatment, we will continue to have a health care system that is wasteful of resources and not very effective at preventing unnecessary morbidity and mortality.

REFERENCES

Allender, P. S., Cutler, J. A., Gollmann, D., Cappuccio, F. P., Pryer, J., & Elliott, P. (1996). Dietary calcium and blood pressure: A meta-analysis of randomized trials. *Annals of Internal Medicine, 124,* 825–831.

Amery, A., Birkenhager, W., Brixko, P., Bulpitt, C., Clement, D., Deruyttere, M., et al. (1985, June 15). Mortality and morbidity results from the European Working Party on high blood pressure in the elderly trial. *Lancet, 15,* 1349–1370.

Anholm, A. C. (1974). The relationship of a vegetarian diet and blood pressure. *Preventive Medicine, 4,* 35.

Appel, L. J., Moore, T. J., Obarzanek, E., Vollmer, W. M., Svetkey, L. P., Sacks, F. M., et al. (1997). A clinical trial of the effects of dietary patterns on blood pressure. *New England Journal of Medicine, 336,* 1117–1124.

Armstrong, B., Clarke, H., Martin, C., Ward, W., Norman, N., & Masarei, J. (1979). Urinary sodium and blood pressure in vegetarians. *American Journal of Clinical Nutrition, 32,* 2472–2476.

Armstrong, B., Van Merwyk, A. J., & Coates, H. (1977). Blood pressure in Seventh-day Adventis vegetarians. *American Journal of Epidemiology, 105,* 444–449.

Aro, A., Pietinen, P. K., Valsta, L. M., Salminen, I., Turpeinen, A. M., Virtanen, M., et al. (1998). Lack of effect on blood pressure by low fat diets with different fatty acid compositions. *Journal of Human Hypertension, 12,* 383–389.

Beilin, L. J. (1994). Vegetarian and other complex diets, fats, fiber, and hypertension. *American Journal of Clinical Nutrition, 59,* 1130S–1135S.

Beilin, L. J., Puddey, I. B., & Burke, V. (1999). Lifestyle and hypertension. *American Journal of Hypertension, 12*(9, Pt. 1), 934–945.

Beresford, S. A., Curry, S. J., Kristal, A. R., Lazovich, D. A., Feng, Z., & Wagner, E. (1997). A dietary intervention in primary care practice: The eating patterns study. *American Journal of Public Health, 87,* 610–616.

Bodenheimer, T., Wagner, E. H., & Grumback, K. (2002). Improving primary care for patients with chronic illness: The chronic care model, Part 2. *Journal of the American Medical Association, 288,* 1909–1914.

Calfas, K. J., Long, B. J., Sallis, J. F., Wooten, W. J., Pratt, M., & Patrick, K. (1997). A controlled trial of physician counseling to promote the adoption of physical activity. *Preventive Medicine, 25,* 225–233.

Cappuccio, F. P., & MacGregor, G. A. (1991). Does potassium supplementation lower blood pressure? A meta-analysis of published trials. *Journal of Hypertension, 9,* 465–473.

Chobanian, A. V. (1996). Calcium channel blockers: Lessons learned from the MIDAS and other clinical trials. *Journal of the American Medical Association, 276,* 829–830.

Conlin, P. R., Erlinger, T. P., Bohannon, A., Miller, E. R., III, Appel, L. J., Svetkey, L. P., et al. (2003). The DASH diet enhances the blood pressure response to losartan in hypertensive patients. *American Journal of Hypertension, 16*(5, Pt. 1), 337–342.

Cruickshank, C. (2003). The J-curve in hypertension. *Current Cardiology Reports, 5*(6), 441–452.

Cutler, J. A., Follmann, D., & Allender, P. S. (1997). Randomized trials of sodium restriction: An overview. *American Journal of Clinical Nutrition, 65*(2 Suppl.), S643–S651.

Diaz, V., Cumsille, M. A., & Bevilacqua, J. A. (2003). Alcohol and hemorrhagic stroke in Santiago, Chile: A case-control study. *Neuroepidemiology, 22,* 339–344.

Elliott, P. (2003). Protein intake and blood pressure in cardiovascular disease. *The Proceedings of the Nutrition Society, 62,* 495–504.

Ewbank, P. P., Darga, L. L., & Lucas, C. P. (1995). Physical activity as a predictor of weight maintenance in previously obese subjects. *Obesity Research, 3,* 257–263.

Farnett, L., Mulrow, C. D., Linn, W. D., Lucey, C. R., & Tuley, M. R. (1991). The J-curve phenomenon and the treatment of hypertension. Is there a point beyond which pressure reduction is dangerous? *Journal of the American Medical Association, 265,* 489–495.

Fortmann, S. P., Haskell, W. L., Vranizan, K., Brown, B. W., & Farquhar, J. W. (1983). The association of blood pressure and dietary alcohol: Differences by age, sex, and estrogen use. *American Journal of Epidemiology, 118,* 497–507.

Fujita, T., Henry, W. L., Bartter, F. C., Lake, C. R., & Delea, C. S. (1980). Factors influencing blood pressure in salt-sensitive patients with hypertenions. *American Journal of Medicine, 69,* 334–344.

Glasgow, R. E., La Chance, P. A., Toobert, D. J., Brown, J., Hampson, S. E., & Riddle, M. C. (1997). Long-term effects and costs of brief behavioral dietary intervention for patients with diabetes delivered from the medical office. *Patient Education and Counseling, 32,* 175–184.

Grobbee, D. E., & Hofman, A. (1986). Does sodium restriction lower blood pressure? *British Medical Journal, 293,* 27–29.

Haines, A. P., Chakabarti, R., Fisher, D., Meade, T. W., North, W. R. S., & Stirling, Y. (1980). Haemosstatic variables in vegetarians and non-vegetarians. *Thrombosis Research, 19,* 139–148.

Hajjar, I., & Kotchen, T. (2003). Regional variations of blood pressure in the United States are associated with regional variations in dietary intakes: The NHANES-III data. *Journal of Nutrition, 133,* 211–214.

Hardy, R., Kuh, D., Langenberg, C., & Wadsworth, M. E. (2003). Birthweight, childhood social class, and change in adult blood pressure in the 1946 British birth cohort. *Lancet, 362,* 1178–1183.

He, J., Whelton, P. K., Appel, L. J., Charleston, J., & Klag, M. J. (2000). Long-term effects of weight loss and dietary sodium reduction on incidence of hypertension. *Hypertension, 35,* 544–549.

Held, P. H., Usuf, S., & Furberg, C. D. (1989). Calcium channel blockers in acute myocardial infarction and unstable angina: An overview. *British Medical Journal, 299,* 1187–1199.

Henriksson, K. M., Lindblad, U., Gullberg, B., Agren, B., Nilsson-Ehle, P., & Rastam, L. (2003). Body composition, ethnicity, and alcohol consumption as determinants for the development of blood pressure in a birth cohort of young middle-aged men. *European Journal of Epidemiology, 18,* 955–963.

Hollis, J. F., Lichtenstein, E., Mount, K., Vogt, T. M., & Stevens, V. J. (1993). Nurse-assisted counseling for smokers in primary care. *Annals of Internal Medicine, 118,* 521–525.

Hypertenion Detection and Follow-Up Program. (1979). Five-year findings of the hypertension detection and follow-up program. I: Reduction in mortality of persons with high blood pressure, including mild hypertension. Hypertension Detection and Follow-Up Program Cooperative Group. *Journal of the American Medical Association, 242,* 2562–2571.

Iacono, J. M., Dougherty, R. M., & Puska, P. (1990). Dietary fat and blood pressure in humans. *Klinische Wochenschrift, 68*(S20), 23–32.

Ishikawa-Takata, K., Ohta, T., & Tanaka, H. (2003). How much exercise is required to reduce blood pressure in essential hypertensives: A dose-response study. *American Journal of Hypertension, 16,* 629–633.

Joossens, J. V., & Geboers, J. (1983). Salt and hypertension. *Preventive Medicine, 12,* 53–59.

Kelley, G. A., & Kelley, K. S. (2000). Progressive resistance exercise and resting blood pressure: A meta-analysis of randomized controlled trials. *Hypertension, 35,* 838–843.

Klatsky, A. L., Friedman, G. D., Siegelaub, A. B., & Gerard, M. J. (1977). Alcohol consumption and blood pressure: Kaiser-Permanente multiphasic health examination data. *New England Journal of Medicine, 296,* 1194–1200.

Knapp, H. R., & FitzGerald, G. A. (1989). The antihypertensive effects of fish oil: A controlled study of polyunsaturated fatty acid supplements in essential hypertension. *New England Journal of Medicine, 320,* 1037–1043.

Knowler, W. C., Barrett-Connor, E., Fowler, S. E., Hamman, R. F., Lachin, J. M., Walker, E. A., et al. (2002). Reduction in the incidence of type 2 diabetes with lifestyle intervention or metformin. *New England Journal of Medicine, 346,* 393–403.

Kottke, T. E., Battista, R. N., DeFriese, G. H., & Brekke, M. L. (1988). Attributes of successful smoking interventions in medical practice: A meta-analysis of 39 controlled trials. *Journal of the American Medical Association, 259,* 2883–2889.

Kurtz, T. W., Al-Bander, H. A., & Morris, R. C., Jr. (1987). "Salt-sensitive" essential hypertension in men: Is the sodium ion alone important? *New England Journal of Medicine, 317,* 1043–1048.

Long, B. J., Calfas, K. J., Wooten, W., Sallif, J. F., Patrick, K., Goldstein, M., et al. (1996). A multisite field test of the acceptability of physical activity counseling in primary care: Project PACE. *American Journal of Public Health, 12,* 73–81.

Marcus, B. H., Bock, B. C., & Pinto, B. M. (1997). Initiation and maintenance of exercise behavior. In D. Gochman (Ed.), *Handbook of Health Behavior Research II. Provider Determinants* (pp. 353–377). New York: Plenum Press.

Margetts, B. M., Beilin, L. J., Vandongen, R., & Armstrong, B. K. (1986). Vegetarian diet in mild hypertension: A randomised controlled trial. *British Medical Journal, 293,* 1468–1471.

McCarron, D. A. (1987). The calcium deficiency hypothesis of hypertension. *Annal of Internal Medincine, 107,* 919–922.

Medical Research Council Working Party. (1985). MRC trial of treatment of mild hypertension: Principal results. *British Medical Journal, 291,* 97–104.

Midgley, J. P., Matthew, G., Greenwood, C. M. T., & Logan, A. (1996). Effect of reduced dietary sodium on blood pressure. *Journal of the American Medical Association, 275,* 1590–1597.

Morbidity and Mortality Weekly Reports. (2002). State-specific trends in self-reported blood pressure screening and high blood pressure: United States 1991–1999. *Morbidity and Mortality Weekly Report, 52,* 456–460.

Multiple Risk Factor Intervention Trial Research Group. (1985). Baseline rest electrocardiographic abnormalities, antihypertensive treatment, and mortality in the Multiple Risk Factor Intervention Trial. *American Journal of Cardiology, 55,* 1–15.

Natarajan, S., & Nietert. P. J. (2003). National trends in screening, prevalence, and treatment of cardiovascular risk factors. *Preventive Medicine, 36,* 389–397.

National High Blood Pressure Education Program. (1997). The sixth report of the Joint National Committee on Prevention, Detection, Evaluation and Treatment of High Blood Pressure. *Archives of Internal Medicine, 157,* 2413–2446.

National High Blood Pressure Education Program. (2003). *The seventh report of the Joint National Committee on Prevention, Detection, Evaluation, and Treatment of High Blood Pressure* (NIH Publication No. 03-5233). Rockville, MD: U.S. Department of Health and Human Services.

Neal, B., MacMahon, S., & Chapman, N. (2000). Effects of ACE inhibitors, calcium antagonists, and other blood-pressure-lowering drugs: Results of prospectively designed overviews of randomised trials. Blood pressure lowering treatment trialists' collaboration. *Lancet, 356,* 1955–1964.

Neil, H. A. W., Roe, L., Godlee, R. J. P., Moore, J. W., Clark, G. M. G., Brown, J., et al. (1995). Randomized trial of lipid lowering dietary advice in general practice: The effects on serum lipids, lipoproteins, and antioxidants. *Lancet, 310,* 569–573.

Obarzanek, E., Proschan, M. A., Vollmer, W. M., Moore, T. J., Sacks, F. M., Appel, L. J., et al. (2003). Individual blood pressure responses to changes in salt intake: Results from the DASH-Sodium trial. *Hypertension, 42,* 459–467.

Ockene, J. K., Ockene, I. S., Quirk, M. E., Hebert, J. R., Saperia, G. M., Luippold, R. S., et al. (1995). Physician training for patient-centered nutrition counseling in a lipid intervention trial. *Preventive Medicine, 24,* 5563–5570.

Patel, C., Marmot, M. G., Terry, D. J., Carruthers, M., Hunt, B., & Patel, M. (1985). Trial of relaxation in reducing coronary risk: Four year follow-up. *American Journal of Public Health, 290,* 1103–1106.

Perri, M. G., Nezu, A. M., McKelvey, W. F., Shermer, R. L., Renjilian, D. A., & Viegener, B. J. (2001). Relapse prevention training and problem-solving therapy in the long-term management of obesity. *Journal of Consulting and Clinical Psychology, 69,* 722–726.

Pickering, T. G. (2002). The history and politics of salt. *Journal of Clinical Hypertension, 4,* 226–228.

Plum-Wirell, M., Stegmayr, B. G., & Wester, P. O. (1994). Nutritional magnesium supplementation does not change blood pressure nor serum or muscle potassium and magnesium in untreated hypertension. A double-blind cross-over study. *Magnesium Research, 7,* 277–283.

Rothenberg, R. B., & Aubert, R. E. (1990). Ischemic heart disease and hypertension: Effect of disease coding on epidemiologic assessment. *Public Health Reports, 105,* 47–52.

Rouse, I. L., Beilin, L. J., Armstrong, B. K., & Vandongen, R. (1983, January). Blood-pressure-lowering effect of a vegetarian diet: Controlled trial in normotensive subjects. *Lancet,* 5–9.

Sacks, F. M., Rosner, B., & Kass, E. H. (1974). Blood pressure in vegetarians. *American Journal of Epidemiology, 100,* 390–398.

Sacks, F. M., Svetkey, L. P., Vollmer, W. M., Appel, L. J., Bray, G. A., Harsha, D., et al. (2001). Effects on blood pressure of reduced dietary sodium and the Dietary Approaches to Stop Hypertension (DASH) diet. DASH-Sodium Collaborative Research Group. *New England Journal of Medicine, 344*(1), 3–10.

Saunders, J. B. (1987). Alcohol: An important cause of hypertension. *British Medical Journal, 294,* 1045–1046.

SHEP Cooperative Research Group. (1991). Prevention of stroke by antihypertensive drug treatment in older persons with isolated systolic hypertension. Final results of the Systolic Hypertension in the Elderly Program (SHEP). *Journal of the American Medical Association, 265,* 3255–3264.

Simpson, R. O. (1985). Monovalent and divalent cations in hypertension. *Preventive Medicine, 14,* 436–450.

Smoking Cessation Clinical Practice Guideline Panel & Staff. (1996). The Agency for Healthcare Policy and Research smoking cessation clinical practice guideline. *Journal of the American Medical Association, 275,* 1270–1280.

Soghikian, K., Casper, S. M., Fireman, B. H., Hunkeler, E. M., Hurley, L. B., Tekawa, I. S., et al. (1992). Home blood pressure monitoring: Effect on blood pressure control, use of medical services, and medical care costs. *Medical Care, 30,* 855–865.

Stevens, V. J., Obarzanek, E., Cook, N. R., Lee, I. M., Appel, L. J., Smith West, D., et al. (2001, January). Trials for the Hypertension Prevention Research Group. Long-term weight loss and changes in blood pressure: Results of the Trials of Hypertension Prevention, Phase II. *Annals of Internal Medicine, 134*(1), 1–11.

Taubes, G. (1998). The (political) science of salt. *Science, 281,* 898–907.

Trials of Hypertension Prevention Collaborative Research Group. (1997). Effects of weight loss and sodium reduction intervention on blood pressure and hypertension incidence in overweight people with high-normal blood pressure. The Trials of Hypertension Prevention, Phase II. *Archives of Internal Medicine, 157,* 657–667.

Tuomilehto, J., Lindstrom, J., Eriksson, J. G., Valle, T. T., Hamalainen, H., Ilanne-Parikka, P., et al. (2001). Prevention of Type 2 diabetes mellitus by changes in lifestyle among subjects with impaired glucose tolerance. *New England Journal of Medicine, 344,* 1343–1350.

Veith, I. (1966). *The yellow emperor's classic in internal medicine* (translated from Hauang Ti Nei Ching Su Wen, 2300 B.C.). Berkeley, CA: University of California Press.

Veterans Administration. (1967). Cooperative Study on Antihypertensive Agents. Effects of treatment on morbidity in hypertension: Results in patients with diastolic blood pressures averaging 115 through 129 mm Hg. *Journal of the American Medical Association, 202,* 1028–1034.

Veterans Administration. (1970). Cooperative Study on Antihypertensive Agents. Effects of treatment on morbidity in hypertension: Results in patients with diastolic blood pressures averaging 90 through 114 mm Hg. *Journal of the American Medical Association, 213,* 1143–1151.

Vogt, T. M., Aickin, M., Ahmed, F., & Schmidt, M. (2003). The Prevention Index: Using technology to improve quality assessment. *Health Services Research, 39,* 511–529.

Vogt, T. M., Aickin, M., Ahmed, F., Schmidt, M., & Hornbrook, M. (2001). *Improving prevention in managed care: Final report* [Centers for Disease Control and Prevention, Grant No. UR5/CCU 917124].

Vogt, T. M., Appel, L. J., Obarzanek, E., Moore, T. J., Vollmer, W. M., Svetkey, L. P., et al. (1999). Dietary approaches to stop hypertension: Rationale, design, and methods. *Journal of American Diet Association, 99,* S12–S18.

Vogt, T. M., Hollis, J. F., Lichtenstein, E., Stevens, V., Glasgow, R., & Hornbrook, M. (1998). The medical care system and prevention: The need for a new paradigm. *HMO Practice, 12,* 5–13.

Vogt, T. M., & Stevens, V. J. (2003). Obesity research: Winning the battle, losing the war. *Permanente Journal, 7,* 11–20.

Warram, J. H., Laffel, L. M. B., Valsania, P., Christlieb, A. R., & Krolewski, A. S. (1991). Excess mortality associated with diuretic therapy in diabetes mellitus. *Archives of Internal Medicine, 151,* 1350–1356.

Weinsier, R. L. (1976). Salt and the development of essential hypertension. *Preventive Medicine, 5,* 7–14.

Weisemann, A., Metz, J., Nuessel, E., Scheidt, R., & Scheuermann, W. (1997). Four years of practice-based and exercise-supported behavioral medicine in one community of the German CINDI area: Countrywide integrated non-communicable diseases intervention. *International Journal of Sports Medicine, 18,* 308–315.

Whelton, P. K., He, J., Cutler, J. A., Brancati, F. L., Appel, L. J., Follmann, D., et al. (1997). Effects of oral potassium on blood pressure, meta-analysis of randomized controlled clinical trials. *Journal of the American Medical Association, 277,* 1624–1632.

Whelton, P. K., Kumanyika, S. K., Cook, N. R., Cutler, J. A., Borhani, N. O., Hennekens, C. H., et al. (1997). Efficacy of nonpharmacologic interventions in adults with high-normal blood pressure: Results from phase 1 of the Trials of Hypertension Prevention. *American Journal of Clinical Nutrition, 65*(Suppl. 2), S652–S660.

Whelton, S. P., Chin, A., Xin, X., & He, J. (2002). Effect of aerobic exercise on blood pressure: A meta-analysis of randomized controlled trials. *Annals of Internal Medicine, 136,* 493–503.

Witteman, J. C., Grobbee, D., Valkenburg, H. A., van Hernert, A. M., Stijnen, T., Burger, H., et al. (1994). J-shaped relation between change in diastolic blood pressure and progression of aortic atherosclerosis. *Lancet, 343,* 504–507.

Yamamoto, M. E., Applegate, W. H., Klag, M. J., Borhani, N. O., Cohen, J. D., Kirchner, K. A., et al. (1995). Lack of blood pressure effect with calcium and magnesium supplementation in adults with high-normal blood pressure. Results from Phase I of the Trials of Hypertension Prevention (TOHP). Trials of Hypertension Prevention Collaborative Research Group. *Annuals of Epidemiology, 5,* 96–107.

Chapter 9

HEART DISEASE

J. DAVID CURB, GINA C. BELLEAU, BRADLEY J. WILLCOX, AND
ROBERT D. ABBOTT

Coronary heart disease (CHD) has been the leading cause of death in the United States and many other developed countries for the past several decades. Beginning in the 1970s, there were significant declines in mortality from CHD as technology and scientific knowledge improved. Today, CHD is largely preventable: Research has shown that modifying lifestyle to correct for high risk can prevent the development of much of the pathology underlying heart disease (Kannel, 1990; Kannel & Sytkowski, 1987; Manson et al., 1992).

The rates of decline of heart disease mortality appear to be related to population levels of cholesterol and blood pressure, among other risk factors (Menotti et al., 2003). Although an increasing number of additional factors that contribute to the risk of CHD continue to be identified, the majority of the risk can still be explained by the traditional modifiable risk factors: smoking, abnormal lipids and lipoprotein values, and hypertension (Greenland, Smith, & Grundy, 2001). However, there are major geographic differences in heart disease trends (Levi, Lucchini, Negri, & La Vecchia, 2002). Continued low CHD rates in some countries, such as Japan, where dietary fat intake has increased, blood cholesterol levels have risen markedly, and smoking rates remain high, makes this trend somewhat difficult to explain (Sekikawa et al., 2003). Other conditions associated with heart disease risk factors, such as diabetes and obesity, contribute through their influence on the traditional risk factors and through independent mechanisms. A large number of new risk factors have recently been identified and may contribute to understanding and controlling the CHD epidemic in the future.

Four major risk factors—smoking, diabetes, high blood pressure, and high cholesterol—are responsible for at least 50% of CHD, and recent studies suggest that these four risk factors may be responsible for a much higher percentage of heart disease than previously thought (Canto & Iskandrian, 2003). Treating these risk factors could have staggering effects in reducing the prevalence of heart disease. The knowledge and skills necessary to make such changes is available in the vast majority of cases, but economic factors, medical system failures, deficient individual knowledge, and lack of compliance currently limit our ability to achieve this goal.

DEFINITION OF HEART DISEASE

Atherosclerosis is the result of a buildup of fatty deposits, calcium, cholesterol, cellular waste, and other substances in the lining of an artery. This buildup is called plaque. Over time, plaque accumulates in the arteries and may become significant enough to reduce blood flow. Atherosclerosis is also referred to as subclinical heart disease because it often occurs before any clinical symptoms of heart disease are revealed.

Coronary heart disease is caused by atherosclerotic narrowing of the coronary arteries likely to produce angina pectoris (chest pain) or heart attack. This chapter focuses on the causes and prevention of coronary heart disease.

TRENDS

The rates of CHD reached a peak in the United States in the 1970s. Although the reasons are not entirely clear, there was then a dramatic decline in CHD until the 1990s. Between 1985 and 1992, there was an approximately 4% reduction per year in CHD mortality in the United States (National Heart, Lung, and Blood Institute [NHLBI], 1996). The decline, however, has been primarily in men; in fact, women may have had an increase. Figure 9.1 shows the number of deaths due to heart disease in the United States.

There are a number of theories as to the reasons for these trends; chief among these are a major reduction in the fat intake of the U.S. population, a dramatic decline in the rates of smoking, and a dramatic increase in attention to heart disease in the clinical setting (e.g., treatment of blood pressure and cholesterol). Which of these is most important is difficult to determine; the decline is likely to be due to a combination of these and other changes that have occurred in our society. Countering these changes have been decreases in physical activity and the dramatic rise in the rate of obesity in the United States.

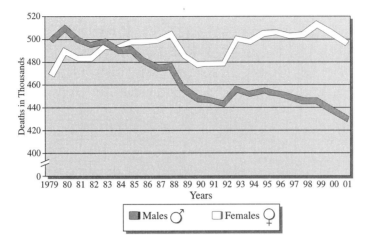

Figure 9.1   Cardiovascular disease mortality trends for males and females in the United States from 1979 to 2001. From *Heart Disease and Stroke Statistics: 2004 Update,* by American Heart Association, 2003, Dallas, TX: Author. Used with permission.

RISK FACTORS

Risk factors for heart disease can be broadly placed into two categories: modifiable and nonmodifiable. Nonmodifiable risk factors are those the individual or physician does not have control over; modifiable risk factors can be altered through lifestyle changes or medical interventions.

In many cases, a given risk factor can be influenced by changes in one or more other risk factors; for example, obesity may have a strong influence on the development of hypertension, abnormal lipid values, and diabetes. In addition, the influence of risk factors may differ by gender and age; for example, the increased risk of a heart attack for a woman with diabetes is higher than for a man with diabetes.

Nonmodifiable Risk Factors

Non-modifiable risk factors include a person's sex, age, family history, and genetics. Though risk cannot be modified, prior knowledge of the risk may help in developing prevention and treatment plans.

Sex and Age

Though heart disease can occur at any age, older people are at a much higher risk for developing heart disease or having a heart attack.

Differences in risk of heart disease between men and women are pronounced, especially at younger ages. For this reason, CHD was thought to be a more significant problem for men than women up to the mid-1900s. More recent studies have dismissed this misconception. On average, women develop heart disease 10 years later than men, but the risk factors for heart disease are very similar in men and women (Kannel & Wilson, 1995). Women's risk of heart attack rises quickly after menopause, resulting in a considerable narrowing of CHD risk between the sexes with age. These data, and other confirmatory data from observational studies, gave rise to the hypothesis that estrogen replacement after menopause would reduce risk in women. As a result, estrogen use in clinical practice was widespread until very recently. The trend of estrogen replacement is changing rapidly after recent reports from the Women's Health Initiative clinical trial. This study did not show a benefit of estrogens on heart disease; instead, findings indicated that estrogen increased the risk for stroke and breast cancer (Chlebowski et al., 2003; Manson et al., 2003; Rossouw et al., 2002; Wassertheil-Smoller et al., 2003).

Family History and Genetics

Familial predisposition can greatly increase the risk of all types of heart disease for an individual. Though genetic risk cannot be currently modified, prior knowledge of the risk can help to determine treatment and prevention plans. In addition, genetics almost always work in concert with environmental and behavioral factors to modify the level of risk. Thus, an individual may be predisposed by his or her genetic makeup for high serum cholesterol, which in turn increases the risk for CHD due to inefficiencies in the body's processing of saturated fats consumed in the diet. However, individuals such as vegetarians and those from cultures where fish is the primary source of animal protein, and who thus habitually consume a low-fat diet or a diet higher in omega-3 fat, may never become aware of that genetic predisposition.

Several large family studies have shown the importance of genetics in heart disease. A Swedish twin study with a 26-year follow-up of 21,004 twins found that males with a monozygotic (identical) twin who died of CHD before the age of 55 had 8.1 times greater risk of developing CHD than males whose twin did not die of CHD. Females had 15 times greater risk (Marenberg, Risch, Berkman, Floderus, & de Faire, 1994). In the same study, dizygotic (nonidentical) male twins had a 3.8 relative risk and females a 2.6 relative risk. Though it is impossible to completely rule out environmental factors that are also shared by siblings, such twin studies do give weight to the evidence that at least some of the risk is genetic.

Genetic studies of chronic disease have proven difficult and complex. Studies related to the genetics of heart disease have primarily focused on lipid disorders, essential hypertension, type 2 diabetes, and obesity. Most of the definitive findings have been for less common disorders; genes linked to more common disorders often have only small effects or affect only a small proportion of people or a specific ethnic group. For example, the first gene linked to common essential hypertension in humans was the angiotensinogen gene (AGT). One allele of the gene was demonstrated to be linked with hypertension (Jeunemaitre et al., 1992), and most subsequent studies have confirmed this finding (Bloem et al., 1997; Borecki et al., 1997; Caulfield et al., 1994; Hegele et al., 1997; Johnson et al., 1996; Kunz, Kreutz, Beige, Distler, & Sharma, 1997). These findings have not been replicated in all studies, however (Brand et al., 1998). It is possible that combinations of genes would be more accurate in predicting complex traits, such as high blood pressure, than single genes.

Modifiable Risk Factors

Modifiable risk factors are those that can be altered through lifestyle changes or medical interventions. Examples of modifiable risk factors include cigarette smoking, obesity, physical activity, diabetes, cholesterol, diet, and inflammation.

Cigarette Smoking

Approximately 4.2 million people worldwide died prematurely from death attributable to tobacco use in the year 2000 (World Health Organization [WHO], 2003). In the United States, smoking has declined greatly over the past several decades. However, this decline has not been as great for women, and smoking rates have actually increased in younger women in the United States. In addition, prevalence rates of smoking are still high in other countries, especially among males. For example, in the year 2000, 54% of males in Japan were smokers (WHO, 2003).

An average of 442,398 Americans died each year of smoking-related illnesses between 1995 and 1999. Approximately one-third of these deaths were cardiovascular-related (Centers for Disease Control and Prevention & National Center for Health Statistics, 2002). Cigarette smoking has been strongly linked to major cardiovascular diseases; for example, smokers are twice as likely to have a heart attack as nonsmokers (U.S. Department of Health and Human Services, 1997; U.S. Public Health Service, 1983). Moreover, the negative effects of smoking are found across age, gender, and ethnicity in the United States (U.S. Public Health Service, 1983) and other countries (Keys et al., 1984). The ill effects of smoking are greater in younger people, though they are still significant in older age groups. In one study, smoking was the only factor that predicted sudden death in those thought to be disease-free (Escobedo & Peddicord, 1997).

Cigarette smoking adds to the effects of other CHD risk factors (Miettinen & Gylling, 1988; Mishell, 1988; Pooling Project Research Group, 1978; Suarez & Barrett-Connor, 1984; Williams et al., 1986), and can also increase the risk of cardiovascular disease in individuals with no other apparent risk factors (U.S. Department of Health and Human Services, 1997). Another example of potential interaction is seen in the rates of heart disease and smoking in Japan. As previously noted, smoking rates among males in Japan are high; interestingly, rates of CHD are low. One potential explanation is that fish consumption may protect heavy smokers from heart disease (Rodriguez et al., 1996), although other factors are almost certainly involved.

Cigarette smoking has both long-term and immediate effects on heart disease. The carbon monoxide and nicotine found in tobacco smoke reduce the amount of oxygen in the blood. These chemicals also damage blood vessel walls, causing plaque buildup and increasing plaque instability. In a study of 1,443 men and women age 15 to 34 who died of external causes such as car accidents, smoking was associated with more fatty streaks and raised lesions in the abdominal aorta in these otherwise healthy individuals (McGill, McMahan, Malcom, Oalmann, & Strong, 1997). The fact that cigarette smoking has an immediate effect on heart disease is supported by the known short-term vascular effects of nicotine and by the rapid improvement of prognosis with smoking cessation. Adults who quit smoking significantly reduce their risk of CHD and cardiovascular disease (Centers for Disease Control and Prevention, 1990; Kawachi et al., 1994).

Though the effect is not as dramatic as for smokers, environmental tobacco smoke (ETS) also increases the chance of heart disease. The risk of death from CHD for those exposed to ETS at home or work increases by up to 30%. Two meta-analyses found that the majority of studies show increased risk for fatal and nonfatal CHD from ETS (Lam & He, 1997; Steenland, Thun, Lally, & Heath, 1996). The 2001 surgeon general's report concluded that there is a casual relationship between ETS exposure from the spouse and CHD mortality (Women and Smoking, 2001). The role of ETS on health has become a significant issue, because those exposed may not have a choice. It is estimated by some that 35,000 to 40,000 yearly deaths from acute myocardial infarction are associated with ETS. In light of these estimates, efforts to reduce exposure of nonsmokers to tobacco smoke should be a high priority (Weiss, 1996).

Obesity

Obesity, or excessive body fat, has become a major health problem in Western cultures, especially in the United States. Data from the National Health and Nutrition Examination Survey (NHANES) show an increasing prevalence of overweight and obesity since the 1960s (Kuczmarski, Carroll, Flegal, & Troiano, 1997). In fact, in 2001, data from NHANES and the Centers for Disease Control showed that 64.5% of U.S. adults were either overweight or obese (American Heart Association, 2003).

Obesity leads to a higher risk of developing some of the major contributors to heart disease, such as hypertension, diabetes, and hyperlipidemia (Sjostrom, 1992). Several studies have linked obesity and hypertension. The Nurses' Health Study found that weight gain increased the risk of hypertension (Huang et al., 1998). The INTERSALT study and National Heart Foundation of Australia both found that body mass index (a measure of obesity defined as weight in kg/height in m^2) was correlated with blood pressure (Dyer & Elliott, 1989; MacMahon, Blacket, Macdonald, & Hall, 1984). Obesity also is an important risk factor in the development of type 2 diabetes; this has been shown in several populations with varying rates of diabetes incidence (Knowler, Pettitt, Savage, & Bennett, 1981; Larsson, Bjorntorp, & Tibblin, 1981; Lee et al., 1995).

Even without other risk factors, obese people are at a greater risk of heart disease (Curb & Marcus, 1991). In response to the evidence linking obesity and CHD, the American Heart Association has reclassified obesity as a major modifiable risk factor for CHD (Eckel & Krauss, 1998).

Cholesterol and Other Lipids

High total cholesterol increases the risk of CHD, especially in the presence of other risk factors such as high blood pressure and smoking. Because high cholesterol, like high blood pressure, often has no symptoms, many people are unaware that they have it. The low-density lipoprotein (LDL) molecule carries most of the cholesterol in the blood. LDL is commonly referred to as the "bad" cholesterol, because high levels of LDL cholesterol increase risk for CHD. The negative effects of LDL and total cholesterol on CHD risk have been demonstrated by numerous studies both across and within populations (Kannel, Castelli, & Gordon, 1979; Keys, 1980; Rhoads, Gulbrandsen, & Kagan, 1976; Robertson et al., 1977).

High-density lipoprotein (HDL) cholesterol carries excess cholesterol back to the liver to be removed from the body. High levels of HDL cholesterol protect from CHD (Curb et al., 2004; Gordon, Castelli, Hjortland, Kannel, & Dawber, 1977; Kannel et al., 1979; Rhoads, Morton, Gulbrandsen, & Kagan, 1978), and for this reason HDL is known as "good" cholesterol. People with low levels of HDL cholesterol have a higher risk of heart attack.

Triglycerides are a common type of fat found in the body and are the major component of stored body fat. The relationship between CHD and triglycerides is not as well understood. Several studies have shown a significant relationship between elevated triglyceride levels and CHD (Gaziano, Hennekens, O'Donnell, Breslow, & Buring, 1997; Gotto, 1998; Jeppesen, Hein, Suadicani, & Gyntelberg, 1998), but others have shown that triglycerides increase risk only in those who have very low HDL or high LDL cholesterol (Burchfiel et al., 1995; Criqui et al., 1993).

Some recent studies have implied that the size of the particles that make up LDL and HDL cholesterol may predict risk of CHD (Austin et al., 2000; Blake, Otvos, Rifai, & Ridker, 2002). A larger HDL particle size seems to reduce the risk of heart disease (Colhoun et al., 2002).

Hypertension

A number of studies have demonstrated the high risk of cardiovascular disease associated with hypertension, or high blood pressure, as well as a reduction in CHD risk when hypertension is treated (Keys, 1980; Stamler, Stamler, & Neaton, 1993; Yano, McGee, & Reed, 1983). Hypertension is the leading cause of congestive heart failure, hemorrhagic stroke, ischemic coronary disease, and cerebrovascular disease (The sixth report of the Joint National Committee on prevention, detection, evaluation, and treatment of high blood pressure, 1997).

There is a direct relationship between an increase in systolic and diastolic blood pressure and coronary death rates. Data from the Seven Countries Study show a doubling in risk for every increment of 10 mmHG in the population's median systolic blood pressure (Keys, 1980). The direct relationship between blood pressure and mortality from CHD was demonstrated in an 11.6-year follow-up of men initially free of CHD. In this study, the relative risk increased more than three times for people with a systolic blood pressure higher than 150 mmHG, as compared to those with a systolic blood pressure of 111 mmHG (Stamler et al., 1993). In a pooling of observational studies including over 400,000 persons initially free of CHD, it was found that CHD mortality begins to increase when diastolic blood pressure is between 73 and 78 mmHg (MacMahon et al., 1990).

Diabetes

Diabetes and impaired glucose tolerance greatly increases the risk of heart disease and stroke (Curb et al., 1995; Donahue, Abbott, Reed, & Yano, 1987). In the Framingham study, diabetes doubled the risk of heart disease in men and tripled it in women (Kannel & McGee, 1979). Diabetes is linked with several other CHD risk factors, such as increased blood pressure, low HDL cholesterol levels, and high triglyceride levels. Yet, even when all other CHD risk factors are adjusted for, diabetes continues as an independent risk factor for heart disease. The cause of death for most people with diabetes is heart or blood vessel disease.

Physical Activity

In past centuries, normal work and daily living required hard physical labor, but in modern society, the majority of people do not do hard physical labor as part of their work. As a result, our lifestyle has become increasingly sedentary. Only an estimated 15% of adult Americans get regular vigorous activity (Physical activity and health: A report of the Surgeon General, 1996). (Regular activity is defined as three times a week for at least 20 minutes.) This trend toward a sedentary lifestyle is worrying in the context of heart disease because lack of exercise is associated with an increased risk of heart disease (Fletcher et al., 1996; Rodriguez et al., 1994).

Many studies have shown that increases in both occupational and leisure-time physical activity reduce the chance of CHD. Occupational studies have shown that those with more sedentary jobs have a higher CHD risk (Berlin & Colditz, 1990). In a study of male civil servants, Morris et al. reported a three times higher risk of fatal myocardial infarction or heart attack among sedentary men as opposed to those who participated in exercise or sports (Morris, Everitt, Pollard, Chave, & Semmence, 1980). Results from this study also indicated that past exercise did not improve risk of CHD; that is, those who had been involved in sports previously but were no longer involved had the same rate of CHD as those who had never been involved (Morris, Clayton, Everitt, Semmence, & Burgess, 1990). Low-level aerobic activity may be protective; among elderly Japanese American men, walking was found to be protective from CHD (Hakim et al., 1999).

Because physical activity obviously affects other CHD risk factors, such as obesity, there is some controversy over whether physical activity alone will reduce risk of CHD. Some studies report that physical activity reduces risk of CHD independent of other risk factors (Eaton et al., 1995; Rosengren & Wilhelmsen, 1997), but other data suggest that the difference in risk between those who are physically active and those who are sedentary disappears after adjustment for other risk factors (Folsom et al., 1997; Rodriguez et al., 1994). Whether directly or indirectly, the positive effects of physical activity on cardiovascular health indicate that a physically active lifestyle is an effective way to reduce risk of heart disease.

Inflammation and Blood Clotting

Thrombosis is the formation of a clot that blocks a blood vessel. The formation of a thrombus is often a critical factor leading to a heart attack. In recent decades, it has been found that markers of thrombosis can be predictive of heart disease. One such marker is fibrinogen, which has been shown to be independently associated with CHD death (Maresca, Di Blasio, Marchioli, & Di Minno,

1999; Yano et al., 2001). Fibrinogen levels are also influenced by factors such as inflammation. For example, smoking, a mediator of inflammation, is correlated with increased fibrinogen levels (Meade, Imeson, & Stirling, 1987; Yano et al., 1999), whereas niacin lowers fibrinogen levels (Ernst & Resch, 1995).

C-reactive protein (CRP), a marker of inflammation, has also been suggested as a predictive factor for heart disease. Many studies have shown that CRP is predictive of future vascular events in individuals without any apparent symptoms (Curb et al., 2003; Danesh et al., 2000; Ridker, Rifai, Rose, Buring, & Cook, 2002; Sakkinen et al., 2002). At this point, it is not apparent whether fibrinogen and CRP actually cause heart disease or are merely markers of the degree of damage taking place (Hackam & Anand, 2003).

PREVENTING HEART DISEASE IN THE GENERAL POPULATION

The rates of heart disease vary greatly from country to country (NHLBI, 1996). In the past, heart disease was more prevalent in Westernized societies such as the United States and certain European countries, whereas economically underdeveloped countries and Asian cultures with lower fat intake, less obesity, and higher levels of physical activity had relatively low rates of heart disease. Although we still do not understand all the causes for the differences in rates of heart disease, in general, they reflect differences in diet, smoking, and other risk factors.

Prevention of heart disease in the general population is classically termed "primary prevention." Specifically, it refers to the prevention of heart disease in individuals without prior symptoms or signs of disease. The majority of individuals who will eventually suffer from heart disease are in this group.

There are at least two possible approaches to such a prevention effort. One, often driven by limited resources, is to focus on lowering risk in a relatively small number of individuals who are at high risk due to known risk factors such as cigarette smoking, hypertension, or high cholesterol. Although this approach would significantly lower the number of heart-related events in a population, many cases of heart disease would still occur in individuals in lower-risk groups. This is because although the rates of heart disease are much higher in individuals with significantly elevated risk factors, many individuals who eventually develop heart disease in a population are not those at the highest level of risk. Individuals with normal or modestly elevated risk make up a large proportion of those who eventually develop heart disease. However, recent data indicate that antecedent major cardiovascular risk exposures are more common than previously believed. In the three large cohorts studied by Greenland et al.

(2003), 87% to 94% of 40- to 59-year-olds had exposure to at least one major CHD risk factor.

This suggests that an approach to prevention of CHD aimed at lowering the average risk of the entire population may be appropriate. This is sometimes referred to as a public health approach. For example, a 10% decrease in total cholesterol levels (populationwide) may result in an estimated 30% reduction in the incidence of CHD (Centers for Disease Control and Prevention & National Center for Health Statistics, 2000). This approach would theoretically prevent normal individuals, those without significant risk factor levels, from moving to abnormal levels. This is often referred to as "primordial prevention," especially when the target is young individuals or children. Examples are programs aimed at keeping children from smoking and those promoting lifelong habits of healthy eating or physically active lifestyles.

Although all are reasonable approaches to lowering the rates of heart disease in the population, perhaps the one with the most appeal is *primordial prevention* as it is most likely to keep the burden of illness and suffering at its lowest level by preventing the population from becoming at risk for developing heart disease. In any society, however, the approach taken must take cost, and the society's ability to pay that cost, into consideration.

Over recent decades, the differences between these approaches have blurred as new technology has made it possible to diagnose disease at earlier stages. Thus, asymptomatic individuals who a decade ago might have been pronounced free of disease and not eligible for intervention may today be revealed to have significant disease burdens when subclinical end points are investigated. Examples of subclinical end points are the amount of calcium in the coronary arteries as measured by the new electron beam CT scan and the thickness of the wall of the carotid arteries as visualized by ultrasound. In addition, newly discovered risk factors such as high CRP levels and the size of the particles that make up LDL and HDL cholesterol may detect increased risk in individuals previously thought to be normal by other risk measures.

Genetic testing offers to push the detection of risk even earlier by identifying genetic markers for potential cardiovascular risk; these risk factors may develop as an individual ages or they may develop only when the genetic predisposition is coupled with specific lifestyle choices such as cigarette smoking, eating a high-fat diet or lack of physical activity. For example, it may be possible to identify individuals who are genetically susceptible to the development of high blood pressure when they ingest increased amounts of sodium as part of their diet. If these individuals live in cultures with normally low-sodium diets or are taught to avoid high-sodium foods early in their lives, they might never develop high blood pressure. On the other hand, if these same individuals were brought up on a high-sodium diet, their genetic predisposition would put them at high risk for heart disease. In the future, such genetic typing is likely to allow precise risk factor stratification even before birth. However, such technology could lead to decisions regarding whether to test for such predisposing genetic factors at birth and whether it is ethical to program an individual to avoid certain behaviors that may be more risky than others.

Among individuals who already have established risk factors, genetic testing may allow for the identification of patients who are most likely to gain from specific behavior change or treatment strategies, thus avoiding the expense and trouble of implementing preventive strategies in whole populations. On the other hand, genetic factors present in the majority of the population that can be treated by low-risk methods could be more economically treated using populationwide strategies that would avoid mass testing and tailoring interventions. Lowering the fat content in the diet of the whole population may be one such intervention. Public health strategies aimed at reducing dietary sodium are likely to benefit the individual who is genetically susceptible to blood pressure increase secondary to high sodium intake. Other individuals may be genetically resistant to such strategies; for them, devoting our limited resources to drug therapy or alternative strategies may be more prudent.

Preventive practices are also driven by more practical considerations. Interventions that can have profound effects on the disease burden to the society may have only a marginal benefit to the individual. For example, a small shift in the average blood pressure in a population could reduce the number of myocardial infarctions substantially (He & Whelton, 1997). To date, although nonpharmacologic means offer some promise (Srinath & Katan, 2004), this type of change would most reliably be accomplished through drug treatment.

For example, in the Systolic Hypertension in the Elderly Program (SHEP), the average participant on active treatment had a 26 mmHg lowering of systolic blood pressure during the study compared to 15 mmHg lowering in the control group. This resulted in a 27% reduction in the rate of CHD. However, only 16 cases of heart disease per 1,000 people per 5 years treated would be prevented (SHEP Cooperative Research Group, 1993). Even the safest drugs carry with them the risk of side effects, for a given individual, so drugs that are helpful for the population as a whole may not benefit a specific individual. Therefore, public health approaches are more likely to impact a larger number of individuals before they have symptomatic heart disease, and drug therapy is usually prescribed by doctors on an individual basis.

There are a number of lifestyle changes that would lower CHD risk in the general population. These include weight reduction, other dietary changes such as lowering fat and sodium intake, increased levels of physical activity, and smoking cessation. If these lifestyle changes were implemented in the population, it would unquestionably result in large reductions in heart disease while simultaneously improving overall health. However, the challenges of motivating individuals to change their established lifestyle are profound. In general, the success of such approaches has been limited without the commitment of significant resources to develop an infrastructure to support such interventions.

A new tactic of prevention, which mixes the public health approach and the clinical approach, has recently been proposed. The success of statins in lowering the risk of heart disease in apparently normal individuals has stimulated the concept of the "polypill." Given the difficulty of stimulating large numbers of individuals to make long-lasting changes in their lifestyle, a pill has been proposed that combines low doses of relatively safe drugs aimed simultaneously at reducing four cardiovascular risk factors (LDL cholesterol, blood pressure, serum homocysteine, and platelet function) regardless of pretreatment levels (Wald & Law, 2003). It is proposed that vast numbers of heart attacks could be prevented at a relatively low cost to society, because the cost of massive screening needed for tailoring such interventions could be avoided and individuals would be more likely to comply with the simple daily single pill approach than lifestyle changes. Certainly some portion of the cost would be incurred treating drug side effects that would not have occurred in the absence of such a massive intervention. But the proponents of this plan argue that the small numbers of serious adverse reactions, such as hemorrhagic strokes, gastrointestinal bleeding, and a relatively larger number but less severe side effects would be a small price to pay for the overall societal benefit. Proponents argue that these could be limited by using some selectivity in determining who should take the polypill. Indeed, any drug intervention involves such trade-offs of risk versus benefit. The real difference in the approaches is the societal scale proposed for the polypill approach.

Perhaps the greatest potential for large changes in population risk are those that change the cultural values of whole societies. However, in a free society, such changes are difficult to initiate and to maintain. They do, however, occur. For example, the percentage of calories from total fat and saturated fat in the American diet has steadily declined over the past 30 years (Kennedy, Bowman, & Powell, 1999), most likely in response to research pointing to an association of blood cholesterol with heart disease coupled with changes in public health policy and medical care. Unfortunately, increases in overall caloric intake and reductions in physical activity levels have also occurred. The end result has been an epidemic of obesity (Ogden, Carroll, & Flegal, 2003). Other possible interventions such as increased alcohol intake, which has been associated with lower rates of heart disease in multiple studies, have obvious dangers when implemented populationwide.

PREVENTING HEART DISEASE IN HIGH-RISK INDIVIDUALS

Secondary prevention involves intervention for those who already have symptomatic heart disease to prevent further progression of the disease. Even if the proportional benefit to normalizing a risk factor is the same as that in a lower-risk person (for example, both interventions might reduce risk for heart attack by 50%), the absolute likelihood of benefit for such individuals is increased over that of the general population because of higher basal risk for that individual. In addition, these individuals often have symptoms or other reasons for being more compliant to recommendations than low-risk, symptom-free individuals. There are also, in general, a smaller number of such higher-risk individuals, making group interventions more practical.

Risk factor assessment in the population is an important method for bringing high-risk individuals to the notice of the medical establishment. It is not unusual for individuals at relatively high risk from high cholesterol or high blood pressure to be unaware of their condition. High-risk individuals are often identified in medical settings. Thus, the medical care system is likely to be a more important part of interventions in such individuals.

PRACTICE AND POLICY IMPLICATIONS

Heart disease and other vascular diseases are the leading causes of death in the United States and many other countries with a Western lifestyle. As lifestyles become more Westernized in countries where heart disease is not yet a significant problem, it may become a public health problem. Heart disease is also a major cause of disability and health expenditures in many countries. In the United States, the cost of cardiovascular diseases and stroke in 2004 is estimated to be $368.4 billion (American Heart Association, 2003). This does not include the cost of human suffering.

Many developed and some less developed populations around the world are rapidly aging, with the number of individuals over 65 projected to increase dramatically (Kinsella & Velkoff, 2001). Therefore, even as the age-adjusted rates of CHD are falling, the actual numbers of cases may rise due to the higher number of aged individuals. Most clinical practitioners dealing with adults will have already experienced an aging of their patient population. These shifts have enormous policy implications because the rate of heart disease rapidly increases with age. Thus, along with the aging of the population we can expect an increasing demand for health care secondary to heart disease. In the United States, these conditions can be expected to increase dramatically as the baby boom generation ages (U.S. Department of Health and Human Services, 2003).

FUTURE DIRECTIONS

We have sufficient knowledge about most of the major risk factors for heart disease to create public policy and clinical practice guidelines that will greatly reduce the burden of heart disease in the United States and worldwide. Implementation of these policies and guidelines should be the primary focus in the prevention of heart disease for the near future. Research aimed at discovering the barriers to translating our current knowledge into practice is needed. There remain significant questions about the reasons for differences in heart disease across populations to justify investing in research aimed at these questions. The advances in the human genome project and human genetics and proteomics offer the promise of new understanding and potential preventive and therapeutic advances that could not have been contemplated a decade ago. Research in markers of inflammation, the components that make up lipids in the blood, and thrombosis as well as continued advances in therapeutics and diagnostic imaging are other areas that offer promise for the future.

REFERENCES

American Heart Association. (2003). *Heart disease and stroke statistics: 2004 update.* Dallas, TX: Author.

Austin, M. A., Rodriguez, B. L., McKnight, B., McNeely, M. J., Edwards, K. L., Curb, J. D., et al. (2000). Low-density lipoprotein particle size, triglycerides, and high-density lipoprotein cholesterol as risk factors for coronary heart disease in older Japanese-American men. *American Journal of Cardiology, 86,* 412–416.

Berlin, J. A., & Colditz, G. A. (1990). A meta-analysis of physical activity in the prevention of coronary heart disease. *American Journal of Epidemiology, 132,* 612–628.

Blake, G. J., Otvos, J. D., Rifai, N., & Ridker, P. M. (2002). Low-density lipoprotein particle concentration and size as determined by nuclear magnetic resonance spectroscopy as predictors of cardiovascular disease in women. *Circulation, 106,* 1930–1937.

Bloem, L. J., Foroud, T. M., Ambrosius, W. T., Hanna, M. P., Tewksbury, D. A., & Pratt, J. H. (1997). Association of the angiotensinogen gene to serum angiotensinogen in blacks and whites. *Hypertension, 29,* 1078–1082.

Borecki, I. B., Province, M. A., Ludwig, E. H., Ellison, R. C., Folsom, A. R., Heiss, G., et al. (1997). Associations of candidate loci angiotensinogen and angiotensin-converting enzyme with severe hypertension: The NHLBI Family Heart Study. *Annals of Epidemiology, 7,* 13–21.

Brand, E., Chatelain, N., Keavney, B., Caulfield, M., Citterio, L., Connell, J., et al. (1998). Evaluation of the angiotensinogen locus in human essential hypertension: A European study. *Hypertension, 31,* 725–729.

Burchfiel, C. M., Laws, A., Benfante, R., Goldberg, R. J., Hwang, L. J., Chiu, D., et al. (1995). Combined effects of HDL cholesterol, triglyceride, and total cholesterol concentrations on 18-year risk of atherosclerotic disease. *Circulation, 92,* 1430–1436.

Canto, J. G., & Iskandrian, A. E. (2003). Major risk factors for cardiovascular disease: Debunking the "only 50%" myth. *Journal of the American Medical Association, 290,* 947–949.

Caulfield, M., Lavender, P., Farrall, M., Munroe, P., Lawson, M., Turner, P., et al. (1994). Linkage of the angiotensinogen gene to essential hypertension. *New England Journal of Medicine, 330,* 1629–1633.

Centers for Disease Control and Prevention. (1990). *The health benefits of smoking cessation: A report of the Surgeon General* (Rep. No. CDC90-8416). Washington, DC: Public Health Service, Office on Smoking and Health.

Centers for Disease Control and Prevention & National Center for Health Statistics. (2000). State-specific cholesterol screening trends—United States, 1991–1999. *Morbidity and Mortality Weekly Report, 49,* 750–755.

Centers for Disease Control and Prevention & National Center for Health Statistics. (2002). Annual smoking-attributable mortality, years of potential life lost, and economic costs. *Morbidity and Mortality Weekly Report, 51,* 300–303.

Chlebowski, R. T., Hendrix, S. L., Langer, R. D., Stefanick, M. L., Gass, M., Lane, D., et al. (2003). Influence of estrogen plus progestin on breast cancer and mammography in healthy postmenopausal women: The Women's Health Initiative Randomized Trial. *Journal of the American Medical Association, 289,* 3243–3253.

Colhoun, H. M., Otvos, J. D., Rubens, M. B., Taskinen, M. R., Underwood, S. R., & Fuller, J. H. (2002). Lipoprotein subclasses and particle sizes and their relationship with coronary artery calcification in men and women with and without type 1 diabetes. *Diabetes, 51,* 1949–1956.

Criqui, M. H., Heiss, G., Cohn, R., Cowan, L. D., Suchindran, C. M., Bangdiwala, S., et al. (1993). Plasma triglyceride level and mortality from coronary heart disease. *New England Journal of Medicine, 328,* 1220–1225.

Curb, J. D., Abbott, R. D., Rodriguez, B. L., Masaki, K., Chen, R., Sharp, D. S., et al. (2004). A prospective study of HDL cholesterol and cholesteryl ester transfer protein gene mutations and the risk of coronary heart disease in the elderly. *Journal of Lipid Research, 45,* 948–953.

Curb, J. D., Abbott, R. D., Rodriguez, B. L., Sakkinen, P., Popper, J. S., Yano, K., et al. (2003). C-reactive protein and the future risk of thromboembolic stroke in healthy men. *Circulation, 107,* 2016–2020.

Curb, J. D., & Marcus, E. B. (1991). Body fat, coronary heart disease, and stroke in Japanese men. *American Journal of Clinical Nutrition, 53,* 1612S–1615S.

Curb, J. D., Rodriguez, B. L., Burchfiel, C. M., Abbott, R. D., Chiu, D., & Yano, K. (1995). Sudden death, impaired glucose tolerance, and diabetes in Japanese American men. *Circulation, 91,* 2591–2595.

Danesh, J., Whincup, P., Walker, M., Lennon, L., Thomson, A., Appleby, P., et al. (2000). Low grade inflammation and coronary heart disease: Prospective study and updated meta-analyses. *British Medical Journal, 321,* 199–204.

Donahue, R. P., Abbott, R. D., Reed, D. M., & Yano, K. (1987). Postchallenge glucose concentration and coronary heart disease in men of Japanese ancestry: Honolulu Heart Program. *Diabetes, 36,* 689–692.

Dyer, A. R., & Elliott, P. (1989). The INTERSALT study: Relations of body mass index to blood pressure (INTERSALT Co-operative Research Group). *Journal of Human Hypertension, 3,* 299–308.

Eaton, C. B., Medalie, J. H., Flocke, S. A., Zyzanski, S. J., Yaari, S., & Goldbourt, U. (1995). Self-reported physical activity predicts long-term coronary heart disease and all-cause mortalities: Twenty-one-year follow-up of the Israeli Ischemic Heart Disease Study. *Archives of Family Medicine, 4,* 323–329.

Eckel, R. H., & Krauss, R. M. (1998). American Heart Association call to action: Obesity as a major risk factor for coronary heart disease (AHA Nutrition Committee). *Circulation, 97,* 2099–2100.

Ernst, E., & Resch, K. L. (1995). Therapeutic interventions to lower plasma fibrinogen concentration. *European Heart Journal, 16*(Suppl. A), 47–52.

Escobedo, L. G., & Peddicord, J. P. (1997). Long-term trends in cigarette smoking among young U.S. adults. *Addictive Behaviors, 22,* 427–430.

Fletcher, G. F., Balady, G., Blair, S. N., Blumenthal, J., Caspersen, C., Chaitman, B., et al. (1996). Statement on exercise: Benefits and recommendations for physical activity programs for all Americans [A statement for health professionals by the Committee on Exercise and Cardiac Rehabilitation of the Council on Clinical Cardiology, American Heart Association]. *Circulation, 94,* 857–862.

Folsom, A. R., Arnett, D. K., Hutchinson, R. G., Liao, F., Clegg, L. X., & Cooper, L. S. (1997). Physical activity and incidence of coronary heart disease in middle-aged women and men. *Medicine and Science in Sports and Exercise, 29,* 901–909.

Gaziano, J. M., Hennekens, C. H., O'Donnell, C. J., Breslow, J. L., & Buring, J. E. (1997). Fasting triglycerides, high-density lipoprotein, and risk of myocardial infarction. *Circulation, 96,* 2520–2525.

Gordon, T., Castelli, W. P., Hjortland, M. C., Kannel, W. B., & Dawber, T. R. (1977). High density lipoprotein as a protective factor against coronary heart disease: The Framingham Study. *American Journal of Medicine, 62,* 707–714.

Gotto, A. M., Jr. (1998). Triglyceride as a risk factor for coronary artery disease. *American Journal of Cardiology, 82,* 22Q–25Q.

Greenland, P., Knoll, M. D., Stamler, J., Neaton, J. D., Dyer, A. R., Garside, D. B., et al. (2003). Major risk factors as antecedents of fatal and nonfatal coronary heart disease events. *Journal of the American Medical Association, 290,* 891–897.

Greenland, P., Smith, S. C., Jr., & Grundy, S. M. (2001). Improving coronary heart disease risk assessment in asymptomatic people: Role of traditional risk factors and noninvasive cardiovascular tests. *Circulation, 104,* 1863–1867.

Hackam, D. G., & Anand, S. S. (2003). Emerging risk factors for atherosclerotic vascular disease: A critical review of the evidence. *Journal of the American Medical Association, 290,* 932–940.

Hakim, A. A., Curb, J. D., Petrovitch, H., Rodriguez, B. L., Yano, K., Ross, G. W., et al. (1999). Effects of walking on coronary heart disease in elderly men: The Honolulu Heart Program. *Circulation, 100,* 9–13.

He, J., & Whelton, P. K. (1997). Epidemiology and prevention of hypertension. *The Medical Clinics of North America, 81,* 1077–1097.

Hegele, R. A., Harris, S. B., Hanley, A. J., Sun, F., Connelly, P. W., & Zinman, B. (1997). Angiotensinogen gene variation associated with variation in blood pressure in aboriginal Canadians. *Hypertension, 29,* 1073–1077.

Huang, Z., Willett, W. C., Manson, J. E., Rosner, B., Stampfer, M. J., Speizer, F. E., et al. (1998). Body weight, weight change, and risk for hypertension in women. *Annals of Internal Medicine, 128,* 81–88.

Jeppesen, J., Hein, H. O., Suadicani, P., & Gyntelberg, F. (1998). Triglyceride concentration and ischemic heart disease: An eight-year follow-up in the Copenhagen Male Study. *Circulation, 97,* 1029–1036.

Jeunemaitre, X., Soubrier, F., Kotelevtsev, Y. V., Lifton, R. P., Williams, C. S., Charru, A., et al. (1992). Molecular basis of human hypertension: Role of angiotensinogen. *Cell, 71,* 169–180.

Johnson, A. G., Simons, L. A., Friedlander, Y., Simons, J., Davis, D. R., & MaCallum, J. (1996). M235—>T polymorphism of the angiotensinogen gene predicts hypertension in the elderly. *Journal of Human Hypertension, 14,* 1061–1065.

Kannel, W. B. (1990). Contribution of the Framingham Study to preventive cardiology (Bishop lecture). *Journal of the American College of Cardiology, 15,* 206–211.

Kannel, W. B., Castelli, W. P., & Gordon, T. (1979). Cholesterol in the prediction of atherosclerotic disease: New perspectives based on the Framingham study. *Annals of Internal Medicine, 90,* 85–91.

Kannel, W. B., & McGee, D. L. (1979). Diabetes and cardiovascular disease: The Framingham study. *Journal of the American Medical Association, 241,* 2035–2038.

Kannel, W. B., & Sytkowski, P. A. (1987). Atherosclerosis risk factors. *Pharmacology and Therapeutics, 32,* 207–235.

Kannel, W. B., & Wilson, P. W. (1995). Risk factors that attenuate the female coronary disease advantage. *Archives of Internal Medicine, 155,* 57–61.

Kawachi, I., Colditz, G. A., Stampfer, M. J., Willett, W. C., Manson, J. E., Rosner, B., et al. (1994). Smoking cessation and time course of decreased risks of coronary heart disease in middle-aged women. *Archives of Internal Medicine, 154,* 169–175.

Kennedy, E. T., Bowman, S. A., & Powell, R. (1999). Dietary-fat intake in the U.S. population. *Journal of the American College of Nutrition, 18,* 207–212.

Keys, A. (1980). *Seven countries: A multivariate analysis of death and coronary heart disease.* Cambridge, MA: Harvard University Press.

Keys, A., Menotti, A., Aravanis, C., Blackburn, H., Djordevic, B. S., Buzina, R., et al. (1984). The seven countries study: 2,289 deaths in 15 years. *Preventive Medicine, 13,* 141–154.

Kinsella, K., & Velkoff, V. A. (2001). *An aging world.* Washington, DC: U.S. Government Printing Office.

Knowler, W. C., Pettitt, D. J., Savage, P. J., & Bennett, P. H. (1981). Diabetes incidence in Pima indians: Contributions of obesity and parental diabetes. *American Journal of Epidemiology, 113,* 144–156.

Kuczmarski, R. J., Carroll, M. D., Flegal, K. M., & Troiano, R. P. (1997). Varying body mass index cutoff points to describe overweight prevalence among U.S. adults: NHANES III (1988 to 1994). *Obesity Research, 5,* 542–548.

Kunz, R., Kreutz, R., Beige, J., Distler, A., & Sharma, A. M. (1997). Association between the angiotensinogen 235T-variant and essential hypertension in whites: A systematic review and methodological appraisal. *Hypertension, 30,* 1331–1337.

Lam, T. H., & He, Y. (1997). Passive smoking and coronary heart disease: A brief review. *Clinical and Experimental Pharmacology and Physiology, 24,* 993–996.

Larsson, B., Bjorntorp, P., & Tibblin, G. (1981). The health consequences of moderate obesity. *International Journal of Obesity, 5,* 97–116.

Lee, E. T., Howard, B. V., Savage, P. J., Cowan, L. D., Fabsitz, R. R., Oopik, A. J., et al. (1995). Diabetes and impaired glucose tolerance in three American Indian populations aged 45–74 years: The Strong Heart Study. *Diabetes Care, 18,* 599–610.

Levi, F., Lucchini, F., Negri, E., & La Vecchia, C. (2002). Trends in mortality from cardiovascular and cerebrovascular diseases in Europe and other areas of the world. *Heart, 88,* 119–124.

MacMahon, S. W., Blacket, R. B., Macdonald, G. J., & Hall, W. (1984). Obesity, alcohol consumption and blood pressure in Australian men and women: The National Heart Foundation of Australia Risk Factor Prevalence Study. *Journal of Human Hypertension, 2,* 85–91.

MacMahon, S. W., Peto, R., Cutler, J., Collins, R., Sorlie, P., Neaton, J., et al. (1990). Blood pressure, stroke, and coronary heart disease: Part 1. Prolonged differences in blood pressure: Prospective observational studies corrected for the regression dilution bias. *Lancet, 335,* 765–774.

Manson, J. E., Hsia, J., Johnson, K. C., Rossouw, J. E., Assaf, A. R., Lasser, N. L., et al. (2003). Estrogen plus progestin and the risk of coronary heart disease. *New England Journal of Medicine, 349,* 523–534.

Manson, J. E., Tosteson, H., Ridker, P. M., Satterfield, S., Hebert, P., O'Connor, G. T., et al. (1992). The primary prevention of myocardial infarction. *New England Journal of Medicine, 326,* 1406–1416.

Marenberg, M. E., Risch, N., Berkman, L. F., Floderus, B., & de Faire, U. (1994). Genetic susceptibility to death from coronary heart disease in a study of twins. *New England Journal of Medicine, 330,* 1041–1046.

Maresca, G., Di Blasio, A., Marchioli, R., & Di Minno, G. (1999). Measuring plasma fibrinogen to predict stroke and myocardial infarction: An update. *Arteriosclerosis, Thrombosis, and Vascular Biology, 19,* 1368–1377.

McGill, H. C., Jr., McMahan, C. A., Malcom, G. T., Oalmann, M. C., & Strong, J. P. (1997). Effects of serum lipoproteins and smoking on atherosclerosis in young men and women: Pathobiological determinants of atherosclerosis in youth [The PDAY Research Group]. *Arteriosclerosis, Thrombosis, and Vascular Biology, 17,* 95–106.

Meade, T. W., Imeson, J., & Stirling, Y. (1987). Effects of changes in smoking and other characteristics on clotting factors and the risk of ischaemic heart disease. *Lancet, 2*, 986–988.

Menotti, A., Puddu, P. E., Lanti, M., Kromhout, D., Blackburn, H., & Nissinen, A. (2003). Twenty-five-year coronary mortality trends in the seven countries study using the accelerated failure time model. *European Journal of Epidemiology, 18*, 113–122.

Miettinen, T. A., & Gylling, H. (1988). Mortality and cholesterol metabolism in familial hypercholesterolemia: Long-term follow-up of 96 patients. *Arteriosclerosis, 8*, 163–167.

Mishell, D. R., Jr. (1988). Use of oral contraceptives in women of older reproductive age. *American Journal of Obstetrics and Gynecology, 158*, 1652–1657.

Morris, J. N., Clayton, D. G., Everitt, M. G., Semmence, A. M., & Burgess, E. H. (1990). Exercise in leisure time: Coronary attack and death rates. *British Heart Journal, 63*, 325–334.

Morris, J. N., Everitt, M. G., Pollard, R., Chave, S. P., & Semmence, A. M. (1980). Vigorous exercise in leisure-time: Protection against coronary heart disease. *Lancet, 2*, 1207–1210.

National Heart, Lung, and Blood Institute. (1996). *Morbidity and mortality: 1996 chartbook on cardiovascular, lung, and blood diseases.* Bethesda, MD: National Institutes of Health.

Ogden, C. L., Carroll, M. D., & Flegal, K. M. (2003). Epidemiologic trends in overweight and obesity. *Endocrinology and metabolism clinics of North America, 32*, vii, 741–760.

Physical activity and health: A report of the Surgeon General. (1996). Washington, DC: Department of Health and Human Services, Centers for Disease Control and Prevention, National Center for Chronic Disease Prevention Health Promotion, The President's Council on Physical Fitness and Sports.

Pooling Project Research Group. (1978). Relationship of blood pressure, serum cholesterol, smoking habit, relative weight, and ECG abnormalities to incidence of major coronary events: Final report of the Pooling Project (Rep. No. 31). *Journal of Chronic Diseases*, 201–306.

Rhoads, G. G., Gulbrandsen, C. L., & Kagan, A. (1976). Serum lipoproteins and coronary heart disease in a population study of Hawaii Japanese men. *New England Journal of Medicine, 294*, 293–298.

Rhoads, G. G., Morton, N. E., Gulbrandsen, C. L., & Kagan, A. (1978). Sinking prebeta lipoprotein and coronary heart disease in Japanese-American men in Hawaii. *American Journal of Epidemiology, 108*, 350–356.

Ridker, P. M., Rifai, N., Rose, L., Buring, J. E., & Cook, N. R. (2002). Comparison of C-reactive protein and low-density lipoprotein cholesterol levels in the prediction of first cardiovascular events. *New England Journal of Medicine, 347*, 1557–1565.

Robertson, T. L., Kato, H., Gordon, T., Kagan, A., Rhoads, G. G., Land, C. E., et al. (1977). Epidemiologic studies of coronary heart disease and stroke in Japanese men living in Japan, Hawaii, and California: Coronary heart disease risk factors in Japan and Hawaii. *American Journal of Cardiology, 39*, 244–249.

Rodriguez, B. L., Curb, J. D., Burchfiel, C. M., Abbott, R. D., Petrovitch, H., Masaki, K., et al. (1994). Physical activity and 23-year incidence of coronary heart disease morbidity and mortality among middle-aged men: The Honolulu Heart Program. *Circulation, 89,* 2540–2544.

Rodriguez, B. L., Sharp, D. S., Abbott, R. D., Burchfiel, C. M., Masaki, K., Chyou, P. H., et al. (1996). Fish intake may limit the increase in risk of coronary heart disease morbidity and mortality among heavy smokers: The Honolulu Heart Program. *Circulation, 94,* 952–956.

Rosengren, A., & Wilhelmsen, L. (1997). Physical activity protects against coronary death and deaths from all causes in middle-aged men: Evidence from a 20-year follow-up of the primary prevention study in Goteborg. *Annals of Epidemiology, 7,* 69–75.

Rossouw, J. E., Anderson, G. L., Prentice, R. L., LaCroix, A. Z., Kooperberg, C., Stefanick, M. L., et al. (2002). Risks and benefits of estrogen plus progestin in healthy postmenopausal women: Principal results From the Women's Health Initiative randomized controlled trial. *Journal of the American Medical Association, 288,* 321–333.

Sakkinen, P., Abbott, R. D., Curb, J. D., Rodriguez, B. L., Yano, K., & Tracy, R. P. (2002). C-reactive protein and myocardial infarction. *Journal of Clinical Epidemiology, 55,* 445–451.

Sekikawa, A., Horiuchi, B. Y., Edmundowicz, D., Ueshima, H., Curb, J. D., Sutton-Tyrrell, K., et al. (2003). A "natural experiment" in cardiovascular epidemiology in the early 21st century. *Heart, 89,* 255–257.

SHEP Cooperative Research Group. (1993). Implications of the systolic hypertension in the elderly program: The systolic hypertension in the Elderly Program Cooperative Research Group. *Hypertension, 21,* 335–343.

The sixth report of the Joint National Committee on prevention, detection, evaluation, and treatment of high blood pressure. (1997). *Archives of Internal Medicine, 157,* 2413–2446.

Sjostrom, L. V. (1992). Mortality of severely obese subjects. *American Journal of Clinical Nutrition, 55,* 516S–523S.

Srinath, R. K., & Katan, M. B. (2004). Diet, nutrition, and the prevention of hypertension and cardiovascular diseases. *Public Health and Nutrition, 7,* 167–186.

Stamler, J., Stamler, R., & Neaton, J. D. (1993). Blood pressure, systolic and diastolic, and cardiovascular risks: U.S. population data. *Archives of Internal Medicine, 153,* 598–615.

Steenland, K., Thun, M., Lally, C., & Heath, C., Jr. (1996). Environmental tobacco smoke and coronary heart disease in the American Cancer Society CPS-II cohort. *Circulation, 94,* 622–628.

Suarez, L., & Barrett-Connor, E. (1984). Interaction between cigarette smoking and diabetes mellitus in the prediction of death attributed to cardiovascular disease. *American Journal of Epidemiology, 120,* 670–675.

U.S. Department of Health and Human Services. (1997). *Changes in cigarette-related disease risks and their implication for prevention and control* (Rep. No. NIH 97-4213). Rockville, MD: U.S. Department of Health and Human Services, Public Health Services, National Institutes of Health, National Cancer Institute.

U.S. Department of Health and Human Services. (2003). *A public health action plan to prevent heart disease and stroke.* Atlanta, GA: U.S. Department of Health and Human Services, Centers for Disease Control and Prevention.

U.S. Public Health Service. (1983). *The health consequences of smoking: Cardiovascular disease: A report of the Surgeon General* (Rep. No. PHS 84-50204). Rockville, MD: U.S. Department of Health and Human Services.

Wald, N. J., & Law, M. R. (2003). A strategy to reduce cardiovascular disease by more than 80%. *British Medical Journal, 326,* 1419.

Wassertheil-Smoller, S., Hendrix, S. L., Limacher, M., Heiss, G., Kooperberg, C., Baird, A., et al. (2003). Effect of estrogen plus progestin on stroke in postmenopausal women: The women's health initiative: A randomized trial. *Journal of the American Medical Association, 289,* 2673–2684.

Weiss, S. T. (1996). Cardiovascular effects of environmental tobacco smoke. *Circulation, 94,* 599.

Williams, R. R., Hasstedt, S. J., Wilson, D. E., Ash, K. O., Yanowitz, F. F., Reiber, G. E., et al. (1986). Evidence that men with familial hypercholesterolemia can avoid early coronary death. An analysis of 77 gene carriers in four Utah pedigrees. *Journal of the American Medical Association, 255,* 219–224.

Women and smoking: A report of the Surgeon General. (2001). Rockville, MD: U.S. Department of Health and Human Services, Public Health Service, Office of the Surgeon General.

World Health Organization. (2003). *Tobacco Atlas.* Geneva, Switzerland: Author.

Yano, K., Grove, J. S., Chen, R., Rodriguez, B. L., Curb, J. D., & Tracy, R. P. (2001). Plasma fibrinogen as a predictor of total and cause-specific mortality in elderly Japanese-American men. *Arteriosclerosis, Thrombosis, and Vascular Biology, 21,* 1065–1070.

Yano, K., Kodama, K., Shimizu, Y., Chyou, P. H., Sharp, D. S., Tracy, R. P., et al. (1999). Plasma fibrinogen and its correlates in elderly Japanese men living in Japan and Hawaii. *Journal of Clinical Epidemiology, 52,* 1201–1206.

Yano, K., McGee, D., & Reed, D. M. (1983). The impact of elevated blood pressure upon 10-year mortality among Japanese men in Hawaii: The Honolulu Heart Program. *Journal of Chronic Diseases, 36,* 569–579.

Chapter 10

DIABETES MELLITUS

MAYTE LOPEZ-SANDRIN AND JAY S. SKYLER

Modernization of our world has brought us convenience, abundance, and diabetes. Our way of life is challenged by this chronic disease, which poses an obstacle to the quality of longevity. During the past 50 years, diabetes mellitus has become an increasing health problem, affecting industrialized nations worldwide and contributing to rising health care costs.

There are two main types of diabetes mellitus, simply named type 1 and type 2. The two types differ from each other in many ways. In addition, there are other varieties of diabetes, which will not be discussed here, such as gestational diabetes, drug-induced diabetes, and mixed types with features of both type 1 and type 2. Although both type 1 and type 2 evolve in genetically susceptible individuals as a result of environmental triggers, the populations at risk for each differ immensely. Furthermore, the pathophysiology for each disease is as unique and distinctive as their potential etiologies.

Therefore, when we speak of diabetes mellitus, we are actually discussing different conditions that have certain key features in common, namely, insulin insufficiency (absolute in type 1 and relative in type 2), the state of hyperglycemia, and many of the end-stage complications of the disease. Patients from each group may differ greatly from each other in many other aspects. To discuss prevention, each form of diabetes mellitus must be scrutinized separately, even though once the disease is present, the therapeutic goals of all forms of diabetes mellitus tend to converge.

TRENDS AND INCIDENCE

The proportion of the population with diabetes mellitus continues to increase. Some consider it one of the main threats to human health in the twenty-first century (Zimmet, Alberti, & Shaw, 2001, p. 782). Between 1970 and 1994, there was a smaller decline in mortality among those with diabetes than among those without the condition (Zimmet et al., 2001). According to the Centers for Disease Control (CDC) *National Diabetes Fact Sheet* (Thomas, Palumbo, Melton, Roger, et al., 2003), as of 2002 the prevalence of diabetes mellitus in the United States was 6.3% or 18.2 million people. Included in this number are the undiagnosed persons, estimated to be 5.2 million. By comparison, in 1994, the prevalence of diabetes mellitus was 2.98% or 7.7 million people (CDC, 2003). Including only adults 20 years and older, current prevalence is 8.7% as of 2002, which is a significant increase from the 5.1% prevalence seen in adults between 1988 and 1994 (CDC, 2003). Based on 2002 data, the yearly incidence among those 20 years and older is 1.3 million. Among those younger than 20, there are approximately 206,000 with diagnosed diabetes mellitus (CDC, 2003).

Worldwide, the number of diabetes patients has also risen. Approximately 30 million people had diabetes mellitus in 1985; 10 years later, there were 135 million, and, as of 2000, the latest estimate is 177 million (Harris, Flegal, Cowie, et al., 1998).

Like other chronic diseases, diabetes mellitus is expensive. Cost of diabetes care in the United States during 2002 totaled $132 billion, including $92 billion of direct medical costs plus $40 billion of indirect costs such as disability, work loss, and premature mortality (Thomas et al., 2003). These costs are significantly higher than those incurred only 5 years earlier. In 1997, the total cost of diabetes in the United States was estimated to be $98 billion, $44 billion direct and $54 billion indirect (World Health Organization [WHO], 2002). On an individual level, the economic burden is formidable. In the United States, people with diabetes spend two to three times more money on health care than those without the condition (WHO, 2002).

The protean complications of this disease are partly to blame for the excess costs incurred. For example, those with diabetes mellitus are more likely to suffer from heart disease; in fact, the risk is the same as for those with known coronary heart disease (American Diabetes Association, 2003; WHO, 2002). In the United States, diabetes is the leading cause of new blindness in adults 20 to 65 years old, the leading cause of end-stage renal disease, and the leading cause of nontraumatic lower extremity amputations (Skyler & Oddo, 2002). People with obesity or diabetes mellitus also tend to develop liver disease, due to steatohepatitis or "fatty liver," termed nonalcoholic fatty liver disease (Li, Clark, & Diehl, 2002). Also, diabetes is associated with neurological damage and small-vessel disease, leading to lacunar brain infarcts, especially among those with type 2 diabetes (Kernan et al., 2002).

Diabetes mellitus is the fifth leading cause of death in the United States (CDC, 1997). Epidemiological data obtained over the past 10 years shows the vulnerability of those with diabetes. While coronary heart disease deaths declined by 36% among men without diabetes, only a 13% reduction occurred in men with diabetes, and among women with diabetes there was actually a 23% increase in mortality when those without diabetes had a 27% decrease in coronary heart disease death (Rennert & Charney, 2003).

Due to the comprehensive nature of this illness, the difficulties encountered with even the best treatments, and its overwhelming effects on our society, the need for prevention has come to be of utmost importance. The search for a cure is the focus of intense research, but with the increasing numbers of newly affected persons, such a milestone cannot come soon enough. Prevention of the disease is our strongest and least used weapon.

IDENTIFYING RISK FACTORS TO FOCUS PREVENTION

Depending on an individual's stage in the disease spectrum, the prevention prescription will vary. Because genetic susceptibility often plays a strong role, for some individuals prevention means not allowing disease progression or the development of complications. Some forms of diabetes mellitus are more susceptible to prevention than others. The classic subdivisions are type 1 and type 2, but, as noted, there are others as well. Approximately 15% have type 1 and about 85% have type 2 (Bate & Jerums, 2003).

The increasing obesity epidemic is associated with increased susceptibility to insulin resistance and the development of type 2 diabetes mellitus, which also has a strong genetic association. Blacks, Latinos, and American Indians (especially the Pima Indians of Arizona) have increased susceptibility to type 2 diabetes, which tends to increase in incidence after the age of 45 years. Type 1 is associated with certain immune susceptibilities that have a genetic predisposition. This condition is more common among Europoid Caucasians, with the highest incidence in those of Scandinavian origin, and the peak age of onset is 10 to 14 years. Although much research has been done in the search for the triggers of type 1 diabetes, it is less clear how this form of diabetes mellitus may be prevented.

THE SEARCH FOR PREVENTION OF TYPE 1
DIABETES MELLITUS

Type 1 diabetes mellitus (T1DM), previously known as insulin-dependent or juvenile-onset diabetes, usually develops before age 30 and is marked by insulinopenia. T1DM is an autoimmune disease that causes the gradual inflammation and destruction of the insulin-secreting pancreatic beta cells and eventually leads to complete insulin deficiency. Patients are dependent on exogenous injections of insulin for survival. T1DM is the result of a genetic predisposition, certain environmental triggers, and immune activation targeted against the insulin-producing pancreatic islet beta cells (Bate & Jerums, 2003). Preventive strategies are the focus of intense research, but a definite recommendation is not yet possible. At this time, there are no known effective universal preventive interventions.

Accurate identification of those at risk remains a crucial challenge. Some of the genes involved in T1DM are part of the major histocompatability complex on the short arm of chromosome 6 (Bate & Jerums, 2003). Several other genetic markers have been identified, but even when all known markers are present, susceptibility to disease is still not greater than 60% (Skyler, 2002). First-degree relatives of patients with T1DM have a 10- to 20-fold increase in risk for developing the disease (3% to 6% incidence) compared to the general population (0.2% to 0.3% incidence), but among those who develop the disease, 80% to 90% do not have a family history of T1DM at the time of diagnosis (Sperling, 1997).

The environmental triggers implicated are diverse, but none has been found to be a definite cause. An ongoing study, Trial to Reduce Incidence of Diabetes in the Genetically at Risk (TRIGR), was designed for the purpose of determining whether exposure to cow milk protein in early infancy may be a trigger for T1DM (Skyler & Marks, 2004). This may provide important preventive information on a topic that has been the focus of polarized debates. Also, so-called pancreotropic viruses have been implicated, including mumps, Coxsackie B4, and some enteroviruses. A proposed mechanism for viral involvement is molecular mimicry (Bate & Jerums, 2003). Data obtained from epidemiological studies suggest an association between enterovirus exposure and positive autoantibodies (Sadeharju, 2003). Molecular mimicry may also explain the relationship to exposure to cow milk protein early in infancy, which may be a diabetes trigger due to the similarity between an epitope of bovine serum albumin and certain beta cell surface proteins (Bate & Jerums, 2003). The proposed pathophysiology is that a beta cell-like antigen instigates an immune cascade mediated by T lymphocytes, specifically Th1 cells and related cytokines (Rabinovitch & Skyler, 1998).

Often, patients with T1DM present with acute symptoms of diabetic-ketoacidosis, preceded by a brief period of polydipsia, polyuria, polyphagia, and weight loss. Before this acute presentation, the disease process is ongoing but patients are asymptomatic (Gale, 2002; Skyler, 2002). Usually at the time of presentation, only about 10% to 20% of pancreatic beta cells remain (Skyler, 2002). Shortly after the initial presentation, there is an improvement in function of the remaining beta cells, until finally these, too, are destroyed (Rabinovitch & Skyler, 1998).

Early in the disease process, autoantibodies may be present. These include islet cell antibodies (ICA), insulin autoantibodies, antibodies to glutamic acid decarboxylase (GAD), and antibodies to islet antigen-2 (an abortive islet tyrosine phosphatase; Sperling, 1997). The presence of these antibodies may be used to predict the risk of T1DM, especially among the siblings of those already affected by the condition, but not everyone with all four autoantibodies develops T1DM (Skyler, 2002).

Those at risk, with T1DM-affected first-degree relatives and with presence of autoantibodies, may be screened with the intravenous glucose tolerance test to evaluate early or first-phase insulin release (FPIR). Loss of FPIR indicates that the asymptomatic individual is at an early stage in the disease process or has prediabetes (Skyler, 2002). Preventing disease progression at this stage was the focus of a multicenter trial using nicotinamide. A meta-analysis published in 1996 reviewed the effects of nicotinamide, a B-group vitamin, when given at diagnosis of T1DM, and found that it has an apparent effect in preserving beta cell function when given in addition to insulin (Pozzilli, Browne, & Kolb, 1996). This led to the European Nicotinamide Diabetes Intervention Trial (ENDIT). ENDIT evaluated this B-vitamin in asymptomatic first-degree relatives of T1DM patients who were positive for ICA (ENDIT Group, 2003). Unfortunately, preliminary results suggest that there is no preventive effect (ENDIT Group, 2004).

Prior studies aimed at preventing progression of disease have focused on treatments started at the stage of acute presentation, when 10% to 20% of beta cells may remain. Cellular immunity suppressants, cyclosporine (Canadian-European Randomized Control Trial Group, 1988; Skyler & Rabinovitch, 1992) and azathioprine (Silverstein et al., 1988), initially showed promising results, but effects were not long lasting (Bougneres et al., 1990) and the side effect profiles made them prohibitive (Skyler, 2002; Skyler & Marks, 2004).

Regulation of T lymphocyte action has been the focus of some research. Linomide, a synthetic immunomodulator, which has been demonstrated to down-regulate Th1 cells and shift the balance of T-cell activation in favor of Th2 cytokines leading to inhibition of autoimmunity and inflammation (Karussis, Abramsky, Rosenthal, Mizrachi-Koll, & Ovadia, 1999), showed some encouraging data when given at low dose for 1 year to patients with newly diagnosed T1DM (Coutant, Landais, Rosilio, Johnsen, et al., 1998). In animal studies, linomide has demonstrated efficacy in preventing autoimmune insulitis, islet cell destruction, and progression to diabetes (Gross, Weiss, Reibstein, Van den Brand, et al., 1998). However, linomide has been withdrawn from the market due to adverse effects noted in other trials not related to diabetes care or prevention. Another immunomodulator, the peptide p277 from the heat-shock protein hsp60, appears to preserve endogenous beta cell insulin production when administered to those newly diagnosed with T1DM, according to findings from a small randomized, double-blind study (Raz, Elias, Avron, et al., 2001). This requires confirmation, which has not yet been forthcoming.

Anti-CD3 monoclonal antibody has been tested with some success in the management of new-onset T1DM (Herold, Hagopian, Auger, Poumian-Ruiz, et al., 2002). CD3 is a surface molecule found on activated human T cells; anti-CD3 binds to it and results in re-regulation of the immune response (Herold et al., 2003). In animal models, disease reversal has been achieved (Chatenoud, Thervet, Primo, et al., 1994). In small human trials, this treatment has been found to mollify the decline in insulin secretion and enhance metabolic control for as long as 1 year after a daily 14-day course, without severe side effects (Herold et al., 2002). More studies are needed to confirm these positive findings.

Antigen exposure to divert the immune system's response has been tried with the administration of insulin, which is considered one of the main antigens propelling the immune reaction in T1DM. The oral administration of insulin has been studied in two randomized, double-blind, placebo-controlled studies involving newly diagnosed T1DM patients as well as in one study involving at-risk or prediabetes subjects. Even though prior animal models suggested efficacy, the human trials showed no effect (Chaillous, Lefevre, Thivolet, Boitard, et al., 2000; Pozzilli, Pitocco, Visalli, Cavallo, et al., 2000; Skyler & Marks, 2004).

Inducing beta cell rest by administration of exogenous insulin may be beneficial for slowing progression of new-onset T1DM. Two studies (one from Tampa, Florida, and the other from Munich, Germany) found that intensive treatment with insulin during the first 2 weeks after diagnosis results in greater preservation of beta cell function after 1 year (Schnell, Eisfelder, Standl, & Ziegler, 1997; Shah, Malone, & Simpson, 1989). In the nonobese diabetic (NOD) mouse model of T1DM, prolonged administration of exogenous insulin has been shown to reduce the development of diabetes mellitus and of insulitis (Skyler & Marks, 2004). In a very small pilot study with human beings, five individuals at high risk for T1DM based on the presence of autoantibodies and diminished FPIR received intravenous insulin infusions for 5 days every 9 months plus twice-daily injections of low-dose insulin. They were compared to seven similar individuals who refused such treatment. After 3 years, all seven subjects who declined to participate had developed diabetes, whereas only one of the five in the treatment group developed diabetes (Keller, Eisenbarth, & Jackson, 1993). These observations led to a full-scale randomized controlled clinical trial, the Diabetes Prevention Trial-Type 1 (DPT-1). In DPT-1, more than 84,000 first- and second-degree relatives of T1DM patients were screened for the presence of autoantibodies, genetic markers, and deficient FPIR. Among those eligible, 339 were randomly assigned to undergo close follow-up or receive low-dose subcutaneous ultralente insulin plus annual 4-day intravenous insulin infusions. After a median follow-up of 3.7 years, the two groups had a similar incidence of T1DM, indicating that either the use of insulin in the prediabetic state is ineffective for prevention or the amount used in this study was not sufficient (Diabetes Prevention Trial-Type 1 Diabetes Study Group, 2002).

On another front, immunological vaccines are being developed using antigens thought to be involved in the autoimmune process. Candidate antigens are insulin and GAD. An example is use of an insulin peptide analog using amino acids 9 to 23 of the B-chain of insulin (Alleva et al., 2002). This has been tested in NOD mice and is undergoing early trials in human beings, as is a vaccine using GAD with an adjuvant. If the environmental triggers for T1DM were known, it might be possible to develop vaccines using them as well.

In summary, although there are no current recommendations on prevention of T1DM, ongoing research efforts aimed at identifying triggers, seeking new targets for beta cell preservation, and finding ways for immune modulation may eventually show that T1DM may be prevented, delayed, or hindered.

PREVENTION OF TYPE 2 DIABETES MELLITUS

Diabetes mellitus type 2 (T2DM) is much more common than type 1 diabetes and quickly growing in incidence and prevalence. As the percentage of obese persons has increased, so has the incidence of T2DM. In fact, obesity seems to be the largest environmental influence on the development of diabetes (Herold, 2004). Unlike type 1, T2DM has known preventive strategies that have been demonstrated in randomized controlled clinical trials.

T2DM is associated with other deleterious health conditions, namely, hypertension, dyslipidemia, and obesity (American Diabetes Association and National Institute of Diabetes, Digestive and Kidney Diseases, 2002). The obesity in these persons tends to be central in nature, otherwise known as the "apple shape." This combination is known as the "metabolic syndrome," which is strongly linked to heart disease. In fact, there is a three-fold increase in risk for coronary heart disease and stroke in those with the metabolic syndrome (Haffner & Cassells, 2003; Scott, 2003). A recent study that evaluated the individual components of the metabolic syndrome among Pima Indians without diabetes found that hyperinsulinemia, body weight, and hyperlipidemia were the best predictors of eventual development of T2DM (Hanson, Imperatore, Bennet, & Knowler, 2002).

The unifying factor of the metabolic syndrome is insulin resistance; therefore, T2DM may be just one of the manifestations of this syndrome, and obesity,

Table 10. 1   The Metabolic Syndrome

Metabolic syndrome considered if patient has any three of the following components:
1. Obesity: BMI > 28, or
   Increased waist circumference:
   Men > 40 inches (102 cm)
   Women > 35 inches (88 cm)

2. Blood pressure: systolic > 130 mmHg or diastolic > 85 mmHg

3. HDL cholesterol: in men < 40 mg/dL (1.0 mmol/L), in women < 50 mg/dL
   (1.3 mmol/L)

4. Triglycerides > 150 mg/dL (1.7 mmol/L)

5. Fasting blood glucose > 110 mg/dL (6.1 mmol/L)

Not required for definition but may be part of the syndrome:
   Hyperuricemia
   Hypercoagulability
   Hyperleptinemia
   Elevated C-reactive protein (CRP) levels

Adapted from "Global and Societal Implications of the Diabetes Epidemic," by P. Zimmet, K. G. M. Alberti, and J. Shaw, 2001, *Nature, 414,* pp. 782–787; and "Metabolic Syndrome: A New Risk Factor of Coronary Heart Disease?" by S. M. Haffner and H. B. Cassells, 2003, *Diabetes, Obesity, and Metabolism, 5,* pp. 359–370.

which increases insulin resistance, may be one of the triggers. Table 10.1 details the components of the metabolic syndrome.

By the time T2DM develops, significant damage to the coronary arteries may already be present. Approximately half of those diagnosed with T2DM also have hypertension, defined as blood pressure above 140/90 mmHg; as blood pressure levels rise, so do increases in complications associated with diabetes, including cardiovascular disease (Bate & Jerums, 2003). Among those with diabetes without a history of heart disease, the risk of myocardial infarction is just as high as among those not affected by diabetes but with a prior history of myocardial infarction (Haffner et al., 1998). For this reason, the Adult Treatment Panel III executive summary from the National Cholesterol Education Program considers diabetes mellitus a coronary artery disease risk equivalent; thus, those with diabetes should be treated as intensely and with the same goals as patients with prior myocardial infarction (Grundy et al., 2004; Scott, 2003). In addition to maintaining normal glucose levels, desired goals include blood pressure less than 125/75 mmHg, low-density lipoprotein (LDL) cholesterol less than 100 mg/dL (less than 70 mg/dL if there are other high-risk factors), triglyceride level less than 150 mg/dL, and high-density lipoprotein (HDL) cholesterol greater than 40 mg/dL in men and greater than 50 mg/dL in women (Grundy et al., 2004; Scott, 2003).

Often, this requires multidrug therapy along with interventions that change modifiable risk factors.

Approximately 47 million Americans are estimated to have the metabolic syndrome (Scott, 2003). This figure is based on U.S. census figures for 2000 and the Third National Health and Nutrition Examination Survey, which determined the prevalence of the metabolic syndrome in almost 9,000 adults between 1988 and 1994 in the United States, and found it to be 24% (Haffner & Cassells, 2003). This includes those who have not yet manifested impaired glucose tolerance or impaired fasting glucose, yet, insulin resistance is present and so is the risk of T2DM. Treating this many people with medications implies classifying a large portion of the population with a chronic illness and mandates a large budget.

The adoption of "a healthier lifestyle" may be the single most important preventive strategy (Hu, Manson, Stampfer, Colditz, et al., 2001). Nonetheless, the genetic predisposition is an important aspect of the disease. Identifying those most at risk early on, before the devastating effects of the numerous complications start having any effect, seems to be the key.

The question of cost-effectiveness remains an issue. Our current screening methods for detecting diabetes mellitus or prediabetes states involve laboratory tests and follow-up visits to a health care provider. Two tests meet the American Diabetes Association (ADA) criteria as being "safe, acceptable, and predictive" (ADA and National Institute of Diabetes, Digestive and Kidney Diseases, 2002). These are the fasting plasma glucose (FPG) and the 2-hour value in the oral glucose tolerance test. A value greater than 126 mg/dL in FPG confers a diagnosis of diabetes mellitus; a value less than 126 mg/dL but greater than 100 mg/dL indicates impaired fasting glucose (IFG) and an increased risk for the development of diabetes mellitus (Expert Committee on the Diagnosis and Classification of Diabetes Mellitus, 2003). A value greater than 200 mg/dL at two hours after a 75-gram oral glucose challenge is diagnostic for diabetes mellitus; a value less than 200 mg/dL but greater than 140 mg/dL indicates impaired glucose tolerance (IGT). Currently, there is no published evidence on the cost-effectiveness of identifying those with IFG or IGT, nor is there any published study indicating that early interventions to prevent or delay diabetes and its complications are cost-effective (ADA and National Institute of Diabetes, Digestive and Kidney Diseases, 2002). Notwithstanding, it seems rational that early prevention is preferable to the current state of affairs.

The number of those with diabetes continues to grow, but the existent quality of care remains suboptimal. A report card study that analyzed national population-based cross-sectional surveys of more than 4,000 persons with diabetes found that 18.9% of participants had hemoglobin A1c levels greater than 9.5% (Saaddine, Engelgau, Beckels, Gregg, et al., 2002). Normal hemoglobin A1c is less than 6%, and the ADA-recommended target for diabetes patients is less than 7%. This study also found that 58% of the survey participants had poor lipid control and 34.3% had poor blood pressure control (Saaddine et al., 2002). Moreover, 36.7% did not receive annual eye examinations (as recommended for the early detection of diabetic retinopathy, a common cause of blindness) and 45.2% did not have frequent foot examinations (as recommended due to the high incidence of neuropathy leading to complications resulting in lower limb amputations; Saaddine et al., 2002). This indicates that a large portion of patients are not being treated adequately; therefore, many patients would be expected to develop serious complications and as a result become disabled. This in turn leads to fewer people in the workforce and more disability payments. Still, the number of those affected with diabetes is expected to remain on the upsurge worldwide. Among those with IGT, currently 200 million in the world, 40% will progress to diabetes over 5 to 10 years (Zimmet et al., 2001).

The reasons for the deficient care are unclear but may be due to the excess number of patients with diabetes combined with the inadequate insurance coverage of many, in addition to the limited time available for health care providers to care for each patient. Accordingly, aiming for decreasing the burden on the current health care system by focusing more on prevention would be beneficial. To allay costs, the least possible invasive parameters for screening should be used.

With this aim in mind, Finnish researchers developed the diabetes risk score as a predictive method (Lindstrom & Tuomilehto, 2003). They gathered information from a random population sample of people without baseline diabetes mellitus. They assigned scores to certain variables assessed in these patients and followed them for 10 years for the development of drug-treated T2DM. The validity of the scores was then tested in an independent population survey with a 5-year follow-up. This method showed sensitivity and specificity of approximately 0.8 for the score value greater than or equal to 9. The categorical variables tested were age, body mass index (BMI), waist circumference, hypertension, prior hyperglycemia, physical inactivity, and daily consumption of berries, fruits, or vegetables (Lindstrom & Tuomilehto, 2003). Table 10.2 shows the categories and scores used.

This appears to be a useful tool and should be further tested. Perhaps we will one day be able to aim for certain fasting glucose measurements to prevent disease in certain patients with elevated scores. With further development, we may be able to use this or a scoring system similar to what is currently used for recommendations for cholesterol goals based on certain risk scores. For example, the fasting glucose goal for someone with the metabolic syndrome may be lower than for those without the metabolic syndrome and otherwise healthy. As scoring systems such as this one or similar ones are implemented, we may be

Table 10.2   The Diabetes Risk Score

Category	Score
Age (Years)	
45–54	2
55–64	3
BMI	
25–30	1
> 30	3
Waist circumference	
Men, 94 to < 102 cm (37 to 40 inches)	3
Women, 80 to < 88 cm (31 to 35 inches)	3
Men, ≥ 102 cm (40 inches)	4
Women, ≥ 88 cm (35 inches)	4
Use of blood pressure medication	2
History of high blood glucose	5
Physical activity < 4 hours per week	2
Daily consumption of vegetables, fruits, or berries	1

Adapted from "The Diabetes Risk Score: A Practical Tool to Predict Type 2 Diabetes Risk," by J. Lindstrom and J. Tuomilehto, 2003, *Diabetes Care, 26,* pp. 725–731.

able to obtain objective goals for certain at-risk groups for the prevention of in-sulin resistance and T2DM.

Laboratory tests are the most direct ways of identifying those at risk for T2DM. Glucose testing in the fasting state or a two-hour postglucose challenge identifies those with IFG and IGT, respectively. The most current ADA guidelines state that fasting glucose of 100 mg/dl or greater but less than 126 mg/dl indicates impaired fasting glucose (Expert Committee on the Diagnosis and Classification of Diabetes Mellitus, 2003). Historically, the oral glucose tolerance has been used to identify the at-risk patients. However, this test is cumbersome and more costly than a sim-ple fasting glucose. There has been a greater emphasis in recent years on eliminat-ing this test completely because the fasting glucose measurement seems to provide sufficient information. A study by Stern et al. showed that there is only a minimal increase in prediction potential when the oral glucose tolerance test is added to fasting glucose (Stern, Williams, & Haffner, 2002). According to a study by Shaw et al., the current definition of IGT (glucose 140 mg/dl or greater but less than 200 mg/dl) classifies more people at risk than when using IFG using 110 mg/dl as the cut-off based on earlier criteria (Shaw et al., 2000). Identification of more people at risk may lead to greater consideration of preventive strategies. This may include medications, which could result in more individuals being labeled ill, causing them to incur additional medical expenses. However, such individuals might be prevented from developing a more serious condition and its accompanying multitude of complications.

To prevent excessive testing, a positive family history or the diabetes risk score may be used to determine who should be screened for T2DM. The ADA recommends screening to detect IFG or IGT be considered in individuals older than 45 years and strongly recommended in those who are older than 45 years and overweight (BMI > 25). Among those persons younger than 45 years, ADA suggests that screening should be considered if BMI is greater than 25 and one additional risk factor is present. Table 10.3 lists these risk factors. Although lifestyle modifications should be recommended to all patients, more specific counseling and other therapies should be reserved for those at risk or with positive screens for IFG or IGT. Several large studies have supported the idea that T2DM is a disease triggered by unhealthy habits, and a few large trials have shown that prevention is possible by correcting these habits.

Using data from the Nurses' Health Study, researchers conducted a 16-year follow up of nearly 85,000 women without prior diagnosis of diabetes, heart disease, or cancer (Hu et al., 2001). At the end of the 16 years, 3,300 new cases of T2DM were identified, approximately 4%. BMI was the most important risk factor. Obese women, defined by BMI greater than 30, had a significant increased risk of developing T2DM. The risk increased further when BMI was greater than 35. In fact, 61% of the women with T2DM were overweight (BMI of 25 or higher). More important, this study found that other lifestyle factors, independent of obesity, were also independently associated with increased risk of T2DM. These other factors were physical inactivity, poor diet, use of tobacco and alcohol. Obese women who did not have any of these other risk factors, and in fact

Table 10.3   Risk Factors for Diabetes Mellitus

Criteria for Screening

1. Age > 45 years and BMI > 25

2. Age < 45 years and BMI > 25, plus at least one of the following risk factors:
   Ethnic background other than Caucasian
   First-degree relative has diabetes mellitus
   History of gestational diabetes
   Gave birth to baby weighing more than 9 lbs
   Presence of hypertension or dyslipidemia

Adapted from "Follow-Up Report on the Diagnosis of Diabetes Mellitus," by Expert Committee on the Diagnosis and Classification of Diabetes Mellitus, 2003, *Diabetes Care, 26,* pp. 3160–3167.

were engaged in an exercise program and had a healthy diet, had less chance of development of T2DM than other obese women.

Multiple studies have shown that physical exercise may delay or prevent the development of T2DM. Additionally, aerobic exercise for at least 30 minutes with sustained heart rate of no more than 60% of predetermined maximum has several beneficial effects, including increased energy expenditure, decreased body fat, increased insulin sensitivity, improved long-term glycemic control and lipid profiles, lower blood pressure, and increased cardiovascular fitness (Hamdy, Goodyear, & Horton, 2001).

No vitamin, mineral, or herbal supplementation is known to reduce the risk of T2DM. Data extracted from the Women's Health Study suggest that magnesium supplementation may play a role in the prevention of T2DM among obese women (Song, Manson, Buring, & Liu, 2004). However, this was a weak association. Similar results were found in a large cohort of health professionals, but this study was limited in that the data were based on surveys (Lopez-Ridaura, Willet, Rimm, & Liu, 2004). Other studies have found that insulin resistance is associated with lower erythrocyte magnesium content (Paolisso & Ravussin, 1995; Roth, 2002). Although the current evidence suggests a role for magnesium, more studies are needed to determine whether treatment or supplementation with magnesium prevents the development of T2DM.

Interventional studies have shown that lifestyle modifications may indeed prevent T2DM. Thus far, there have been several important studies showing the direct effects of lifestyle modifications in selected patients. The first of these was the Malmo, Sweden, study, published in 1991. In this study, Swedish men between 47 and 49 years old with impaired glucose tolerance and diabetes were placed in an intervention group that received dietary advice for 6 months and supervised physical training for 6 months, followed by continued small group training or self-training. After 6 years, there was a relative risk reduction of 63% for developing diabetes among IGT subjects in the intervention group when compared to controls (Eriksson & Lidgarde, 1991). Also, more than 50% of those with diabetes were in remission by the end of the follow-up (Eriksson & Lidgarde, 1991). The Da Qing Study, published in 1997, selected clinics with 577 individuals with IGT and randomized the clinics into four groups (control, diet only, exercise only, and diet plus exercise; Pan, Li, Hu, Wang, et al., 1997). Each of the intervention groups was associated with reductions in risk of developing T2DM by 31% to 46% at 6 years. The Finnish Diabetes Prevention Study Group studied 522 overweight subjects with IFG. Subjects placed in the intervention group received individualized counseling regarding weight reduction, improvement of diet, and increase in physical activity. When compared to the control group, the risk of diabetes was reduced by 58% in the intervention group after an average follow-up period of just 3.2 years (Finnish Diabetes Prevention Study Group, 2001). Five goals of intervention were assessed: greater than 5% weight reduction, less than 30% fat intake, less than 10% saturated fat intake, high fiber intake, and at least 4 hours of exercise per week. Those subjects who met at least four out of five goals did not develop diabetes (49 in the intervention group and 15 in the control group). In the United States, the Diabetes Prevention Program (DPP) Research Group studied 3,234 subjects classified as having elevated fasting glucose and impaired glucose tolerance as per the 1997 criteria from the ADA. After an average follow-up period of 2.8 years, high-risk persons placed on a rigorous exercise regimen (150 minutes per week) had a 58% reduction in T2DM incidence when compared to controls (Diabetes Prevention Program Research Group, 2002). The DPP also studied metformin, which had a risk reduction of 31% compared to placebo (Diabetes Prevention Program Research Group, 2002). The effects of metformin were more pronounced for those with a higher baseline BMI, but there was greater weight loss among those in the lifestyle modification group. Metformin was most effective among those who were younger (age 24 to 44 years) and more obese (BMI at least 35; Diabetes Prevention Program Research Group, 2002).

Metformin has not been the only medication shown to play a role in the prevention of T2DM. The STOP-NIDDM trial showed that acarbose, an alpha-glucosidase inhibitor, may decrease the risk of development of T2DM among those with impaired glucose tolerance and elevated fasting glucose (Chiasson et al., 2002). Acarbose reduces postprandial hyperglycemia, which is considered to be a risk factor for cardiovascular disease. Subjects were given acarbose 100 mg before each meal three times daily, or placebo. After 3.3 years, the risk of progression to diabetes was reduced by 25% in the treatment group. Acarbose also caused reversal of IGT (Chiasson et al., 2002). Further, acarbose was found to be associated with significant reductions in incidence of newly diagnosed hypertension and cardiovascular events, thus supporting the theory of postprandial hyperglycemia as a cardiovascular risk factor (Chiasson et al., 2002).

The TRIPOD (troglitazone in prevention of diabetes) trial introduced the potential preventive benefits of thiazolidinedione drugs (Buchanan, Xiang, Peters, Kjos, et al., 2002). Hispanic women with a prior history of gestational diabetes received a placebo or the now discontinued drug troglitazone for 3 months. Women treated with troglitazone 400 mg daily had an 88% increase in insulin sensitivity, with a proportional decrease in insulin output. At the end of the 3-month trial, women in the treatment group required less endogenous insulin to maintain stable glucose tolerance. These changes persisted 8 months after the end of treatment, as assessed by a follow-up visit. By this point, the incidence of diabetes in the placebo group was 12.1%, and only 6% in the troglitazone group, without significant differences in weight between the two groups. Posttrial follow-up data revealed that the annual incidence rate of T2DM in the placebo group was 21.2% and in the troglitazone group was 3.1%. Thus, the researchers concluded that the brief intervention with troglitazone must have preserved beta cell function, leading to long-term benefits such as delay or prevention of diabetes (Buchanan et al., 2002). The TRIPOD study showed that the natural history of glucose intolerance may be affected by troglitazone, leading to prevention of diabetes mellitus (Buchanan et al., 2002). Troglitazone, however, was removed from the market due to associations with liver failure. Nevertheless, other thiazolidinediones (pioglitazone and rosiglitazone) remain in use with better safety profiles and are being studied for effects on preventing T2DM.

The average follow-up time in most of the studies described was 2 to 6 years, which means that the interventions are effective within a relatively short period. In fact, even for those who are still euglycemic but have insulin resistance, an intensive lifestyle modification, including 150 minutes per week of exercise and improved dietary habits, may improve insulin sensitivity after only a few months (McAuley, Williams, Mann, Goulding, et al., 2002). McAuley et al. studied 79 subjects who were normoglycemic but had insulin resistance as measured by the euglycemic insulin clamp. They were divided into three groups, one serving as control, one following the standard recommendations, and the third following a more intense dietary and exercise program. Only the group following the intense intervention program had reduction in insulin resistance, as measured by euglycemic insulin clamp, after 4 months, even though amount of weight loss was similar in both lifestyle modification groups. Other significant changes in the intense group were in waist circumference, BMI, body fat, and blood pressure (McAuley et al., 2002). These findings are neither surprising nor based on any novel ideas. In fact, since 1970, several studies have shown that physical training results in lower insulin concentrations and improved insulin sensitivity (Hamdy et al., 2001). Because insulin resistance often leads to T2DM, McAuley's study supports the notion that a healthy lifestyle, more rigorous than the current recommendations, should be promoted to the general public as part of a public campaign for diabetes prevention.

Intensive lifestyle modification, including both improvement of diet and increase in exercise, makes good sense as a preventive strategy for at-risk or prediabetic patients (those with elevated fasting glucose and those with impaired glucose tolerance). However, because physicians usually more easily write a prescription than provide counseling and education, just as some patients would sooner take a pill than make drastic lifestyle changes, the results of the DPP should be emphasized whenever there is a discussion of prevention options.

Treatment with medication—metformin, acarbose, or a thiazolidinedione—as part of a preventive regimen may turn out to be useful, but currently there is reluctance to initiate such a strategy.

The ADA recommends that initial goals focus on modest weight loss, 5% to 10% of body weight, and modest physical activity, 30 minutes daily, for nearly all patients who are either overweight or sedentary. Currently, the ADA does not recommend drug therapy for prevention of diabetes due to insufficient evidence of benefits and the recent data showing the superiority of lifestyle modifications in the short term (American Diabetes Association and National Institute of Diabetes, Digestive and Kidney Diseases, 2002). Nonetheless, the studies mentioned previously suggest that there is likely a role for medications in selected groups. More studies are needed to determine long-term effects of prevention via medications because side effects will have to be taken into account in any risk-benefit analysis. The ADA position statement emphasizes that of the available drugs, only the biguanide metformin has outcome data suggesting possible effectiveness in reducing the incidence of macrovascular complications (American Diabetes Association and National Institute of Diabetes, Digestive and Kidney Diseases, 2002).

When the metabolic syndrome is present with or without IFG or IGT, certain drug therapies have been shown to be beneficial. However, glycemic control has not been evaluated independently in this setting. The HMG CoA reductase inhibitors, antilipid agents otherwise known as statins, and antihypertensive agents—namely, angiotensin-converting-enzyme (ACE) inhibitors or angiotensin receptor blockers—have been shown to improve outcomes (Haffner & Cassells, 2003).

Weight loss, when appropriate, is a critical step for the prevention of diabetes. Medical treatment of obesity may also play a role in the management of metabolic syndrome to reduce the risk of diabetes. Recent studies have focused on orlistat, a gastrointestinal lipase inhibitor that reduces fat absorption. In a group of 120 IGT subjects who were placed on either orlistat or placebo, after 1.5 years there was a decreased incidence of diabetes in the orlistat group when compared to placebo (3% versus 7.6%), and more of those in the orlistat group, 71.6%, returned to normal glucose tolerance than those in the placebo group, 49.1% (Heymsfield, 2000). Studies evaluating the effects of surgical treatment of obesity have also shown that weight loss is directly linked to decreased incidence of diabetes (Sjöström, Peltonen, Wedel, & Sjöström, 2000).

Thus far, one study has found an association with use of pravastatin and decreased incidence of diabetes (Freeman, 2001). In this study, the development of diabetes was a secondary end point in a study for the evaluation of coronary event prevention. A small percentage of the subjects developed diabetes. Those who had been placed on pravastatin had a 30% reduction in the risk of developing diabetes.

The cardiovascular benefits of ACE-inhibitors have been noted in many trials (Gottlieb, Leor, Shotan, Harpaz, et al., 2003). In the Heart Outcomes Prevention Evaluation (HOPE) Study, patients 55 years and older, identified as high-risk because of evidence of vascular disease or diabetes, received ramipril 10 mg or placebo (vitamin E) daily for 5 years (Heart Outcomes Prevention Evaluation Study Investigators, 2000a). The risk of myocardial infarction, stroke, and all causes of mortality was significantly reduced in the ramipril group. In addition, secondary end points, such as the risk of new diagnosis of diabetes mellitus or the development of diabetes complications, were reduced in the ramipril group (Heart Outcomes Prevention Evaluation Study Investigators, 2000b). Other studies have shown that ACE-inhibitors, as well as angiotensin receptor blockers (ARBs), prevent diabetes via increased insulin sensitivity (McFarlane, Kumar, & Sowers, 2003). In addition, ACE-inhibitors and ARBs have shown efficacy in reducing proteinuria and microalbuminuria (Goldberg, 2003; Skyler, 2001). Because microalbuminuria is closely associated with cardiovascular morbidity and mortality, ACE-inhibitors and ARBs have important roles in the treatment of hypertension as well as in the prevention of diabetes and its complications.

The metabolic syndrome, the prediabetic state, and diabetes mellitus are all pro-coagulant and pro-inflammatory states with increased risk of cardiovascular morbidity and mortality. Specifically, those who have diabetes have multiple abnormalities in platelet function, coagulation, and fibrinolysis (Goldberg, 2003). Therefore, aspirin therapy should always be part of the preventive regimen (Colwell, 1997).

Oral hypoglycemic agents should be instituted if the hemoglobin A1c level is greater than 7%. Although this is the ADA recommendation, there actually is increased risk for adverse outcomes even at A1c levels greater than 6%. According to a study from the United Kingdom, the predictive value of hemoglobin A1c for all-cause mortality was stronger than for cholesterol concentration, BMI, and blood pressure. Men with levels above 5% had greater risk than men with levels below 5% (Khaw, Wareham, Luben, Bingham, et al., 2001). Furthermore, a hemoglobin A1c elevation of 1% among men without diabetes was associated with a 28% increased risk of death independent of other risk factors.

Conclusions about Type 2 Diabetes Mellitus

In summary, there is ample evidence that T2DM may be prevented in certain circumstances, namely, among those with obesity or the metabolic syndrome. Most studies on prevention have focused on patients with prediabetes, that is, IFG or

IGT. The preventive strategies may be even more efficacious among those who are at risk of developing prediabetes. Currently, we have no proven screening methods for detecting those at risk for prediabetes, but we may use parameters that are associated with insulin resistance, such as the criteria for metabolic syndrome, the diabetes risk score, and family history.

Given the available evidence, obesity should be considered a serious medical condition and must be treated with evidenced-based interventions, although not necessarily with medications unless other risk factors are present. Lifestyle modifications must be rigorous and continuous. This may involve additional costs for prevention modalities, such as dietitian counseling, supervised exercise programs, and other interventions designed to modify behavior such as psychological counseling or support groups. Knowing the devastating consequences and progressive nature of prediabetes, the metabolic syndrome, and T2DM, using medications with proven efficacy in prevention (the biguanide metformin, thiazolidinediones, the alpha glucosidase inhibitor acarbose, ACE inhibitors, statins, and orlistat) should not be delayed when lifestyle modifications are not successful.

PREVENTION OF COMPLICATIONS IN DIABETES MELLITUS

Those already affected by diabetes mellitus also benefit from intense lifestyle modification. Often, when medications seem to have failed to achieve goals, the culprits remain poor dietary and exercise habits. Physical exercise results in improved utilization of glucose, which may last between 2 to 7 days after cessation of exercise, and habitual physical training is linked to lower glycosylated hemoglobin concentrations. This occurs because exercise, via contraction of muscle, results in the translocation of the glucose transporter GLUT4 to the surface of cells, thus facilitating the mobilization of glucose. Insulin has a similar effect on muscle (Hamdy et al., 2001). A Swedish study showed that patients with uncontrolled diabetes had improved management after 31 weeks of a dedicated exercise program and dietary education. Glycohemoglobin came down by approximately 1%, and there were significant reductions in weight and blood pressure. Also, HDL cholesterol increased significantly (Krook, Holm, Pettersson, & Wallberg-Henriksson, 2003).

Once diabetes mellitus develops, strict control of hypertension and cholesterol, as well as tight glucose control, are the main goals. Besides the important lifestyle modifications, including education about glycemic content of foods, specific interventions that affect cardiovascular risk should be implemented. For example, smoking cessation is essential because, in addition to its effects on cardiovascular disease and peripheral vascular disease, it is implicated in the progression of nephropathy in T2DM patients (Chuahirun, Khanna, Kimball, & Wesson, 2003). Weight loss, when appropriate (BMI > 25), should be a major aim. The benefits of weight loss include improved glycemic control and lipid profile, reduced fasting insulin, increased insulin sensitivity, and reduced blood pressure (Herold, 2004). There are certain medications that confer benefits beyond their specific use. These medications include the statins and the ACE-inhibitors. Statins provide protection against cardiovascular disease while bringing LDL cholesterol levels to goal (Gotto, 2002), and some studies suggest that ACE-inhibitors also provide cardiovascular protection in addition to reducing blood pressure (Goldberg, 2003). ACE-inhibitors also provide protection against progression of nephropathy (Skyler, 2001). ARBs provide renal protection in addition to lowering blood pressure among patients with T2DM (Raij, 2003).

Some oral hypoglycemic agents also have beneficial uses beyond their glycemic control. Metformin improves insulin sensitivity while promoting weight loss in some obese patients, and it may provide a reduction in mortality, including cardiovascular mortality (U.K. Prospective Diabetes Study [UKPDS] Group, 1998a). Thiazolidinediones, via anti-inflammatory properties, may improve endothelial function. Studies have shown reduction in carotid intimal wall thickness, decreased episodes of silent ischemia, and improved vascular reactivity (Koshiyama, Shimono, Kuwamura, Minamikawa, & Nakamura, 2001).

The Diabetes Control and Complications Trial showed that patients who had more intense glycemic control had less risk of retinopathy and nephropathy, as well as preservation of residual endogenous insulin secretion (Diabetes Control and Complications Trial Research Group, 1993). The UKPDS also showed reduced retinopathy and nephropathy among those with tighter glucose control (UKPDS Group, 1998b; Stratton et al., 2000).

Preventing the complications of diabetes becomes paramount to treat this disease in the most cost-effective way. Diabetes complications often lead to permanent disability and dramatic increase in health care costs. Therefore, frequent screening for these complications is necessary. This includes at least yearly assessment for fasting lipid levels, urinary excretion of albumin, retinal eye exams for evaluation of proliferative retinopathy, and foot exams. Starting the medications that have been shown to slow progression of disease (such as aspirin, ACE-inhibitors, and statins) in a timely manner is crucial. In addition, thorough education on a regular basis is important. Prevention of infection is necessary;

this includes yearly dental care and administration of vaccines such as for influenza and tetanus. Patients must be active participants in their care and must be aware of all the potential complications of diabetes.

Once complications occur, the same goals should be sought to minimize progression in addition to focusing on secondary prevention. Additional medications may be needed at this stage.

PRACTICE AND POLICY IMPLICATIONS

In light of the medical costs involved in treating diabetes mellitus and its complications, the increasing incidence and prevalence, the resulting high rates of disability and mortality among those affected, and the difficulties in reversing disease progression, greater focus must be placed on prevention of the two main forms of the disease. Public awareness campaigns and continued research funding must become higher priorities.

For the prevention of type 1 diabetes, trials will have to continue in search of the environmental triggers that may be avoided, the medications that may be used in the early stages, and the vaccines that may one day offer immunity. The public, especially parents, must be educated about this condition and its implications. The importance of study participation should be emphasized. Further, other animal models in addition to the nonobese diabetic mice should be considered for the development of new treatments. NOD mice have shown response to treatments that were later found to be ineffective in humans. The identification of individuals at risk may not be occurring early enough to demonstrate efficacy in preventive strategies. Thus, better identification methods must be developed.

For the prevention of type 2 diabetes, education of the public is crucial. This is a disease that is centered around behavioral and lifestyle problems. Type 2 diabetes affects those with high caloric intake habits and sedentary lives. This behavior pattern is becoming more prevalent in the industrialized, developed nations, and its impact is increasingly affecting younger generations. Obesity leading to insulin resistance is the main mechanism of T2DM, and both obesity and T2DM have risen dramatically in the past decade. The health care costs and complications associated with T2DM warrant urgent attention to prevention. Evidence strongly supports dietary discretions and cardiovascular physical exercise for a total of 150 minutes weekly leading to weight reduction for those with BMI of 25 or greater. For those with the metabolic syndrome, itself a risk factor for cardiovascular disease, the addition of medications shown to delay the progression to T2DM should also be considered. Although this may mean labeling someone ill who may not even develop T2DM, the fact remains that obesity with insulin resistance, the metabolic syndrome, and prediabetes (IFG, IGT) are all associated with adverse outcomes. There may be better promotion of healthy lifestyle modifications when this is part of a serious medical intervention regimen.

FUTURE DIRECTIONS

New knowledge about type 1 diabetes should expand in the next decade as large trials provide a large database of information, inspiring further research. In addition, efforts to develop a vaccine or a way to control the immune system's attack on beta cells may provide more effective tools in the prevention and early treatment of this disease.

Detailed instruction on diet and exercise, along with safe medications for metabolism control and prevention or delay of type 2 diabetes, should be part of the usual office visit. As the recent trials become the mainstay in public policy, the primary care visit may become more multifaceted, meaning more time and greater active patient involvement. For this to be done effectively, it will have to be reflected on insurance policies in the form of health provider compensation for more time spent on counseling and education.

REFERENCES

Alleva, D. G., Gaur, A., Jin, L., Wegmann, D., Gottlieb, P. A., Pahuja, A., et al. (2002). Immunological characterization and therapeutic activity of an altered-peptide ligand, NBI-6024, Based on the immunodominant type 1 diabetes autoantigen insulin B-Chain (9–23). *Peptide Diabetes, 51,* 2126–2134.

American Diabetes Association. (2003). Economic costs of diabetes in the U.S. in 2002. *Diabetes Care, 26,* 917–932.

American Diabetes Association and National Institute of Diabetes, Digestive and Kidney Diseases. (2002). The prevention or delay of type 2 diabetes: Position statement. *Diabetes Care, 25,* 742–749.

Bate, K. L., & Jerums, G. (2003). Preventing complications of diabetes. *Medical Journal of Australia, 179*(9), 498–503.

Bougneres, P. F., Landais, P., Boisson, C., Carel, J. C., Frament, N., Boitard, C., et al. (1990). Limited duration of remission of insulin dependency in children with recent overt type 1 diabetes treated with low-dose cyclosporine. *Diabetes, 39,* 1264–1272.

Buchanan, T. A., Xiang, A. H., Peters, R. K., Kjos, S. L., et al. (2002). Preservation of pancreatic Beta-cell function and prevention of type 2 diabetes by pharmacological treatment of insulin resistance in high-risk Hispanic women. *Diabetes, 51,* 2796–2803.

Canadian-European Randomized Control Trial Group. (1988). Cyclosporin-induced remission of IDDM after early intervention: Association of 1 year of cyclosporin treatment with enhanced insulin secretion. *Diabetes, 37,* 1574–1582.

Centers for Disease Control and Prevention. (1997, October). Trends in the prevalence and incidence of self-reported diabetes mellitus: United States 1980–1994. *Morbidity and Mortality Weekly Report,* 46:1014–1018.

Centers for Disease Control and Prevention. (2003, November). National Diabetes Fact Sheet. Rockville, MD: U.S. Department of Health and Human Services.

Chaillous, L., Lefevre, H., Thivolet, C., Boitard, C., Lahlou, N., Atlan-Gepner, C., et al. (2000). Oral insulin administration and residual beta cell function in recent onset type 1 diabetes: A multicentre randomized controlled trial. *Lancet, 356,* 545–549.

Chatenoud, L., Thervet, E., Primo, J., & Bach, J. F. (1994). Anti-CD3 antibody induces long-term remission of overt autoimmunity in nonobese diabetic mice. *Proceedings of the National Academy of Sciences, USA, 91*(1), 123–127.

Chiasson, J. L., Josse, R. G., Gomis, R., Hanefeld, M., Karasik, A., & Laakso, M. (2002). Acarbose for prevention of type 2 diabetes mellitus: The STOP-NIDDM randomized trial. *Lancet, 359,* 2072–2077.

Chuahirun, T., Khanna, A., Kimball, K., & Wesson, D. E. (2003). Cigarette smoking and increased urine albumin excretion are interrelated predictors of nephropathy progression in type 2 diabetes. *American Journal of Kidney Diseases, 41,* 13–21.

Colwell, J. A. (1997). Aspirin therapy in diabetes (Technical Review). *Diabetes Care, 20,* 1767–1771.

Coutant, R., Landais, P., Rosilio, M., Johnsen, C., Lahlou, N., Chatelain, P., et al. (1998). Low dose linomide in type 1 diabetes of recent onset: A randomized placebo-controlled double blind trial. *Diabetologia, 41,* 1040–1046.

Diabetes Control and Complications Trial Research Group. (1993). The effect of intensive treatment of diabetes on the development and progression of long-term complications in insulin-dependent diabetes mellitus. *New England Journal of Medicine, 329,* 683–689.

Diabetes Prevention Program Research Group. (2002). Reduction in the incidence of type 2 diabetes with lifestyle intervention or metformin. *New England Journal of Medicine, 346,* 393–403.

Diabetes Prevention Trial—Type 1 Diabetes Study Group. (2002). Effects of insulin in relatives of patients with type 1 diabetes mellitus. *New England Journal of Medicine, 346,* 1685–1691.

Eriksson, K. F., & Lidgarde, F. (1991). Prevention of type 2 (non-insulin-dependent) diabetes mellitus by diet and physical exercise: The 6-year Malmo feasibility study. *Diabetologia, 34*(12), 891–898.

European Nicotinamide Diabetes Intervention Trial Group. (2003). Intervening before the onset of Type 1 diabetes: Baseline data from the European Nicotinamide Diabetes Intervention Trial (ENDIT). *Diabetologia, 46,* 339–346.

European Nicotinamide Diabetes Intervention Trial Group. (2004). European Nicoti-namide Diabetes Intervention Trial (ENDIT): A randomised controlled trial of in-tervention before the onset of type 1 diabetes. *Lancet, 363,* 925–931.

Expert Committee on the Diagnosis and Classification of Diabetes Mellitus. (2003). Follow-up report on the diagnosis of diabetes mellitus. *Diabetes Care, 26,* 3160–3167.

Finnish Diabetes Prevention Study Group. (2001). Prevention of type 2 diabetes melli-tus by changes in lifestyle among subjects with impaired glucose tolerance. *New England Journal of Medicine, 344,* 1343–1350.

Freeman, D. J. (2001). Pravastatin and the development of diabetes mellitus: Evidence for a protective treatment effect in the West of Scotland Coronary Prevention Study. *Circulation, 103*(3), 346–347.

Gale, E. A. M. (2002). Can we change the course of beta cell destruction in type 1 di-abetes? *New England Journal of Medicine, 346*(22), 1740–1742.

Goldberg, R. B. (2003). Cardiovascular disease in patients who have diabetes. *Cardiol-ogy Clinics, 21*(3), 399–413.

Gottlieb, S., Leor, J., Shotan, A., Harpaz, D., Boyko, V., Rott, D., et al. (2003). Com-parison of effectiveness of angiotensin-converting enzyme inhibitors after acute myocardial infarction in diabetic versus nondiabetic patients. *American Journal of Cardiology, 92*(9), 1020–1025.

Gotto, A. M. (2002). Lipid management in diabetic patients: Lessons from prevention trials. *American Journal of Medicine, 112*(8A), 19S–26S.

Gross, D. J., Weiss, L., Reibstein, I., Van den Brand, J., et al. (1998). Amelioration of diabetes in nonobese diabetic mice with advanced disease by linomide-induced immunoregulation combined with reg protein treatment. *Endocrinology, 139,* 2369–2374.

Grundy, S. M., Cleeman, J. I., Merz, C. N., Brewer, H. B., Jr., Clark, L. T., Hunning-hake, D. B., et al. (2004). Implications of recent clinical trials for the National Cholesterol Education Program Adult Treatment Panel III guidelines. *Circulation, 110,* 227–239.

Haffner, S. M., & Cassells, H. B. (2003). Metabolic syndrome: A new risk factor of coronary heart disease? *Diabetes, Obesity, and Metabolism, 5,* 359–370.

Haffner, S. M., Lehto, S., Ronnemaa, T., Pyorala, K., & Laakso, M. (1998). Mortality from coronary heart disease in subjects with type 2 diabetes and in nondiabetic subjects with and without prior myocardial infarctions. *New England Journal of Medicine, 339,* 229–234.

Hamdy, O., Goodyear, L. J., & Horton, E. S. (2001). Diet and exercise in type 2 dia-betes mellitus. *Endocrinology and Metabolism Clinics, 30*(4), 883–907.

Hanson, R. L., Imperatore, G., Bennet, P. H., & Knowler, W. C. (2002). Components of the "metabolic syndrome" and incidence of type 2 diabetes. *Diabetes, 51,* 3120–3127.

Harris, M. I., Flegal, K. M., Cowie, C. C., et al. (1998). Prevalence of diabetes, im-paired fasting glucose, and impaired glucose tolerance in U.S. adults: The Third

National Health and Nutrition Examination Survey, 1988–1994. *Diabetes Care, 21*(4), 475–476.

Heart Outcomes Prevention Evaluation Study Investigators. (2000a). Effects of an angiotensin converting enzyme inhibitor, ramipril, on cardiovascular events in high risk patients. *New England Journal of Medicine, 342*, 145–153.

Heart Outcomes Prevention Evaluation Study Investigators. (2000b). Effects of ramipril on cardiovascular and microvascular outcomes in people with diabetes mellitus: Results of the HOPE study and MICRO-HOPE substudy. *Lancet, 355*, 253–259.

Herold, K. C. (2004). Achieving antigen specific immune regulation. *Journal of Clinical Investigation, 113*, 346–349.

Herold, K. C., Burton, J. B., Francois, F., Poumian-Ruiz, E., Glandt, M., & Bluestone, J. A. (2003). Activation of human T cells by FcR non-binding anti-CD3 mAb, hOKT3γ1(Ala-Ala). *Journal of Clinical Investigation, 11*, 409–418.

Herold, K. C., Hagopian, W., Auger, J. A., Poumian-Ruiz, E., et al. (2002). Anti-CD3 monoclonal antibody in new-onset type 1 diabetes mellitus. *New England Journal of Medicine, 346*(22), 1692–1698.

Heymsfield, S. B. (2000). Effects of weight loss with orlistat on glucose tolerance and progression to type 2 diabetes in obese adults. *Archives of Internal Medicine, 160*(9), 1321–1326.

Hu, F. B., Manson, J. E., Stampfer, M. J., Colditz, G., et al. (2001). Diet, lifestyle, and the risk of type 2 diabetes mellitus in women. *New England Journal of Medicine, 345*, 790–797.

Karussis, D., Abramsky, O., Rosenthal, Y., Mizrachi-Koll, R., & Ovadia, H. (1999). Linomide downregulates autoimmunity through induction of Th2 cytokine production by lymphocytes. *Immunology Letters, 67*, 203–208.

Keller, R. J., Eisenbarth, G. S., & Jackson, R. A. (1993). Insulin prophylaxis in individuals at high risk of type 1 diabetes. *Lancet, 341*, 927–928.

Kernan, W. N., Inzucchi, S. E., Viscoli, C. M., Brass, L. M., Bravata, D. M., & Horwitz, R. I. (2002). Insulin resistance and risk for stroke. *Neurology, 59*(6), 809–815.

Khaw, K. T., Wareham, N., Luben, R., Bingham, S., et al. (2001). Glycated haemoglobin, diabetes, and mortality in men in Norfolk cohort of European prospective investigation of cancer and nutrition (EPIC-Norfolk). *British Medical Journal, 322*, 1–6.

Koshiyama, H., Shimono, D., Kuwamura, N., Minamikawa, J., & Nakamura, Y. (2001). Rapid communication: Inhibitory effect of pioglitazone on carotid arterial wall thickness in type 2 diabetes. *Journal of Clinical Endocrinology and Metabolism, 86*, 3452–3456.

Krook, A., Holm, I., Pettersson, S., & Wallberg-Henriksson, H. (2003). Reduction of risk factors following lifestyle modification program in subjects with type 2 (non-insulin dependent) diabetes mellitus. *Clinical Physiology and Functional Imaging, 23*, 21–30.

Li, Z., Clark, J., & Diehl, A. M. (2002). The liver in obesity and type 2 diabetes mellitus. *Clinics in Liver Disease, 6*(4), 867–877.

Lindstrom, J., & Tuomilehto, J. (2003). The diabetes risk score: A practical tool to predict type 2 diabetes risk. *Diabetes Care, 26,* 725–731.

Lopez-Ridaura, R., Willet, W. C., Rimm, E. B., & Liu, S. (2004). Magnesium intake and risk of type 2 diabetes in men and women. *Diabetes Care, 27,* 134–140.

McAuley, K. A., Williams, S. M., Mann, J. I., Goulding, A., Chisholm, A., Wilson, N., et al. (2002). Intensive Lifestyle changes are necessary to improve insulin sensitivity: A randomized controlled trial. *Diabetes Care, 25,* 445–452.

McFarlane, S. I., Kumar, A., & Sowers, J. R. (2003). Mechanisms by which angiotensin-converting enzyme inhibitors prevent diabetes and cardiovascular disease. *American Journal of Cardiology, 91*(Suppl. 12A), 30H–37H.

Pan, X. R., Li, G. W., Hu, Y. H., Wang, J. X., Yang, W. Y., An, Z. X., et al. (1997). Effects of diet and exercise in preventing NIDDM in people with impaired glucose tolerance: The Da Qing IGT and Diabetes Study. *Diabetes Care, 20,* 537–544.

Paolisso, G., & Ravussin, E. (1995). Intracellular magnesium and insulin resistance: Results in Pima Indians and Caucasians. *Journal of Clinical Endocrinology and Metabolism, 80*(4), 1382–1385.

Pozzilli, P., Browne, P. D., & Kolb, H. (1996). Meta-analysis of nicotinamide treatment in patients with recent-onset IDDM. The nicotinamide trialists. *Diabetes Care, 19*(12), 1357–1363.

Pozzilli, P., Pitocco, D., Visalli, N., Cavallo, M. G., et al. (2000). No effect of oral insulin on residual beta-cell function in recent-onset type 1 diabetes (the IMDIAB VII). *Diabetologia, 43,* 1000–1004.

Rabinovitch, A. R., & Skyler, J. S. (1998). Prevention of type 1 diabetes. *Medical Clinics of North America, 82*(4), 739–755.

Raij, L. (2003). Recommendations for the management of special populations: Renal disease in diabetes. *American Journal of Hypertension, 16,* 46S–49S.

Raz, I., Elias, D., Avron, A., et al. (2001). B-cell function in new-onset type 1 diabetes and immunomodulation with a heat-shock protein peptide (DiaPep277): A randomized, double-blind, phase II trial. *Lancet, 358,* 1749–1753.

Rennert, N. J., & Charney, P. (2003). Preventing cardiovascular disease in diabetes and glucose intolerance: Evidence and implications of care. *Primary Care: Clinics in Office Practice, 30*(3), 569–592.

Roth, A. (2002). Diabetes mellitus and obesity. *Primary Care: Clinics in Office Practice, 29*(2), 279–295.

Saaddine, J. B., Engelgau, M. M., Beckels, G. L., Gregg, E. W., et al. (2002). A diabetes report card for the United States: Quality of care in the 1990s. *Annals of Internal Medicine, 136,* 565–574.

Sadeharju, K. (2003). Enterovirus infections as a risk factor for type 1 diabetes: Virus analyses in a dietary intervention trial. *Clinical and Experimental Immunology, 132*(2), 271–277.

Schnell, O., Eisfelder, B., Standl, E., & Ziegler, A. G. (1997). High-dose intravenous insulin infusion versus intensive insulin treatment in newly diagnosed IDDM. *Diabetes, 46,* 1607–1611.

Scott, C. L. (2003). Diagnosis, prevention, and intervention for the metabolic syndrome. *American Journal of Cardiology, 92*(Suppl. 1A), 35i–43i.

Shah, S. C., Malone, J. I., & Simpson, N. E. (1989). A randomized trial of intensive insulin therapy in newly diagnosed type i insulin-dependent diabetes mellitus. *New England Journal of Medicine, 320,* 550–554.

Shaw, J. E., Zimmet, P. Z., Hodge, A. M., De Courten, M., Dowse G. K., Chitson, P., et al. (2000). Impaired fasting glucose: How low should it go? *Diabetes Care, 23,* 34–39.

Silverstein, J., Maclaren, N., Riley, W., Spillar, R., Radjenovic, D., & Johnson, S. (1988). Immunosuppression with Azathioprine and Prednisone in recent onset insulin-dependent diabetes mellitus. *New England Journal of Medicine, 319,* 599–604.

Sjostrom, C. D., Peltonen, M., Wedel, H., & Sjostrom, L. (2000). Differentiated long-term effects of intentional weight loss on diabetes and hypertension. *Hypertension, 36,* 20–25.

Skyler, J. S. (2001). Microvascular complications: Retinopathy and nephropathy. *Endocrinology and Metabolism Clinics of North America, 30*(4), 833–856.

Skyler, J. S. (2002). Prevention of type 1 diabetes. In R. Williams, W. Herman, A. L. Kinmouth, & N. J. Wareham (Eds), *The evidence base for diabetes care* (pp. 45–68). West Sussex, England: Wiley.

Skyler, J. S., & Marks, J. B. (2004). Immune intervention: Diabetes mellitus. Immune Intervention. In D. LeRoith, S. I. Taylor, & J. M. Olefsky (Eds.), *Diabetes mellitus: A fundamental and clinical text* (3rd ed., pp. 701–709). Philadelphia: Lippincott-Williams & Wilkins.

Skyler, J. S., & Oddo, C. (2002). Diabetes trends in the USA. *Diabetes/Metabolism Research and Reviews, 18,* S21–S26.

Skyler, J. S., Rabinovitch, A., & Miami Cyclosporine Diabetes Study Group. (1992). Cyclosporine in recent onset type 1 diabetes mellitus: Effects on Islet Beta Cell function. *Journal of Diabetes and Its Complications, 6,* 77–88.

Song, Y., Manson, J. E., Buring, J. E., & Liu, S. (2004). Dietary magnesium intake in relation to plasma insulin levels and risk of type 2 diabetes in women. *Diabetes Care, 27,* 59–65.

Sperling, M. A. (1997). Aspects of the etiology, prediction, and prevention of insulin-dependent diabetes mellitus in childhood. *Pediatric Clinics of North America, 44*(2), 269–284.

Stern, M. P., Williams, K., & Haffner, S. M. (2002). Identification of persons at high risk for type 2 diabetes mellitus: Do we need the oral glucose tolerance test? *Annals of Internal Medicine, 136,* 575–581.

Stratton, I. M., Adler, A. I., Neil, H. A. W., Matthews, D. R., Manley, S. E., Cull, C. A., et al. (2000). Association of glycaemia with macrovascular and microvascular complications of type 2 diabetes (UKPDS 35): Prospective observational study. *British Medical Journal, 321,* 405–412.

Thomas, R. J., Palumbo, P. J., Melton, J., Roger, V. L., et al. (2003). Trends in the mortality burden associated with diabetes mellitus. *Archives of Internal Medicine, 163,* 445–451.

U.K. Prospective Diabetes Study Group. (1998a). Effect of intensive blood-glucose control with metformin on complications in overweight patients with type 2 diabetes (UKPDS 34). *Lancet, 352,* 854–865.

U.K. Prospective Diabetes Study Group. (1998b). Intensive blood glucose control with sulphonylureas or insulin compared with conventional treatment and risk of complications in patients with type 2 diabetes (UKPDS 33). *Lancet, 352,* 837–853.

World Health Organization. (2002, September). *The cost of diabetes* [Fact Sheet No. 236]. Geneva, Switzerland: Author.

Zimmet, P., Alberti, K. G. M., & Shaw, J. (2001). Global and societal implications of the diabetes epidemic. *Nature, 414,* 782–787.

Chapter 11

BREAST CANCER

CINDY DAVIS

Breast cancer is the most common cancer among women in the United States, excluding skin cancer (American Cancer Society [ACS], 2003). Breast cancer generally begins in the breast tissues and then can invade the surrounding tissues. It can also spread to other parts of the body and form new tumors, a process called metastasis (Grayson, 2003). Most types of tumors that form in the breast are benign, or not cancerous. Some cancerous breast tumors are in situ breast cancers that are confined within the ducts (ductal carcinom in situ) or lobules (lobular carcinoma in situ). Most breast cancers at this stage can be cured; in fact, many oncologists view this type of cancer as not a "true" cancer but an indicator of increased risk for the development of invasive cancer. Other cancerous breast tumors are invasive and have infiltrated into the surrounding fatty tissues of the breast. The seriousness of invasive breast cancer is determined by the stage of the disease: local stage (tumors confined to the breast), regional stage (tumors that have spread to surrounding tissue or lymph nodes), and distant stage (tumors that have spread to distant organs; ACS, 2003).

Early detection is the most important factor in increasing survival among women with breast cancer; however, early-stage breast cancer, when the tumor is small and most treatable, typically does not produce any symptoms. The most common symptom of breast cancer is a painless mass or lump, which may feel as small as a pea; however, up to 10% of patients have breast pain without a mass. Less common symptoms include a change in the size, shape, or contour of the breast; a lump or thickening in or near the breast or in the underarm that persists through the menstrual cycle; nipple discharge; and a change in the feel or appearance of the nipple (ACS, 2003; Grayson, 2003).

After a diagnosis of breast cancer is made, an optimal treatment plan should be developed by the patient and her physician based on the type of cancer and stage of development. Most women with breast cancer will have some type of surgery and adjunct treatment, such as radiation therapy, chemotherapy, and hormone therapy (National Health and Medical Research Council [NHMRC], 1995). A patient may have just one form of treatment or a combination, depending on her individual needs.

TRENDS AND INCIDENCE

More women in the United States are living with breast cancer than any other cancer (with the exception of skin cancer). A woman in the United States now has a 1 in 8 chance of developing invasive breast cancer during her lifetime, compared to a 1 in 11 chance in 1975 (National Breast Cancer Coalition [NBCC], 2004b). In 2003, an estimated 211,300 new cases of invasive breast cancer and an estimated 55,700 new cases of in situ breast cancer were expected to be diagnosed among women. Breast cancer is the second leading cause of cancer death for women in the United States. In 2003, 39,800 women were expected to die from this disease. Although men account for fewer than 1% of all breast cancers, 1,300 new cases and 400 deaths among men were expected during 2003 (Jemal et al., 2003).

Incidence rates of invasive breast cancer for women have shown three distinct phases since 1973, when systematic monitoring of breast cancer began. Between 1973 and 1980, incidence was basically constant. Between 1980 and 1987, incidence increased by approximately 4% each year due largely to detection from the greater use of mammography screening. Between 1987 and 2000, rates increased by 0.4% each year. The incidence and mortality rates from breast cancer increase with age: 94% of new cases and 96% of deaths reported between 1996 and 2000 occurred in women age 40 and older (ACS, 2003). However, younger women who get breast cancer have a lower survival rate than older women (NBCC, 2004b).

Race and ethnicity impact both the incidence and mortality rates of breast cancer. Caucasian women have a higher incidence than African American women after age 40, and African American women have a slightly higher rate before age 40. Despite incidence rates, African American women have higher mortality rates from breast cancer at every age (ACS, 2003). The 5-year survival rate for Caucasian women diagnosed with invasive breast cancer is 87%; for African American women, it is only 72% (NBCC, 2004b).

The differences in incidence of and mortality from breast cancer in Caucasian and African American women have been attributed, at least in part, to the lower rate of mammography screening among African American women. In 1998, national data revealed that 60% of Caucasian women but only 55% of

African American women had had a mammogram (Centers for Disease Control and Prevention, 2000); in 2000, national data revealed that 57% of Caucasian women and 53% of African American women age 40 and older had had a mammogram within the prior year (ACS, 2003). Although the discrepancy between mammography screening among Caucasian and African American women is decreasing, it is still important to explore the reasons for this discrepancy and for the overall low number of women having an annual mammogram. Studies examining racial differences in mammography screening have found numerous possible factors, such as attitudes, beliefs, and knowledge about breast cancer and screening procedures (Holm, Frank, & Curtin, 1999; Jazieh & Soora, 2001; Makuc, Breen, & Freid, 1999). Incidence and mortality rates are generally even lower among other racial and ethnic groups (ACS, 2003).

Lack of health insurance is also associated with lower survival rates among women with breast cancer (Bradley, Given, & Roberts, 2001). Regardless of race, breast cancer patients with lower income are more likely to be diagnosed with advanced-stage cancer and to have lower 5-year survival rates when compared to higher-income patients (Baquet & Commiskey, 2000; Miller, Hankey, & Thomas, 2002; O'Malley, Le, Glaser, Shema, & West, 2003). This difference in survival rates has been attributed in part to the presence of additional illness, unequal access to medical care, and treatment disparities (Joslyn, 2002; Shavers & Brown, 2002).

RISK FACTORS

Every woman is at risk for breast cancer, but some women have a higher risk than others. Although the exact cause of the vast majority of breast cancers remains unknown, certain characteristics and exposures can contribute to the development of the disease (NBCC, 2004b). The established relative risk factors for breast cancer are listed in Table 11.1 in order of strength of their association (ACS 2003). Some of the risk factors, such as age, family history, early menarche, and late menopause, are not modifiable; others, such as postmenopausal obesity, use of postmenopausal hormones, and alcohol consumption, are modifiable (Fentiman, 2001).

Relative risk compares the risk of disease among people with a particular exposure to the risk among people without that exposure. If the relative risk is above 1, then risk is higher among exposed than unexposed persons; if the relative risk is below 1, then risk is lower among exposed than unexposed persons (ACS, 2003). For example, researchers divide the percentage of alcohol drinkers who got breast cancer (1.4%) by the percentage of non-alcohol drinkers who got

Table 11.1   Factors That Increase the Relative Risk for Breast Cancer in Women

Relative Risk	Factor
> 4	Age (65+)
	Certain inherited genetic mutations (BRCA1 and/or BRCA2)
	Two or more first-degree relatives with breast cancer diagnosed at an early age
	Personal history of breast cancer
	Postmenopausal breast density
2.1–4	One first-degree relative with breast cancer
	Biopsy-confirmed atypical hyperplasia
	High-dose radiation to chest
	High bone density (postmenopausal)
1.1–2 Reproduction factors	Late age at first full-term pregnancy (> 30 years)
	Early menarche (<12 years)
	Late menopause (>55 years)
	No full-term pregnancies
	Never breast-fed a child
Factors that affect circulating hormones	Recent oral contraceptive use
	Recent and long-term use of hormone replacement therapy
	Obesity (postmenopausal)
Other factors	Personal history of cancer of endometrium, ovary, or colon
	Alcohol consumption
	Being tall
	High socioeconomic status
	Jewish heritage

Note: Relative risk compares the risk of disease among people with a particular exposure to the risk among people without that exposure. If the relative risk is >1, then risk is higher than for unexposed persons. However, although relative risks are useful for comparisons, they do not provide information about the absolute amount of additional risk experienced by the exposed group (American Cancer Society, 2003).

Source: Reprinted from American Cancer Society, 2003, and adapted with permission from "Breast Cancer: Hormones and Other Risk Factors," by B. S. Hulka and P. G. Moorman, 2001, *Maturitas, 38*(1), pp. 103–113.

breast cancer (1%), which corresponds to a relative risk of 1.4. Because 1.4 is 40% greater than 1, researchers conclude that women who drink have a 40% increase in risk when compared to women who do not drink (NBCC, 2004c). It is important to note that these risk factors are often misleading in their actual significance. Studies have shown that you would have to drink two to five glasses of alcohol per day to increase your breast cancer risk by 40% (Smith-Warner et al., 1998). Women who drink one glass of alcohol a day have only a small risk increase of 9%, compared to women who do not drink alcohol (Smith-Warner et al., 1998).

The most important risk factors for developing breast cancer are being female and increased age. The probability of developing breast cancer in the next 10 years is 0.4% for women age 30, 2.78% for women age 40, and 3.81% for women age 60 (ACS, 2003). Despite recent media coverage about younger women developing breast cancer, the incidence rate of breast cancer in women under 40 has remained relatively constant for the past 25 years (ACS, 2003).

Another important risk factor is a family history of or genetic predisposition for breast cancer; however, this risk factor accounts for only approximately 10% of women who develop breast cancer (NBCC, 2004b). Women with a family history of breast cancer, especially in a first-degree relative, have an increased risk of developing breast cancer. Approximately 5% to 10% of breast cancer cases result from inherited mutations in breast cancer susceptibility genes, such as BRCA1 and BRCA2 (Domchek et al., 2003). However, it is not yet possible to predict if or when a woman with a specific mutation will develop breast cancer (ACS, 2003).

Hormonal factors are another important concern in addressing risk factors for breast cancer. A woman's risk of breast cancer can be increased by affecting endogenous hormones through early menarche (<12 years), older age at menopause, older age at first full-term pregnancy, and fewer number of pregnancies (Hulka & Moorman, 2001). There is some evidence that the use of oral contraceptive may slightly increase the risk of breast cancer; however, women who stopped using oral contraceptives 10 or more years ago have the same risk as those women who never used oral contraceptives (ACS, 2003). Similarly, use of hormone replacement therapy has been shown to increase breast cancer risk (Olsson, Ingvar, & Bladstrom, 2003; Porch, Lee, Cook, Rexrode, & Burnin, 2003). In contrast, there is some evidence to support the link between breast-feeding and decreased breast cancer risk (ACS, 2003; NBCC, 2004b).

Numerous other factors have been discussed as possible risk factors for breast cancer. For example, some have suggested there may be an increased risk for women who wear underwire bras or who use antiperspirants; however, there is currently no scientific evidence to support these associations (ACS, 2003). Likewise, there is no scientific evidence to support concerns regarding the link between having had an abortion and increased risk of breast cancer (Couzin, 2003).

There is much disagreement in the scientific and advocacy communities about the role of environmental factors in the development of breast cancer (NBCC, 2004a). It is generally believed that the environment plays some role, but the extent of that role is unknown. The incidence of breast cancer in Westernized industrialized countries is much higher than in Africa and Asia, and when women migrate from these countries to Westernized industrialized countries, their daughters experience the breast cancer risk of the host country's population (Buell, 1973; Kelsey & Horn-Ross, 1993). This discrepancy lends support to the role of environmental factors in increased breast cancer risk; however, these factors have not been adequately tested by the scientific community (NBCC, 2004a).

EFFECTIVE UNIVERSAL PREVENTIVE INTERVENTIONS

Although there is valuable information on the relative risk factors for breast cancer,we still cannot predict who will develop the disease. A woman with all known risk factors may never develop breast cancer, and a women with none of the known risk factors may. Because of this unpredictability, and although there is no guaranteed way to prevent breast cancer, all women should engage in universal preventive interventions. Early detection is key to increasing survival rates, which is why regular mammograms (i.e., X-rays of the breasts) are so important. Mammography screening detects breast cancer at earlier stages, resulting in reducing the risk of death from this disease. A mammogram is the single most effective method of early detection, as it can identify cancer several years before physical symptoms develop (ACS, 2003).

The ACS currently recommends all women age 40 and over to have an annual mammogram and annual clinical breast examination, and for women age 20 to 39 to have a clinical breast examination every 3 years. A clinical breast examination is conducted by a trained medical professional. In 2003, the ACS dropped its recommendation that all women perform monthly breast self-examinations; however, they still recommend that women be told of the benefits and limitations of breast self-examinations. Women who choose to perform breast self-examinations should be given instructions by a health care professional. It is recommended that all women become familiar with both the appearance and feel of their breasts so that they can notice any changes and promptly report those changes to a doctor or nurse (ACS, 2003).

EFFECTIVE SELECTIVE PREVENTIVE INTERVENTIONS

Besides regular mammograms and clinical breast examinations, a woman's best overall preventive health strategy is to reduce her known risk factors whenever possible. As mentioned, some of the risk factors for breast cancer, such as age, family history, early menarche, and late menopause, are not modifiable; others, such as postmenopausal obesity, use of postmenopausal hormones, and alcohol consumption, are modifiable (Fentiman, 2001). Women, particularly postmenopausal women, should strive to maintain a healthy body weight to reduce the risk of breast cancer and other diseases. Similarly, women should maintain a reasonable degree of physical activity; however, there is no clear evidence on what type, frequency, duration, or intensity of activity is optimal for risk reduction (ACS, 2003). Reducing alcohol consumption is another strategy for decreasing breast cancer risk. A meta-analysis of more than 40 studies suggests that the equivalent of two drinks a day may increase breast cancer risk by approximately 21%, and this increased risk exists regardless of the type of alcoholic beverage consumed (Ellison, Zhang, McLennan, & Rothman, 2001).

Although not all hormonal factors that increase breast cancer risk can be modified (e.g., early menarche, late menopause), it is possible to control some of the hormonal risk factors. The U.S. Preventive Services Task Force has recommended against the routine use of estrogen and progestin for the prevention of chronic diseases in postmenopausal women (ACS, 2003). The use of hormone replacement therapy must be determined by each woman weighing the benefits and risks for her individual situation. Women should also consider their reproductive choices and the role this may play in increasing their breast cancer risk. Recent oral contraceptive use has been associated with an increased risk of breast cancer; therefore, women may want to consider alternative contraceptive methods. Women should be informed that having their first full-term pregnancy before age 30 and choosing to breast-feed their baby has been found to decrease the risk of breast cancer.

EFFECTIVE INDICATED PREVENTIVE INTERVENTIONS

Women at highest risk for breast cancer are those with inherited genetic mutations (BCRA1 and/or BCRA2), two or more first-degree relatives with breast cancer diagnosed at an early age, a personal history of breast cancer, and postmenopausal breast density. Approximately 5% to 10% of breast cancer cases result from inherited mutations in breast cancer susceptibility genes, such as BRCA1 and BRCA2 (Domchek et al., 2003). Genetic testing is now available to determine if women carry these mutations; thus, women with a strong family history of breast cancer should be referred for genetic counseling to determine the best course of action for their particular situation.

Randomized controlled trials have demonstrated that tamoxifen can reduce the risk of breast cancer in women at high risk for developing the disease (ACS, 2003). Women who are at a high risk should discuss taking tamoxifen with their doctor and weigh the benefits and risks of this drug for their individual situation. It is estimated that over 2 million women in the United States would benefit from taking tamoxifen as a preventive intervention (Freedman et al., 2003).

Another preventive intervention for women at highest risk for breast cancer is prophylactic mastectomy, the removal of one or both breasts before there is a known breast cancer. Several studies have demonstrated that prophylactic mastectomies are highly successful in reducing the risk of developing breast cancer (Hartmann et al., 1999; Meijers-Heijboer et al., 2001). Although this operation reduces the risk of breast cancer, it does not guarantee that cancer will not develop in the small amount of remaining breast tissue (ACS, 2003). Women considering this alternative are strongly encouraged to discuss the pros and cons with their physician and to get a second opinion before making a final decision.

PRACTICE AND POLICY IMPLICATIONS

Despite estimates of relative risk, it is not possible to currently predict who will and will not get breast cancer. At this time, there is no guaranteed way to prevent breast cancer, and early detection is a key factor in increasing survival rates, which is why regular mammograms are so important as a universal preventive intervention. According to data from 2000, only 63% of U.S. women age 40 and older had a recent mammogram, and women with less than a high school education, without health insurance, or who are members of an ethnic minority were least likely to have had a recent mammogram (ACS, 2003). Efforts need to be made to increase use of mammograms among socioeconomically disadvantaged women and minority women. Researchers have demonstrated the effectiveness of community health promotion screening programs in increasing mammography rates among African American women (Altpeter, Earp, & Schopler, 1998; Husaini et al., 2001). Funding for such community awareness programs targeting African American and other minority women is a vital component in ensuring that these populations are adequately screened for breast cancer at an early stage.

It is also important that physicians are educated on the importance of discussing mammography screening with their women patients and making appropriate referrals for screenings. Previous research suggests that physician's assistants or nurse practitioners may be even more effective than physicians in communicating information about mammography screening (Crump, Mayberry, Taylor, Barefield, & Thomas, 2000). For example, a follow-up phone call by a breast care nurse to discuss mammography screening and the particular needs of the woman has been shown to increase mammography rates more than fivefold (Dalessandri, Cooper, & Rucker, 1998).

The evidence is clear that mammography screening detects breast cancer at earlier stages, resulting in reducing the risk of death from this disease. Given this information, it is tragic that socioeconomically disadvantaged women are being hindered from obtaining a mammogram due to lack of insurance coverage. It is essential that health care professionals and policy makers improve the system to ensure that all women have access to mammography screening. For example, randomized trials in the use of vouchers for a free mammogram have been effective in improving mammography rates (Stoner et al., 1998).

A woman's best overall preventive health strategy, besides regular mammograms and clinical breast examinations, is to reduce her known risk factors whenever possible. Thus, it is important that women are educated on their relative risk for developing breast cancer. Many of the risk factors are lifestyle choices (e.g., age to have children, breast-feeding, taking oral contraception, physical activity), which need to be considered prior to middle and older age; therefore, younger women should be educated on breast cancer so that they can make informed choices throughout their lives.

FUTURE DIRECTIONS

Much remains unknown in the fight against breast cancer. There is currently no cure for breast cancer and no clear cause of breast cancer. A woman with all known risk factors may never develop breast cancer; whereas, a women with none of the known risk factors might develop breast cancer. Breast cancer is a complex disease, and about 90% of the women who develop breast cancer do not have a family history of the disease. More research is needed to identify the causes of breast cancer and to find a cure. Specifically, more research is needed on the relationship between environmental factors and the development of breast cancer. Understanding the causes of breast cancer is essential to understanding how to prevent the disease.

In 2000, nearly 40% of women age 40 and older did not have a mammogram. This figure indicates that more education is needed to ensure that all women have an annual mammogram and more intervention research is needed to determine which strategies are most effective in increasing mammography rates among specific target populations. Until we can accurately predict who will get breast cancer, universal preventive intervention strategies targeted to all women are key in fighting this disease. All women, regardless of race and socioeconomic status, need access to universal preventive interventions for breast cancer.

REFERENCES

Altpeter, M., Earp, J. L., & Schopler, J. H. (1998). Promoting breast cancer screening in rural, African American communities: The "science and art" of community health promotion. *Health and Social Work, 23*(2), 104–115.

American Cancer Society. (2003). *Breast cancer facts and figures: 2003–2004.* Atlanta, GA: Author.

Baquet, C. R., & Commiskey, P. (2000). Socioeconomic factors and breast carcinoma in multicultural women. *Cancer, 88*(5), 1256–1264.

Bradley, C. J., Given, C. W., & Roberts, C. (2001). Disparities in cancer diagnosis and survival. *Cancer, 91*(1), 178–188.

Buell, P. (1973). Changing incidence of breast cancer in Japanese-American women. *Journal of the National Cancer Institute, 51,* 1479–1483.

Center for Disease Control and Prevention. (2000). *Behavioral risk factor surveillance system.* Atlanta, GA: U.S. Department of Health and Human Services, Centers for Disease Control and Prevention, National Center for Chronic Disease Prevention & Health Promotion.

Couzin, J. (2003). Cancer risk: Review rules out abortion-cancer link. *Science, 299*(5612), 1498.

Crump, S. R., Mayberry, R. M., Taylor, B. D., Barefield, K. P., & Thomas, P. E. (2000). Factors related to noncompliance with screening mammogram appointments in low-income African American women. *Journal of the National Medical Association, 92*(5), 237–246.

Dalessandri, K. M., Cooper, M., & Rucker, T. (1998). Effect of mammography outreach in women veterans. *Western Journal of Medicine, 169*(3), 150–153.

Domchek, S. M., Eisen, A., Calzone, K., Stopfer, J., Blackwood, A., & Weber, B. L. (2003). Application of breast cancer risk prediction models in clinical practice. *Journal of Clinical Oncology, 21*(4), 593–601.

Ellison, R. C., Zhang, Y., McLennan, C. E., & Rothman, K. J. (2001). Exploring the relationship of alcohol consumption to risk of breast cancer. *American Journal of Epidemiology, 154*(8), 740–747.

Fentiman, I. S. (2001). Fixed and modifiable risk factors for breast cancer. *International Journal of Clinical Practice, 55*(8), 527–530.

Freedman, A. N., Graubard, B. I., Rao, S. R., McCaskill-Stevens, W., Ballard-Barbash, R., & Gail, M. H. (2003). Estimates of the number of US women who could benefit from tamoxifen for breast cancer chemoprevention. *Journal of the National Cancer Institute, 95*(7), 526–532.

Grayson, C. E. (2003). *Breast cancer basics.* Cleveland, OH: Cleveland Clinic.

Hartmann, L. C., Schaid, D. J., Woods, J. E., Crotty, T. P., Myers, J. L., Arnold, P. G., et al. (1999). Efficacy of bilateral prophylactic mastectomy in women with a family history of breast cancer. *New England Journal of Medicine, 340*(2), 77–84.

Holm, C. J., Frank, D. I., & Curtin, J. (1999). Health beliefs, health locus of control, and women's mammography behavior. *Cancer Nursing, 22,* 49–56.

Hulka, B. S., & Moorman, P. G. (2001). Breast cancer: Hormones and other risk factors. *Maturitas, 38*(1), 103–113.

Husaini, B. A., Sherkat, D. E., Bragg, R., Levine, R., Emerson, J. S., Mentes, C. M., et al. (2001). Predictors of breast cancer screening in a panel study of African-American Women. *Women and Health, 34*(3), 35–51.

Jazieh, A. R., & Soora, I. (2001). Mammography utilization pattern throughout the state of Arkansas: A challenge for the future. *Journal of Community Health, 26*(4), 249–252.

Jemal, A., Murray, T., Samuels, A., Ghafoor, A., Ward, E., & Thun, M. J. (2003). Cancer statistics, 2003. *CA Cancer Journal Clinical, 53*(1), 5–26.

Joslyn, S. A. (2002). Racial differences in treatment and survival from early-stage breast carcinoma. *Cancer, 95*(8), 1759–1766.

Kelsey, J. L., & Horn-Ross, P. L. (1993). Breast cancer: Magnitude of the problem and descriptive epidemiology. *Epidemiology Review, 15,* 7–16.

Makuc, D. M., Breen, N., & Freid, V. (1999). Low income, race, and the use a mammography. *Health Services Research, 34*(1), 229–234.

Meijers-Heijboer, H., van Geel, B., van Putten, W. L., Henzen-Logmans, S. C., Seynaeve, C., Menke-Pluymer, M. B., et al. (2001). Breast cancer after prophylactic bilateral mastectomy in women with a BRCA1 or BRCA2 mutation. *New England Journal of Medicine, 345*(3), 159–164.

Miller, B. A., Hankey, B. F., & Thomas, T. L. (2002). Impact of sociodemographic factors, hormone receptor status, and tumor grade on ethnic differences in tumor stage and size for breast cancer in US women. *American Journal of Epidemiology, 155*(6), 534–545.

National Breast Cancer Coalition. (2004a). *Breast cancer and the environment: October 2003.* Washington, DC: Author.

National Breast Cancer Coalition. (2004b). *Facts about breast cancer in the United States: Year 2003.* Washington, DC: Author.

National Breast Cancer Coalition. (2004c). *What is meant by "breast cancer risk?": August 2002.* Washington, DC: Author.

National Health and Medical Research Council. (1995). *The management of early breast cancer.* Canberra, Australia: Author.

Olsson, H. L., Ingvar, C., & Bladstrom, A. (2003). Hormone replacement therapy containing progestins and given continuously increases breast carcinoma risk in Sweden. *Cancer, 97*(6), 1387–1392.

O'Malley, C. D., Le, G. M., Glaser, S. L., Shema, S. J., & West, D. W. (2003). Socioeconomic status and breast carcinoma survival in four racial/ethnic groups. *Cancer, 97*(5), 1303–1311.

Porch, J. V., Lee, I. M., Cook, N. R., Rexrode, K. M., & Burnin, J. E. (2003). Estrogen-progestin replacement therapy and breast cancer risk: The Women's Health Study (United States). *Cancer Causes Control, 13*(9), 847–854.

Shavers, V. L., & Brown, M. L. (2002). Racial and ethnic disparities in the receipt of cancer treatment. *Journal of the National Cancer Institute, 94*(5), 334–357.

Smith-Warner, S. A., Spiegelman, D., Yaun, S. S., van den Brant, P. A., Folsom, A. R., Goldbohm, R. A., et al. (1998). Alcohol and breast cancer in women: Pooled analysis of cohort studies. *Journal of the American Medical Association, 279*(7), 535–540.

Stoner, T. J., Dowd, B., Carr, W. P., Maldonado, G., Church, T. R., & Mandel, J. (1998). Do vouchers improve breast cancer screening rates? Results from a randomized trial. *Health Services Research, 33*(1), 11–18.

Chapter 12

HIV/AIDS AND STDs

ANDRES G. GIL AND JONATHAN G. TUBMAN

The United States has the highest rates of sexually transmitted diseases (STDs) in the industrialized world (Centers for Disease Control and Prevention [CDC], 1996). In 1996, approximately 400,000 chlamydia trachomatis infections were detected and reported to the CDC, making this infectious disease the most common STD reported in the United States (CDC, 1997). Gonorrhea, the second most frequently reported STD in the United States (CDC, 2001a, 2002b), declined nearly 60% between 1980 and 1996, to a rate of 124 per 100,000 persons (CDC, 1996). However, this rate was 26 times higher than the rate in Germany and 50 times higher than the rate in Sweden (CDC, 1996). Rates for other STDs, such as syphilis, are also higher in the United States than in other industrialized countries, as much as 13 times higher than in Germany and 33 times higher than in Sweden. Even more serious is the ethnic disparities in the United States in rates of STDs (CDC, 1997).

In 1999, 65 million Americans were living with an incurable STD (CDC, 2000). An additional 15 million become infected with one or more STDs each year, and roughly half of them contract lifelong incurable infections (Cates, 1999). These statistics illustrate that STDs are a serious public health problem in the United States. However, STDs tend to be under the radar of the public and of professionals working in key health fields, such as social work. The CDC (2000) has described STDs as the "hidden" epidemics because although STDs are extremely common, they are difficult to track, as many individuals with infections are symptom-free and remain unaware and undiagnosed.

More than 25 diseases are spread primarily through sexual activity, and trends vary considerably across these diseases (CDC, 2000). Many share common risk factors, and the level of success in preventing and reducing their incidence varies dramatically. Thus, although syphilis has been brought to all-time lows, other STDs such as genital herpes, gonorrhea, and chlamydia continue to resurge and spread through the population. Similarly, HIV/AIDS continues to spread despite extensive prevention efforts and increasingly effective treatments that have augmented the longevity of many people living with the disease. Nonetheless, HIV/STDs represent a serious public health challenge in the United States. There are geographic, economic, and social challenges to the development and implementation of effective prevention efforts. This chapter provides an overview of the problem, describes the risk factors associated with HIV/STDs, and identifies effective preventive interventions.

TRENDS AND INCIDENCE

In this section we review trends and incidence of STDs, HIV/AIDS, and risk factors from a developmental perspective, encompassing adolescence and adulthood. The section concludes with a brief description of how community contexts interact with risk factors to increase the likelihood of acquiring STDs and HIV/AIDS.

STDs Other Than HIV/AIDS

Table 12.1 presents the incidence and prevalence rates of some of the most serious STDs in the United States, excluding HIV/AIDS. As stated earlier, chlamydia is the most frequently reported STD in the United States, followed by gonorrhea. In the case of gonorrhea, 361,705 cases were reported in 2001, yet rates declined 73.8% during the period 1975 to 1997. However, in 1998, the

Table 12.1   Incidence and Prevalence of Most Common STDs in the United States

STD	Incidence (Annual New Cases)	Prevalence (Number of People Infected)
Chlamydia	3 million	2 million
Gonorrhea	650,000	Not available
Syphilis	70,000	Not available
Herpes	1 million	45 million
Human Papillomavirus (HPV)	5.5 million	20 million
Hepatitis B	120,000	417,000
Trichomoriasis	5 million	Not available

Source: Tracking the Hidden Epidemics: Trends in STDs in the United States, by Centers for Disease Control and Prevention, 2000, Atlanta, GA: U.S. Department of Health and Human Services, Centers for Disease Control and Prevention.

reported rate of gonococcal infections (131.9 cases per 100,000 persons) increased by 7.8% compared with the previous year (122.4 cases per 100,000 persons). Therefore, the 2001 rate of 128.5 cases per 100,000 population represented little change from 1998. Gonorrhea rates are highest among minorities and adolescents (CDC, 2001a, 2002b). The health impact of gonorrhea is largely related to its role as a major cause of pelvic inflammatory disease, which frequently leads to adverse outcomes such as infertility or ectopic pregnancy (McCormack, 1994). In addition, data suggest that gonorrhea facilitates HIV transmission in both men and women (Cohen et al., 1997; Laga et al., 1993).

The reported rate of primary and secondary syphilis in the United States in 2001 was 2.2 cases per 100,000 persons, slightly higher than the rate reported in 2000 (2.1 cases per 100,000; CDC, 2002b). This increase of 2.1%, observed primarily among men, constitutes the first increase since 1990 (CDC, 2001c). Moreover, the rate reported in 2000 was the lowest since 1941 (CDC, 2001b). In contrast, between 2000 and 2001, the overall rate of congenital syphilis decreased by 20.7%, from 14 to 11.1 cases per 100,000 live births (CDC, 2002b). The continuing decrease in the rate of congenital syphilis reflects substantial reductions in rates of primary and secondary syphilis among women that occurred throughout the 1990s. During 1991 to 2001, the average yearly decrease in the rate of primary and secondary syphilis reported among women was 20.8% and the average yearly decrease in the rate of congenital syphilis was 19.8% (CDC, 2001c).

In terms of racial/ethnic disparities in prevalence, rates of STDs for African Americans and Hispanics are significantly higher than for non-Hispanic Whites (CDC, 2002b). For example, 62% of all cases of primary and secondary syphilis reported to the CDC in 2001 occurred among African Americans, a rate 16 times greater than for non-Hispanic Whites. Similarly, 71% of reported cases in 2000 occurred among African Americans, 24 times higher than for non-Hispanic Whites.

HIV/AIDS

Table 12.2 presents key statistics regarding the prevalence of HIV/AIDS in the United States. The CDC (2004) estimates that there are currently 800,000 to 900,000 Americans infected with HIV. Each year there are approximately 40,000 new infections; among these, 70% are men. Categorized by recognized risk groups, men who have sex with men (MSM) represent 42% of new cases, closely followed by men and women engaged in heterosexual sex (33%) and those who were infected through injected drugs (IDU; 25%). More than half of the new HIV infections occur among Blacks (54%), followed by non-Hispanic Whites

Table 12.2   HIV/AIDS Statistics

	HIV Annual New Infections (%)	Through 2002	
		Cases (%)	AIDS Deaths (%)
Gender			
Male	70	81.8	
Female	30	18.2	
Transmission			
MSM	42	48	
Heterosexual	33	15.5	
IDU	25	27.4	
Race/Ethnicity			
Black	54	39.2	35.5
White non-Hispanic	26	41.1	46.2
Hispanic	19	18.5	17.3
Females			
Black	64		
White non-Hispanic	18		
Hispanic	18		
Transmission			
Heterosexual	75		
IDU	25		
Males			
Black	50		
White non-Hispanic	30		
Hispanic	20		
Transmission			
MSM	60		
IDU	25		
Heterosexual	15		
Total number	40,000	886,575	448,060

Sources: From *HIV/AIDS Surveillance Report,* by Centers for Disease Control and Prevention, 2002a; and *HIV/AIDS Update: A Glance at the HIV Epidemic,* by Centers for Disease Control and Prevention, 2004, Atlanta, GA: U.S. Department of Health and Human Services, Centers for Disease Control and Prevention.

(26%) and Hispanics (19%). Infection rates among Blacks and Hispanics are disproportionately higher than their representation in the U.S. population.

Recent estimates of the composition of new infections for women across race/ethnicity are 64% for Black women and 18% each for Hispanic and White non-Hispanic women. For all women, infection by heterosexual transmission was estimated to be 75%, and 25% via IDU. For men, the racial/ethnic distribution of new infection cases is 50% Black, 30% White non-Hispanic, and 20% Hispanic.

Among men, estimates suggest that 60% of new infections are transmitted through men having sex with men, 25% through IDU, and 15% through hetero-sexual transmission (CDC, 2004).

The estimated number of AIDS cases in the United States through 2002 was 886,575; 10,700 of these were adolescents. In terms of gender distribution, 81.8% of cases have been among males. The estimated number of deaths of persons with AIDS is 496,354 adults and 5,315 adolescents. The age group most commonly represented among AIDS cases is 35- to 44-year-olds, with 347,860 cases, or 39.3% of all cases. The second highest age group is 25- to 34-year-olds, with 34% of all cases. In terms of ethnicity, the estimated numbers of cases through December 2002 were distributed as follows: White non-Hispanics were 41.1% of all cases, followed by Black non-Hispanics (39.2%), Hispanics (18.5%), and Native Americans (0.31%; CDC, 2004).

Since the mid-1990s, advances in HIV treatments have led to dramatic declines in AIDS-related deaths and slowed the progression from HIV infection to AIDS. However, in more recent years, the rate of decline for both new AIDS cases and deaths began to slow (CDC, 1998a). For example, between 1997 and 1998, the decline of new AIDS cases was 13% and the decline in deaths was 17%; however, between 1998 and 1999, the declines were 3% and 8%, respectively (CDC, 1998a).

Through the end of 2002, the primary reported sources of infection for those who have contracted HIV ranged from 48% from male-to-male sexual contact, 27.4% from IDU, 15.5% from heterosexual contact, and 6.8% from combined male-to-male sexual contact and IDU. Finally, as of December 2000, the deaths attributed to AIDS were disproportionately high for African Americans, accounting for 35.5% of all deaths, and for Hispanics, who accounted for 17.3% of all deaths. White non-Hispanics accounted for 46.2% of all AIDS-related deaths (CDC, 2002a, 2004).

RISK FACTORS

The outbreak of the AIDS epidemic in the early 1980s has served to highlight research and clinical interest on key risk factors for STDs and HIV/AIDS. A comprehensive examination of risk factors for HIV/STDs must begin with a focus on risk factors during adolescence. HIV has a median incubation period of approximately 10 years. Therefore, a significant proportion of adults diagnosed with AIDS during their twenties were infected through risk behaviors in adolescence (Chesney, 1994; Joseph, 1991; Kotchick, Shaffer, & Forehand, 2001). Furthermore, 15- to 19-year-olds have the highest rates of gonorrhea, syphilis, and chlamydia in the United States (Bowler, Sheon, D'Angelo, & Vermund, 1992;

Kotchick et al., 2001). Thus, we begin the examination of risk factors by examining health risk behaviors that have been associated with HIV/STD transmission, and then proceed to an examination of risk factors for adults. It is important to note that, largely, risk factors for HIV/STD among adolescents are similar to those among adults.

Adolescent Risk Factors Impacting Adult HIV/STDs

Large proportions of Americans initiate sexual activity by early adolescence, with 21% of males having engaged in sexual intercourse by age 15 (Sonenstein, Pleck, & Ku, 1991). Furthermore, close to 50% of high school students engage in sexual intercourse prior to graduation (Kann et al., 1998), and the rates are higher for males and ethnic minorities, particularly for African American and Hispanic youth, who tend to report higher rates of sexual intercourse at younger ages (Christopher, Johnson, & Roosa, 1993; Kann et al., 1998; Leigh, Morrison, Trocki, & Temple, 1994; Romer et al., 1994; Seidman & Reider, 1994; Stanton et al., 1994).

This high prevalence of sexual activity at young ages represents high risk for HIV/STDs due to specific health risk behaviors exhibited by sexually active adolescents. For example, 24.7% of sexually active adolescents reported that they used alcohol or drugs at the time of their most recent sexual experience (Kann et al., 1998). In addition, consistent condom use is rare among adolescents; only 10% to 20% of sexually active adolescents report using them consistently (DiClemente et al., 1992; Kann et al., 1995). The rate is even lower among ethnic minority youth (Airhihenbuwa, DiClemente, Wingood, & Lowe, 1992; Brown, DiClemente, & Park, 1992). Finally, adolescents tend to engage in serial monogamous relationships that are of short duration (Kotchick et al., 2001). The consequence of these sexual behaviors is increased risk for HIV/STD exposure in general (Overby & Kegeles, 1994).

The prevalence and incidence data presented earlier indicate that a portion of the adult cases of HIV/STDs probably have their roots in adolescence and normative sexual risk behaviors that occur during this period. Moreover, psychosocial and behavioral factors arise during adolescence that increase risk for exposure, and primary prevention efforts ought to address these factors. In terms of psychosocial risks, academic performance and cognitive competence have been found to be significant predictors of adolescent sexual activity (East, 1998; Jessor, Van Den Bos, Vanderryn, Costa, & Turbin, 1995; Small & Luster, 1994); for example, low GPA has been associated with greater numbers of sexual partners and lower rates of condom use (Luster & Small, 1994). Self-esteem is another psychosocial factor related to sexual risk behavior during adolescence. Higher self-esteem is associated with greater frequency of condom use among minority females (Overby & Kegeles, 1994) and with greater consistent use of contraceptives among females (Miller, Forehand, & Kotchick, 2000).

Several behavioral factors place individuals at risk for HIV/STD exposure. Most notable among these is substance use. Multiple studies have demonstrated that a history of alcohol and substance use or abuse is correlated with inconsistent condom use (Brown et al., 1992; Cooper, Peirce, & Huselid, 1994; Luster & Small, 1994; Miller, Kotchick, & Forehand, 1999; Shrier, Emans, Woods, & DuRant, 1996) and having multiple sexual partners (Devine, Long, & Forehand, 1993; Duncan, Strycker, & Duncan, 1999; Tubman, Windle, & Windle, 1996). Data from the national Youth Risk Behavior Survey indicate that adolescents who used drugs during the previous year were more likely to have multiple sexual partners and no condom use at last intercourse (Kotchick et al., 2001). More important, however, in terms of the risks posed by substance use, use of alcohol or other drugs immediately prior to or during sexual encounters is related to decreased condom use (Bagnall, Plant, & Warwick, 1990; Fullilove et al., 1993; Jemmott & Jemmott, 1993; Strunin & Hingson, 1992); those with higher frequencies of being high while having sex are more likely to have unprotected sex, greater numbers of sexual partners, and greater numbers of poorly known, risky sexual partners (Jemmott & Jemmott, 1993).

Risk Factors during Adulthood

Key risk factors for the transmission of HIV/STDs among adults are unprotected intercourse, other exchanges of bodily fluids, such as blood via needle sharing, multiple sexual partners or more extensive sexual history, and abuse of alcohol or other drugs in conjunction with sexual behaviors. For HIV, it appears that there is a threshold concentration needed to facilitate transmission between persons; furthermore, HIV is a fragile virus that dies quickly if dried or exposed to disinfecting agents (Kelly, 1995). Thus, risk of contracting HIV is largely limited to several routes.

Key behavioral practices conferring risk for HIV infection can be divided into the sexual activities of MSM, heterosexual men and women, and injection drug users, as well as abuse of alcohol or other drugs in conjunction with sexual behaviors. Among MSM, unprotected anal intercourse is the behavior most predictive of acquiring or transmitting HIV infection (Kelly, 1995; Kingsley et al., 1987). This risk of infection is due to direct contact of sexual fluids with rectal blood vessels that are injured during intercourse. Among heterosexual men and women, unprotected vaginal or oral intercourse permits transmission of HIV as well as other STDs. Transmission to females takes place if semen is absorbed through vaginal capillaries; for males, transmission can occur from vaginal secretions or blood traces entering the penis during intercourse. Oral sex without fluid exchange carries minimal risk for HIV infection, but other STDs can be contracted in this manner (Kelly, 1995). Among intravenous drug users, risk for HIV transmission is through sharing syringes with infected individuals or by engaging in unprotected intercourse once infected through IDU. This means that risk reduction efforts with intravenous drug users involve targeting two risks: injection behaviors and risky sexual practices (Kelly, 1995).

Alcohol and drug abuse constitutes a risk for HIV/STD exposure through its influence on condom use and unprotected sexual intercourse. Multiple studies have shown a relationship between a history of alcohol and drug abuse and the presence of HIV/STDs (Hwang et al., 2000). In particular, the use of drugs prior to or during sex diminishes the likelihood of condom use (Kann et al., 1998), and having sex while high has been found to be significantly related to both sexual risk behaviors and a history of STD (Siegal et al., 1999). Therefore, substance use reduction is an appropriate target for primary and selective prevention of HIV/STD transmission.

Finally, one of the major risk factors for HIV/AIDS is the presence of other STDs. STDs that cause skin lesions (e.g., syphilis, genital herpes) are particularly involved in the increased risk for HIV transmission (Kelly, 1995). Since the beginning of the AIDS epidemic, researchers have consistently noted a strong association between HIV/AIDS and other STD infections (Royce, Sena, Cates, & Cohen, 1997; Wasserheit, 1992). Numerous studies have indicated at least a two- to fivefold increase in risk for HIV infections among persons with other STDs (CDC, 1998a; De Vicenzi, 1994; Kassler et al., 1994; Wasserheit, 1992). The mutually reinforcing nature of these infectious disease processes has been termed *epidemiological synergy* (Wasserheit, 1992).

Contexts Influencing Risks for HIV/STDs

Thus far, we have addressed risk factors for HIV/STD exposure from a developmental perspective. Social and biological contexts also influence behavioral risk factors (National Institutes of Health [NIH], 1997). The prevalence of HIV in a given community or population greatly impacts the influence of any specific risk behavior. Thus, the potential of a given risk behavior to cause exposure to an STD is much greater when the population or community in which the behavior takes place is saturated with potential sex partners who are infected.

As stated earlier, the prevalence of STDs also can impact risk for acquiring HIV/AIDS. Having STDs is an important marker for behaviors associated with HIV transmission, and genital sores (chancres) caused by syphilis make it easier to transmit and acquire HIV infection. In fact, there is an estimated two- to five-fold increased risk for acquiring HIV infection when syphilis is present (CDC, 2002c). In both men and women, inflammatory STDs (e.g., gonococcal and chlamydial infections) appear to increase both the prevalence of HIV shedding and the HIV RNA copy number or "viral load" in genital secretions (Atkins, Carlin, Emery, Griffiths, & Boag, 1996; Clemetson et al., 1993; Cohen et al., 1997). Among HIV-infected men, gonococcal infection increases shedding of HIV RNA in semen tenfold (Cohen et al., 1997). Furthermore, both ulcerative (e.g., due to herpes, syphilis, and chancroid) and nonulcerative (e.g., due to gonorrhea and chlamydia) STDs attract CD4+ lymphocytes to the ulcer surface (Spinola et al., 1996) or the endocervix (Levine et al., 1998), which disrupts epithelial and mucosal barriers to infections and thus establishes the potential to increase susceptibility to HIV infection.

Poverty and cultural factors are other critical social contexts that influence the impact of risk behaviors on STD transmission. Poverty lessens both availability of prevention education and access to high-quality health care. It is notable that rates of seeking treatment for STDs are much greater in countries with access to universal health care (NIH, 1997). In terms of cultural factors, negotiations about safe sex practices are much more difficult for women in populations where there are cultural barriers to doing so (NIH, 1997).

EFFECTIVE UNIVERSAL PREVENTIVE INTERVENTIONS

The primary purpose of universal preventive interventions is to reduce or control the rate at which particular STDs are transmitted in the general population of adults in a specific or wider geographic location (CDC, 1998c). Prevention programs of this type are designed to be applied to a broad range of adults without prior selection of potential participants on the basis of specific individual characteristics demonstrated to increase risk for HIV/STD exposure. Key goals of primary preventive interventions are to lower the levels of putative risk factors for HIV/STD exposure and to increase levels of factors thought to protect sexually active adults from exposure. Therefore, the implementation of comprehensive universal preventive interventions, ideally tailored to the needs of specific communities, can be an effective means of encouraging positive behavioral changes at a population level to slow the pace at which STD epidemics have spread during the past few decades in the United States (CDC, 2000).

Effective comprehensive universal preventive interventions for HIV/STD risk reduction often incorporate a common set of core elements and behavior change strategies (CDC, 1998c). Features of greatest relevance to the advancement of HIV/STD risk reduction goals among adults are community planning and involvement, voluntary anonymous HIV testing and counseling, access to STD treatment services, health education and risk-reduction activities for individuals, groups, and the broader community, public information campaigns, and rigorous evaluation of program activities. In addition, these core features provide clear links between program goals and targets for change in program-related initiatives. For example, key risk factors for HIV and STD transmission identified earlier (i.e., unprotected intercourse, other exchanges of bodily fluids such as blood via needle sharing, multiple sexual partners or more extensive sexual history, and abuse of alcohol or other drugs in conjunction with sexual behaviors) are likely to be systematically influenced by both modifiable psychosocial factors (e.g., knowledge level, condom-related skills, communication or assertiveness, self-efficacy, and risk perception) and contexts in which sexual behavior occurs, including prevalent social norms, poverty and access to health care, and HIV/STD prevalence in a local community (CDC, 1998b). Specific CDC-recommended program features (e.g., public information campaigns, community involvement and mobilization) are often implemented to reduce risk factors such as inaccurate information and lack of access to STD testing or condoms while increasing protective factors such as social norms supporting voluntary testing and condom use and community empowerment.

Exemplar Universal HIV/STD Preventive Interventions

In contrast to school-based prevention programs for adolescents, universal prevention programs for sexually active adults are typically implemented in community settings, focusing on changing community norms, gaining access to accurate information, and clarifying perceptions of risk, or alternatively, accessing difficult-to-reach groups for behavior change efforts. Prevention efforts designed to reduce potential consequences of sexual activity among adults are in sharp contrast to universal prevention programs designed to delay onset of sexual behavior among adolescents or to encourage abstinence. Representative universal prevention modalities include communitywide interventions for HIV/STD risk reduction and health communication interventions (Trickett, 2002). Both strategies have been empirically supported and demonstrate significant efficacy for effectiveness. In each of these types of intervention, social work professionals play significant roles in the implementation process.

Community-based interventions promote universal reductions in HIV risk through activities that impact a broad range of people by changing social norms, social relationships, and community structures associated with HIV transmission.

Key activities may include community outreach, attempts to influence opinion leaders, publicity regarding risk reduction strategies, and the creation of networks focused on HIV risk reduction issues (Kegeles, Hays, & Coates, 1996; Kelly et al., 1991). For example, in the CDC-funded AIDS Community Demonstration Project (Fishbein et al., 1997), health services related to HIV risk reduction (e.g., condoms, bleach for disinfecting needles) were provided to difficult-to-reach groups of adults in community settings by removing barriers to access. Specifically, community outreach volunteers were enlisted to contact vulnerable adult groups, to distribute health care items to these adults, and to promote their proper use via informational flyers and brochures. Results from this community-level intervention documented significant improvements in participants' consistent use of condoms with main and other sex partners. Other community-level programs have used similar outreach strategies for accessing vulnerable minority populations of young adults and women to deliver information, HIV prevention activities, and related services (Feudo, Vining-Bethea, Shulman, Shedlin, & Burleson, 1998; Lauby, Smith, Stark, Person, & Adams, 2000). These programs have generally demonstrated significant effectiveness, increasing condom use and other self-protective behaviors such as discussions with partners regarding condom use.

Universal HIV prevention efforts involving health communications or public health campaigns focus on the delivery of carefully crafted HIV risk reduction messages to individuals within a broader community with high rates of STD/HIV transmission, often in conjunction with other ongoing intervention modalities (Singhal & Rogers, 2003). This intervention strategy involves assessing the values, needs, and goals of specific target audiences (young parents, adolescents, minority group members), constructing and delivering easily accessible health promotion messages that clearly underscore the immediate direct benefits of health behavior change (CDC, 1998b). Successful HIV-related health communication prevention programs deliver developmentally appropriate and culturally competent messages about health risks associated with sexual behavior that tap into core values of targeted groups (e.g., regarding autonomy, physical vitality, responsibility to sexual partners and family). In this regard, the effectiveness of this approach is related to how well-defined the target audience is and how clearly the messages presented parallel or are tailored to the needs of the targeted group.

Successful programs are multimedia (print, visual materials, radio, television, Internet) and multilevel, involving contact with individuals (outreach with brochures and visual materials), neighborhoods (posters, billboards, group activities through agencies), and communities (mass media, contacts with opinion leaders) to disseminate as broadly as possible key health-related messages to a clearly defined target audience (Kiwanuka-Tondo & Snyder, 2002; Witte, Cameron, Lapinski, & Nzyuko, 1998). Such outreach is also flexible enough to adapt to local forms of media in underdeveloped communities (Panford, Nyaney, Amoah, & Aidoo, 2001). To date, however, this promising modality for universal HIV risk reduction intervention lacks consistent, rigorous empirical evaluations (Myhre & Flora, 2000).

EFFECTIVE SELECTIVE PREVENTIVE INTERVENTIONS

The primary purpose of selective preventive interventions is to reduce risk for HIV/STD exposure among adults who are identified as belonging to populations at high risk for transmission (e.g., due to excessive substance abuse, persistent psychopathology, significant history of physical or sexual abuse; Kelly, 1995). As such, these prevention programs are designed to address the needs of targeted groups of adults, screened for particular psychosocial characteristics, rather than general populations of adults. Selective prevention programs attempt to interrupt underlying processes related to the onset or maintenance of behaviors that facilitate the transmission of HIV and reduce exacerbating influences of key risk factors that define specific populations of interest. Within the framework of selective prevention, interventions are designed to shift the balance between dynamically interacting risk and protective factors that influence risk for HIV/STD exposure in a probabilistic manner, while addressing developmentally distal issues (e.g., childhood abuse, ongoing psychopathology) that moderate these processes. In contrast to universal prevention programs, selective programs are typically more labor intensive to implement, tailored to the needs of specific high-risk groups, and, at a minimum, designed to promote behavioral changes to reduce harm (i.e., HIV risk) associated with membership in the target group.

Identified groups targeted by selective prevention programs vary widely and may be defined by stable characteristics (e.g., segment of life span, ethnicity, nativity, gender, or sexual orientation) or by psychological, behavioral, or contextual factors empirically documented as increasing vulnerability to HIV/STD exposure. Programs designed for populations with elevated vulnerability to HIV/STD exposure typically improve behavioral and health-related outcomes in two ways. First, selective interventions are designed to reduce the likelihood of transmission of HIV/STD by targeting directly behaviors associated with transmission (e.g., unprotected intercourse, multiple sexual partners, needle sharing). Second, selective prevention programs are designed to reduce transmission indirectly via their influence on factors that amplify levels of behavioral risk (e.g., substance use, psychopathology, disenfranchisement and powerlessness, abuse history; Benotsch, Kalichman, & Pinkerton, 2001; Gomez, Hernandez, & Faigeles, 1999; Purcell, Malow, Dolezal, & Carballo-Dieguez, 2004). By incorporating program elements that address distal or proximal conditions that serve to maintain psychological variables associated with behavioral risk factors (e.g., cognitions, attitudes, inadequate risk reduction skills, or limited social supports for change; Kelly & Kalichman, 2002), selective prevention efforts address the complex and multiply determined nature of risk behaviors in specific vulnerable client populations.

Exemplar Selective HIV/STD Preventive Interventions

Selective prevention programs for sexually active adults are implemented in a wide variety of community and treatment settings, such as STD clinics or other places in which specific vulnerable adult populations can be recruited and recontacted easily. Vulnerable populations of interest to social work practitioners have included persons seeking reproductive health care, participants in substance abuse treatment, persons with severe and chronic mental health problems, impoverished urban minority women, and homeless adults (Kelly & Kalichman, 2002). Representative selective prevention modalities with demonstrated efficacy typically address deficits in self-protective attitudes, intentions, behaviors, and social norms/supports, or co-occurring factors that maintain or exacerbate HIV risk behaviors (e.g., substance use, psychopathology, perceived powerlessness) via intensive psychoeducational or psychotherapeutic intervention in individual or group formats. Both strategies for implementing selective prevention programs for HIV/STD risk reduction can be tailored to address the needs of specific groups of adults vulnerable to HIV/STD exposure, with attention to the unique systems of risk and protective factors experienced by each group. As these interventions continue to be evaluated empirically and formatted for efficient transfer to community and treatment settings, social work professionals will play key roles in their implementation and ongoing evaluation (CDC, 1999).

A wide range of selective prevention programs have shown significant efficacy for HIV/STD risk reduction with regard to both psychological variables thought to moderate or mediate risk behaviors and key risk behavior outcomes, often through the application of intensive, theory-driven, interactive protocols to modify these factors among vulnerable individuals. For example, a Cognitive-Behavioral Skills Training Group intervention (Kelly et al., 1994) has shown significant efficacy for improving behavioral outcomes (e.g., increased condom use, decreased frequency of unprotected intercourse) among an urban STD clinic sample of young, predominantly minority women. This brief, four-session, small group format intervention used cognitive-behavioral strategies such as interactive skill-building exercises in conjunction with accurate information to enhance behavioral skills associated with HIV risk reduction, accurate perceptions of risk, and a range of competencies related to assertion, communication, and self-efficacy. A similar but more lengthy and comprehensive program designed for gay men has shown significant efficacy for reducing the frequency of unprotected intercourse while increasing the use of condoms (Kelly, St. Lawrence, Hood, & Brasfield, 1989). This prevention program emphasized the use of behavioral self-management strategies and training in assertion skills to enhance self-protective competencies related to risk recognition and negotiation, effective communication and refusal skills, and relationship and problem-solving skills. Comparable selective prevention programs implemented with other samples of adults recruited from clinic settings, women at high risk for HIV transmission, and gay men have demonstrated significant efficacy (e.g., Carey et al., 1997; Kamb et al., 1998; Peterson et al., 1996).

Efficacious selective prevention programs have also been designed to incorporate content or tailored delivery approaches to address specific factors in populations vulnerable to HIV transmission (e.g., psychopathology, substance abuse, perceived disenfranchisement) thought to exacerbate HIV/STD risk behaviors. For example, a recent randomized clinical trial of a 10-session motivational intervention emphasizing skill development and accurate information regarding HIV transmission, designed for outpatients receiving psychiatric treatment, demonstrated significantly greater reductions of HIV risk behaviors than a parallel comparison condition targeting substance abuse or a standard care control condition (Carey et al., 2004). The significance of this study is that it rigorously evaluated a specific intervention approach (i.e., motivational skills development) combined with several delivery strategies for tailored information and interactive exercises designed to provide HIV risk reduction program content to a vulnerable population experiencing developmental systems that maintain HIV risk behavior. A comparable approach has shown efficacy for the reduction of risk behaviors in other client populations vulnerable to HIV exposure, such as inner-city minority women (DiClemente & Wingood, 1995) and adult drug users (McCusker, Stoddard, Zapka, & Lewis, 1993). These empirically supported interventions are designed to address not only sexual risk behaviors directly related to HIV transmission, but also co-occurring risk behaviors or contextual conditions (e.g., IDU, lack of empowerment) associated with the maintenance of sexual risk behaviors.

EFFECTIVE INDICATED PREVENTIVE INTERVENTIONS

Indicated prevention programs, in contrast to universal or selective prevention programs, are designed to be implemented after the onset of a specific pattern of maladaptive behavior (e.g., a psychiatric disorder or disease process, a significant health risk behavior) to (1) increase the likelihood of remission; (2) prevent maintenance, acceleration of severity, or relapse; or (3) minimize harmful consequences associated with the condition. Applied to treatment of HIV and other STDs, indicated prevention programs (also referred to as secondary prevention) are intended to reduce the transmission of STDs, in particular those that may be treated but not cured, from infected adults to other persons who may not have been exposed previously (Kelly & Kalichman, 2002). Indicated prevention programs play a significant role in efforts to improve patient compliance to short- and long-term treatment regimens, especially those that require strict adherence to ensure efficacy. In addition, indicated prevention programs may be used to address key psychological issues that accompany long-term treatment of HIV or other STDs, improving the quality of life for infected clients, their partners, and their families. Therefore, indicated prevention programs, while they can be an additional strategy for slowing rates of STD transmission between infected persons and their partners, are also critical to improving long-term health and psychological outcomes among adults with treatable but incurable STDs (Kelly, Otto-Salaj, Sikkema, Pinkerton, & Bloom, 1998).

In contrast to selective prevention programs, indicated prevention programs target clients who are already identified as infected with an STD, in particular one that can be treated but not cured, that is, HIV/AIDS, herpes, or hepatitis C. While indicated prevention strategies may be targeted to specific groups of clients based on demographic characteristics (e.g., gender, sexual orientation) or issues related to a significant moderating factor (recurring psychopathology, substance abuse) associated with HIV risk behavior, indicated prevention also involves addressing the medical, psychological, and broader social needs of persons already infected. Therefore, indicated prevention programs tend to be more comprehensive than universal or selective prevention programs, because existing HIV infection is necessarily integrated into program content and goals and they are implemented with a more clearly defined target population.

Exemplar Indicated HIV/STD Preventive Interventions

Indicated prevention programs are often implemented in clinical- and community-based settings where clients living with HIV-related conditions routinely access treatment services. One key goal of indicated prevention programs is the improvement of client adherence to the complex and demanding highly active antiretroviral therapy (HAART) regimens required to effectively manage the symptoms of HIV-related diseases and to ensure high-quality prognoses for health outcomes (Schneiderman, 1999). Kelly and Kalichman (2002) list factors that can interfere with clients' ability to adhere to these demanding treatment protocols: treatment intrusiveness and side effects, clients' beliefs about treatment efficacy, cognitive deficits, substance abuse, and literacy levels. Recent efforts to implement and evaluate indicated prevention programs to improve clients' ability to adhere to antiretroviral medication regimens have included cognitive-behavioral stress management (Jones et al., 2003), self-management training (Smith, Rublein, Marcus, Brock, & Chesney, 2003), and a multicomponent, multidisciplinary medication adherence intervention (Murphy, Lu, Martin, Hoffman, & Marelich, 2002). While each of these approaches shows some promise for improving client attitudes or behaviors related to participation in HIV treatment protocols, they do not work equally well for all participating clients or necessarily improve significantly clients' adherence to medication dosage. Therefore, these forms of indicated prevention programs deserve continued refinement and evaluation.

A second key goal of indicated prevention programs for clients who have been identified as HIV-positive is the promotion of attitudinal and behavioral changes to reduce risk for transmission of HIV to regular or casual sex partners (CDC, 2003; Kelly & Kalichman, 2002). As promising antiretroviral treatment regimens such as HAART have become available, many adults have changed their attitudes regarding their risk for HIV transmission and the seriousness of such an event (Demmer, 2002; Ostrow et al., 2002). These changes in attitudes, coupled with misperceptions about the impact of HAART for reducing transmission risk and clients' weariness of safer sex guidelines, are associated with higher levels of sexual risk-taking behavior among sexually active adults. While unprotected sexual intercourse by HIV-positive persons is a significant source of transmission to their regular sex partners, these behaviors are systematically related to modifiable psychosocial factors, and thus amenable to intervention (Parsons et al., 1998; Rosser, Gobby, & Carr, 1999). Recent clinical trials of behavioral risk-reduction interventions for HIV-positive adults have demonstrated significant efficacy for promoting higher rates of protected intercourse, as well as lower estimated rates of transmission of HIV to sex partners (e.g., Kalichman et al., 2001).

Indicated prevention programs may also be designed and implemented for HIV-positive clients for the purpose of addressing key quality of life issues (e.g., psychopathology, stress management), which may also be significant moderators of treatment adherence and sexual risk behaviors (Kelly & Kalichman, 2002). For example, high levels of depressive symptoms and other indicators of distress occur in a significant proportion of persons diagnosed with HIV-related diseases, coupled with associated losses, and are likely to influence clients' perceptions of treatment effectiveness and self-efficacy to adhere to treatment protocol (Ironson et al., 2002; Kelly et al., 1998; Stober, Schwartz, McDaniel, & Abrams, 1997). Increasingly, however, research and practice efforts have resulted in the development and evaluation of programs designed to assist HIV-positive persons to cope more effectively with the experience of long-term survival with HIV-related diseases. For example, results from a recent randomized clinical trial suggest that brief cognitive-behavioral group interventions demonstrate significant short-term efficacy for reductions in both depressive symptoms and psychiatric distress associated with AIDS-related losses, in particular among HIV-positive women (Sikkema, Hansen, Kochman, Tate, & Difranceisco, 2004). Similarly, an empirical evaluation of a 10-session coping effectiveness training intervention for self-identified HIV-positive gay and bisexual men documented significant decreases in perceived stress and burnout, as well as parallel improvements in coping self-efficacy, in comparison to an active informational control condition (Chesney, Chambers, Taylor, Johnson, & Folkman, 2003).

PRACTICE AND POLICY IMPLICATIONS

Efforts to combat the HIV/AIDS epidemic have been oriented above all toward finding biomedical and behavioral solutions, which are no doubt of vital importance. In the United States, the government has played a key role in shaping the course of the epidemic. Although the first federal funds for medical research and community-based services were allocated in the early 1980s, government response was woefully inadequate in the face of a growing epidemic. Not until 1990 did Congress pass the Ryan White CARE Act, which now provides over $1.6 billion in critical funding for services for people living with HIV/AIDS, including drug treatments, primary medical care, and essential supportive services. There have been other high points, such as the 1990 passage of the Americans with Disabilities Act, which prohibits discrimination against persons with HIV. The fiscal year 2005 federal budget request to Congress from the president included an estimated $19.8 billion for domestic and global HIV/AIDS funding. This is less than 1% of the total federal budget; however, it represents a 7% ($1.3 billion) increase over the FY 2004 HIV/AIDS funding of $18.5 billion. Domestic HIV/AIDS funding will be 86% of the total (approximately $17.1 billion) of this FY 2005 request, and $2.7 billion (14%) will be for global HIV/AIDS. Federal funding for HIV/AIDS programs consists of five general categories: care, cash and housing assistance, prevention, research, and international/global outreach. More than half (59%) of the FY 2005 request is for care activities, 15% for research, and only 5% for prevention (NIH, 2004; Henry Kaiser Family Foundation, 2004). With no cure and no vaccine for AIDS currently available, the only way to stop HIV is to prevent its spread. The low proportion of the budget allocated to prevention does not bode well for the future.

Concern with the deeper socioeconomic and political roots of the pandemic is growing. Clearly, HIV/AIDS strikes hardest where poverty is extensive, gender inequality is pervasive, and public services are weak. In fact, the spread of HIV/AIDS at the turn of the twenty-first century is a sign of maldevelopment—an indicator of the failure at both national and international levels to create more equitable and prosperous societies. Similarly, the problem of other STDs is related to poverty and lack of access to health care and education.

A social work perspective on HIV/AIDS and other STDs is one that emphasizes prevention, and such an approach requires policies that confront HIV/STDs as a public health concern. The CDC (1997) has proposed guidelines for prevention case management for HIV that emphasize early identification of infection and assessment of community resources, including other HIV prevention programs and diagnosis and treatment services for substance abuse and for other STDs.

FUTURE DIRECTIONS

As illustrated earlier, there have been numerous successes in the fight against STDs in the United States, despite the relatively high prevalence rates in comparison with other industrialized countries. We have seen declines in population levels of gonorrhea from the 1970s through the late 1990s, as well as declines in syphilis from the 1940s to the 1990s. Community-based HIV prevention programs have taught us that not all interventions work with all populations, and some interventions that may have met with success in the past do not work in the present. Unquestionably, there have been substantial advances in the treatment of HIV infection, as well as other STDs such as gonorrhea and syphilis. There are two key issues in terms of future success in the prevention of HIV/STDs for social work and other health care professionals: the need to refine and evaluate rigorous prevention efforts with populations already infected and the need to implement empirically based interventions with vulnerable ethnically and economically diverse populations.

To date, HIV prevention has largely focused on persons who are not HIV-infected to help them avoid becoming infected through universal and selective preventive interventions. However, given recent treatment successes, further reduction of HIV transmission will require increased emphasis on preventing transmission by infected persons who are aware of their infection via indicated preventive interventions (Janssen, Holtgrave, Valdiserri, Shepherd, & Gayle, 2001). As the number of individuals surviving and living with HIV increases, reversion to risky sexual behavior is as important to trends in transmission as failure to adopt safer sexual behavior immediately after receiving a diagnosis of HIV.

In addition to focusing on indicated prevention through work with individuals who are already infected with HIV and other STDs, future success requires implementation of empirically supported prevention efforts within communities and populations that are culturally diverse and vulnerable. The movement of immigrants and other populations within the United States creates systemic challenges for social workers and others in public health systems in areas such as surveillance, access to care, different health care systems, and varying medical care practices. On an individual level, mistrust of health care systems prevents needed health care seeking because of the legal status of workers or cultural differences between health care providers and persons in need of their services. The stigma associated with STDs imposes an additional impediment for persons steeped in a culture that does not easily deal with risk behaviors related to STD acquisition and transmission.

REFERENCES

Airhihenbuwa, C. O., DiClemente, R. J., Wingood, G. M., & Lowe, A. (1992). Perspective: HIV/AIDS education and prevention among African-Americans: A focus on culture. *AIDS Education and Prevention, 4,* 267–276.

Atkins, M. C., Carlin, E. M., Emery, V. C., Griffiths, P. D., & Boag, F. (1996). Fluctuations of HIV load in semen of HIV positive patients with newly acquired sexually transmitted disease. *British Medical Journal, 313,* 341–342.

Bagnall, G., Plant, M., & Warwick, W. (1990). Alcohol, drugs and AIDS-related risks: Results from a prospective study. *AIDS Care, 2,* 309–317.

Benotsch, E. G., Kalichman, S. C., & Pinkerton, S. D. (2001). Sexual compulsivity in HIV-positive men and women: Prevalence, predictors, and consequences of high-risk behaviors. *Sexual Addiction and Compulsivity, 8*(2), 83–99.

Bowler, S., Sheon, A. R., D'Angelo, L. J., & Vermund, S. H. (1992). HIV and AIDS among adolescents in the United States: Increasing risk in the 1990s. *Journal of Adolescence, 15*(4), 345–371.

Brown, L. K., DiClemente, R. J., & Park, T. (1992). Predictors of condom use in sexually active adolescents. *Journal of Adolescent Health, 13,* 651–657.

Carey, M. P., Carey, K. B., Maisto, S. A., Gordon, C. M., Schroder, K. E. E., & Vanable, P. A. (2004). Reducing HIV-risk behavior among adults receiving outpatient psychiatric treatment: Results from a randomized control trial. *Journal of Consulting and Clinical Psychology, 72,* 252–268.

Carey, M. P., Maisto, S. A., Kalichman, S. C., Forsyth, A. D., Wright, E. M., & Johnson, B. T. (1997). Enhancing motivation to reduce the risk of HIV infection for economically disadvantaged urban women. *Journal of Consulting and Clinical Psychology, 65*(4), 531–541.

Cates, W. (1999). Estimates of the incidence and prevalence of sexually transmitted diseases in the United States. *Sexually Transmitted Diseases, 26*(Suppl), S2–S7.

Centers for Disease Control and Prevention. (1996, November). *The challenge of STD prevention in the United States.* Atlanta, GA: U.S. Department of Health and Human Services, National Center for HIV, STD, and TB Prevention.

Centers for Disease Control and Prevention. (1997). *Sexually transmitted diseases, 1996.* Atlanta, GA: U.S. Department of Health and Human Services, Public Health Service.

Centers for Disease Control and Prevention. (1998a). HIV prevention through early detection and treatment of other sexually transmitted diseases: United States recommendations of the advisory committee for HIV and STD prevention. *Morbidity and Mortality Weekly Report, 47*(PR12), 1–24.

Centers for Disease Control and Prevention. (1998b). *Program operations guidelines for STD prevention: Community and individual behavior change interventions.* Atlanta, GA: U.S. Department of Health and Human Services, Centers for Disease Control and Prevention, National Center for HIV, STD, & TB Prevention.

Centers for Disease Control and Prevention. (1998c, June). *Update: Linking science and prevention programs—The need for comprehensive strategies.* Atlanta, GA: U.S. Department of Health and Human Services, Centers for Disease Control and Prevention, National Center for HIV, STD, & TB Prevention.

Centers for Disease Control and Prevention. (1999). *Compendium of HIV preventive interventions with evidence of effectiveness.* Atlanta, GA: U.S. Department of Health and Human Services, Centers for Disease Control and Prevention, National Center for HIV, STD, & TB Prevention.

Centers for Disease Control and Prevention. (2000). *Tracking the hidden epidemics: Trends in STDs in the United States 2000.* Atlanta, GA: U.S. Department of Health and Human Services, Centers for Disease Control and Prevention.

Centers for Disease Control and Prevention. (2001a). *Control of neisseria gonorrhoeae infection in the United States* (Report of an external consultants' meeting convened by the Division of STD Prevention, National Center for HIV, STD, and TB Prevention). Atlanta, GA: U.S. Department of Health and Human Services, Centers for Disease Prevention.

Centers for Disease Control and Prevention. (2001b, September). *Sexually transmitted disease surveillance 2000.* Atlanta, GA: U.S. Department of Health and Human Services, Centers for Disease Control and Prevention.

Centers for Disease Control and Prevention. (2001c, September). *Sexually transmitted disease surveillance 2001 supplement* (Syphilis Surveillance Report. National Center for HIV, STD, and TB Prevention. Division of STD Prevention). Atlanta, GA: U.S. Department of Health and Human Services, Centers for Disease Control and Prevention.

Centers for Disease Control and Prevention. (2002a). *HIV/AIDS surveillance report.* Atlanta, GA: U.S. Department of Health and Human Services, Centers for Disease Control and Prevention.

Centers for Disease Control and Prevention. (2002b, September). *Sexually transmitted disease surveillance 2001.* Atlanta, GA: U.S. Department of Health and Human Services, Centers for Disease Control and Prevention.

Centers for Disease Control and Prevention. (2002c, September). *Syphilis and msm* (men who have sex with men). Atlanta, GA: U.S. Department of Health and Human Services, Centers for Disease Control and Prevention, National Center for HIV, STD, and TB Prevention, Division of Sexually Transmitted Diseases.

Centers for Disease Control and Prevention. (2003, July). Incorporating HIV prevention into the medical care of persons living with HIV. *Morbidity and Mortality Weekly Report, 52*(PR12), 1–24.

Centers for Disease Control and Prevention. (2004). *HIV/AIDS Update: A glance at the HIV epidemic.* Atlanta, GA: U.S. Department of Health and Human Services, Centers for Disease Control and Prevention.

Chesney, M. A. (1994). Prevention of HIV and STD Infections. *Preventive Medicine, 23,* 655–660.

Chesney, M. A., Chambers, D. B., Taylor, J. M., Johnson, L. M., & Folkman, S. (2003). Coping effectiveness training for men living with HIV: Results from a randomized clinical trial testing a group-based intervention. *Psychosomatic Medicine, 65,* 1038–1046.

Christopher, F. S., Johnson, D. C., & Roosa, M. W. (1993). Family, individual, and social correlates of early Hispanic adolescent sexual expression. *Journal of Sex Research, 30,* 54–61.

Clemetson, D. B. A., Moss, G. B., Willerford, D. M., Hensel, M., Emonyi, W., Holmes, K. K., et al. (1993). Detection of HIV DNA in cervical and vaginal secretions. Prevalence and correlates among women in Nairobi, Kenya. *Journal of the American Medical Association, 269,* 2860–2864.

Cohen, M. S., Hoffman, I. F., Royce, R. A., Kazembe, P., Dyer, J. R., Daly, C. C., et al. (1997). Reduction of concentration of HIV-1 in semen after treatment of urethritis: Implications for prevention of sexual transmission of HIV-1. AIDSCAP Malawi Research Group. *Lancet, 349,* 1868–1873.

Cooper, M. L., Peirce, R. S., & Huselid, R. F. (1994). Substance use and sexual risk taking among Black adolescents and White adolescents. *Health Psychology, 13,* 251–262.

Demmer, C. (2002). Impact of improved treatments on perceptions about HIV and safer sex among inner-city HIV-infected men and women. *Journal of Community Health: The Publication for Health Promotion and Disease Prevention, 27*(1), 63–73.

De Vicenzi, I. (1994). European study group on heterosexual transmission of HIV: A longitudinal study of human immunodeficiency virus transmission by heterosexual partners. *New England Journal of Medicine, 331,* 341–346.

Devine, D., Long, P., & Forehand, R. (1993). A prospective study of adolescent sexual activity: Description, correlates, and predictors. *Advances in Behaviour Research and Therapy, 15,* 185–209.

DiClemente, R. J., Durbin, M., Siegel, D., Krasnovsky, F., Lazarus, N., & Camacho, T. (1992). Determinants of condom use among junior high students in a minority, inner-city school district. *Pediatrics, 89,* 197–202.

DiClemente, R. J., & Wingood, G. M. (1995). A randomized controlled trial of an HIV sexual risk-reduction intervention for young African-American women. *Journal of the American Medical Association, 274*(16), 1271–1276.

Duncan, S. C., Strycker, L. A., & Duncan, T. A. (1999). Exploring associations in developmental trends of adolescent substance use and risky sexual behavior in a high-risk population. *Journal of Behavioral Medicine, 22,* 21–34.

East, P. L. (1998). Racial and ethnic differences in girls' sexual, marital, and birth expectations. *Journal of Marriage and the Family, 60,* 150–162.

Feudo, R., Vining-Bethea, S., Shulman, L. C., Shedlin, M. G., & Burleson, J. A. (1998). Bridgeport's Teen Outreach and Primary Services (TOPS) project: A model for raising community awareness about adolescent HIV risk. *Journal of Adolescent Health, 23*(Suppl. 2), 49–58.

Fishbein, M., Guenther-Grey, C., Johnson, W., Wolitski, R. J., McAlister, A., Rietmeijer, C. A., et al. (1997). Using a theory-based community intervention to reduce AIDS risk behaviors: The CDC's AIDS community demonstration projects. In M. E. Goldberg, M. Fishbein, & S. E. Middlestadt (Eds.), *Social marketing: Theoretical and practical perspectives. Advertising and consumer psychology* (pp. 123–146). Mahwah, NJ: Erlbaum.

Fullilove, M. T., Golden, E., Fullilove, R. E., Lennon, R., Porterfield, D., Schwarcz, S., et al. (1993). Crack cocaine use and high-risk behaviors among sexually active Black adolescents. *Journal of Adolescent Health, 14,* 295–300.

Gomez, C. A., Hernandez, M., & Faigeles, B. (1999). Sex in the new world: An empowerment model for HIV prevention in Latina immigrant women. *Source Health Education and Behavior, 26*(2), 200–212.

Henry Kaiser Family Foundation. (2004, February). Federal funding for HIV/AIDS: The FY 2005 budget request (No. 7029) *HIV/AIDS Policy Fact Sheet.*

Hwang, L. Y., Ross, M. W., Zack, C., Bull, L., Rickman, K., & Holleman, M. (2000). Prevalence of sexually transmitted infections and associated risk factors among populations of drug abusers. *Clinical Infectious Diseases, 31*(4), 920–926.

Ironson, G., Solomon, G. F., Balbin, E. G., O'Cleirigh, C., George, A., Kumar, M., et al. (2002). The Ironson-woods Spirituality/Religiousness Index is associated with long survival, health behaviors, less distress, and low cortisol in people with HIV/AIDS. *Annals of Behavioral Medicine, 24*(1), 24–48.

Janssen, R. S., Holtgrave, D. R., Valdiserri, R. O., Shepherd, M., & Gayle, H. D. (2001). The serostatus approach to fighting the HIV epidemic: Prevention strategies for infected individuals. *American Journal of Public Health, 91,* 1019–1024.

Jemmott, J. B., & Jemmott, L. S. (1993). Alcohol and drug use during sexual activity: Predicting the HIV-risk-related behaviors of inner-city Black male adolescents. *Journal of Adolescent Research, 8,* 41–57.

Jessor, R., Van Den Bos, J., Vanderryn, J., Costa, F. M., & Turbin, M. S. (1995). Protective factors in adolescent problem behavior: Moderator effects and developmental change. *Developmental Psychology, 31,* 923–933.

Jones, D. L., Ishii, M., LaPirriere, A., Stanley, H., Antoni, M., Ironson, G., et al. (2003). Influencing medication adherence among women with AIDS. *AIDS Care, 15*(4), 463–474.

Joseph, S. C. (1991). AIDS and adolescence: A challenge to both treatment and prevention. *Journal of Adolescent Health, 12,* 614–618.

Kalichman, S. C., Rompa, D., Cage, M., DiFonzo, K., Simpson, D., Austin, J., et al. (2001). Effectiveness of an intervention to reduce HIV transmission risks in HIV-positive people. *American Journal of Preventive Medicine, 21*(2), 84–92.

Kamb, M. L., Fishbein, M., Douglas, J. M., Rhodes, F., Rogers, J., Bolan, G., et al. (1998). Efficacy of risk-reduction counseling to prevent human immunodeficiency virus and sexually transmitted diseases: A randomized controlled trial (Project RESPECT Study Group). *Journal of the American Medical Association, 280*(13), 1161–1170.

Kann, L., Kinchen, S. A., Williams, B. I., Ross, J. G., Lowry, R., Hill, C., et al. (1998). Youth risk behavior surveillance—United States, 1997. *Morbidity and Mortality Weekly Report, 47*(SS-3), 1–89.

Kann, L., Warren, C. W., Harris, W. A., Collins, J. L., Douglas, K. A., Collins, M. E., et al. (1995). Youth risk behavior surveillance—United States, 1993. *Morbidity and Mortality Weekly Report, 44,* 1–57.

Kassler, W. J., Zenilman, J. M., Erickson, B., Fox, R., Peterman, T. A., & Hook, E. W. (1994). Seroconversion in patients attending sexually transmitted disease clinics. *AIDS, 8,* 351–355.

Kegeles, S. M., Hays, R. B., & Coates, T. J. (1996). The Mpowerment Project: A community-level HIV prevention intervention for young gay men. *American Journal of Public Health, 86*(8, Pt. 1), 1129–1136.

Kelly, J. A. (1995). *Changing HIV risk behavior: Practical strategies.* New York: Guilford Press.

Kelly, J. A., & Kalichman, S. C. (2002). Behavioral research in HIV/AIDS primary and secondary prevention: Recent advances and future directions. *Journal of Consulting and Clinical Psychology, 70*(3), 626–639.

Kelly, J. A., Kalichman, S. C., Kauth, M. R., Kilgore, H. G., Hood, H. V., Campos, P. E., et al. (1991). Situational factors associated with AIDS risk behavior lapses and coping strategies used by gay men who successfully avoid lapses. *American Journal of Public Health, 81,* 1335–1338.

Kelly, J. A., Murphy, D. A., Washington, C. D., Wilson, T. S., Koob, J. J., Davis, D. R., et al. (1994). The effects of HIV/AIDS intervention groups for high-risk women in urban clinics. *American Journal of Public Health, 84*(12), 1918–1922.

Kelly, J. A., Otto-Salaj, L. L., Sikkema, K. J., Pinkerton, S. D., & Bloom, F. R. (1998). Implications of HIV treatment advances for behavioral research on AIDS: Protease inhibitors and new challenges in HIV secondary prevention. *Health Psychology, 17*(4), 310–319.

Kelly, J. A., St. Lawrence, J. S., Hood, H. V., & Brasfield, T. L. (1989). Behavioral intervention to reduce AIDS risk activities. *Journal of Consulting and Clinical Psychology, 57*, 60–67.

Kingsley, J., Detels, R., Kaslow, R., Polk, B. F., Rinaldo, C. R., Chmiel, D. K., et al. (1987). Risk factors for seroconversion to human immunodeficiency virus among male homosexuals. *Lancet, 1*(8529), 345–349.

Kiwanuka-Tondo, J., & Snyder, L. B. (2002). The influence of organizational characteristics and campaign design elements on communication campaign quality: Evidence from 91 Ugandan AIDS campaigns. *Journal of Health Communication, 7*(1), 59–77.

Kotchick, B. A., Shaffer, A., & Forehand, R. (2001). Adolescent sexual risk behavior: A multi-system perspective. *Clinical Psychology Review, 21*(4), 491–519.

Laga, M., Manoka, A., Kivuvu, M., Malele, B., Tuliza, M., Nzila, N. G. J., et al. (1993). Non-ulcerative sexually transmitted diseases as risk factors for HIV-1 transmission in women: Results from a cohort study. *AIDS, 7*(95–102).

Lauby, J. L., Smith, P. J., Stark, M., Person, B., & Adams, J. (2000). A community-level HIV prevention intervention for inner-city women: Results of the women and infants demonstration projects. *American Journal of Public Health, 90*(2), 216–222.

Leigh, B. C., Morrison, D. M., Trocki, K., & Temple, M. T. (1994). Sexual behavior of American adolescents: Results from a U.S. national survey. *Journal of Adolescent Health, 15*, 117–125.

Levine, W. C., Pope, V., Bhoomkar, A., Tambe, P., Lewis, J. S., Zaidi, A. A., et al. (1998). Increase in endocervical CD4 lymphocytes among women with nonulcerative sexually transmitted diseases. *Journal of Infectious Diseases, 177*, 167–174.

Luster, T., & Small, S. A. (1994). Factors associated with sexual risk-taking behaviors among adolescents. *Journal of Marriage and the Family, 56*, 622–632.

McCormack, W. M. (1994). Pelvic inflammatory disease. *New England Journal of Medicine, 330*, 115–119.

McCusker, J., Stoddard, A. M., Zapka, J. G., & Lewis, B. F. (1993). Behavioral outcomes of AIDS educational interventions for drug users in short-term treatment. *American Journal of Public Health, 83*(10), 1463–1466.

Miller, K. S., Forehand, R., & Kotchick, B. A. (2000). Adolescent sexual behavior in two ethnic minority samples: A multi-system perspective. *Adolescence, 35*, 313–333.

Miller, K. S., Kotchick, B. A., & Forehand, R. (1999). Adolescent sexual behavior in two ethnic minority samples: The role of family variables. *Journal of Marriage and the Family, 61*, 85–98.

Murphy, D. A., Lu, M. C., Martin, D., Hoffman, D., & Marelich, W. D. (2002). Results of a pilot intervention trial to improve antiretroviral adherence among HIV-positive patients. *Journal of the Association of Nurses in AIDS Care, 13*(6), 57–69.

Myhre, S. L., & Flora, J. A. (2000). A theoretically based evaluation of HIV/AIDS prevention campaigns along the trans-African highway in Kenya. *Journal of Health Communication, 5,* 29–45.

National Institutes of Health. (1997). Interventions to prevent HIV risk behaviors. *NIH Consensus Statement Online, 15*(2), 1–41.

National Institutes of Health. (2004). *FY 2005 Budget of the United States.* Rockville, MD: U.S. Department of Health and Human Services, Office of the Budget.

Ostrow, D. E., Fox, K. J., Chmiel, J. S., Silvestre, A., Visscher, B. R., Vanable, P. A., et al. (2002). Attitudes towards highly active antiretroviral therapy are associated with sexual risk taking among HIV-infected and uninfected homosexual men. *AIDS, 16*(5), 775–780.

Overby, K. J., & Kegeles, S. M. (1994). The impact of AIDS on an urban population of high-risk female minority adolescents: Implications for intervention. *Journal of Adolescent Health, 15,* 216–227.

Panford, S., Nyaney, M. O., Amoah, S. O., & Aidoo, N. G. (2001). Using folk media in HIV/AIDS prevention in rural Ghana. *American Journal of Public Health, 91*(10), 1559–1562.

Parsons, J. T., Huszti, H. C., Crudder, S. O., Gage, B., Jarvis, D., Mendoza, J., et al. (1998). Determinants of HIV risk reduction behaviors among female partners of men with hemophilia and HIV infection. *AIDS and Behavior, 2*(1), 1–12.

Peterson, J. L., Coates, T. J., Catania, J., Hauck, W. W., Acree, M., Daigle, D., et al. (1996). Evaluation of an HIV risk reduction intervention among African-American homosexual and bisexual men. *AIDS, 10*(3), 319–325.

Purcell, D. W., Malow, R. M., Dolezal, C., & Carballo-Dieguez, A. (2004). Sexual abuse of boys: Short- and long-term associations and implications for HIV prevention. In J. L. Koenig, L. S. Doll, A. O'Leary, & W. Pequegnat (Eds.), *From child sexual abuse to adult sexual risk: Trauma, revictimization, and intervention* (pp. 93–114). Washington, DC: American Psychological Association.

Romer, D., Black, M., Ricardo, I., Feigelman, S., Kalijee, L., Galbraith, J., et al. (1994). Social influences on the sexual behavior of youth at risk for HIV exposure. *American Journal of Public Health, 84,* 977–985.

Rosser, B. S., Gobby, J. M., & Carr, W. P. (1999). The unsafe sexual behavior of persons living with HIV/AIDS: An empirical approach to developing new HIV preventive interventions targeting HIV-positive persons. *Journal of Sex Education and Therapy, 24*(1/2), 18–28.

Royce, R. A., Sena, A., Cates, W., & Cohen, M. S. (1997). Sexual transmission of HIV. *New England Journal of Medicine, 336,* 1072–1078.

Schneiderman, N. (1999). Behavioral medicine and the management of HIV/AIDS. *International Journal of Behavioral Medicine, 6*(1), 3–12.

Seidman, S. N., & Reider, R. O. (1994). A review of sexual behavior in the United States. *American Journal of Psychiatry, 151,* 330–341.

Shrier, L. A., Emans, S. J., Woods, E. R., & DuRant, R. H. (1996). The association of sexual risk behaviors and problem drug behaviors in high school students. *Journal of Adolescent Health, 20,* 377–383.

Siegal, H. A., Li, L., Leviton, L. C., Cole, P. A., Hook, E. W., Bachmann, L., et al. (1999). Under the influence: Risky sexual behavior and substance abuse among driving under the influence offenders. *Sexually Transmitted Diseases, 26*(2), 87–92.

Sikkema, K. J., Hansen, N. B., Kochman, A., Tate, D. C., & Difranceisco, W. (2004). Outcomes from a randomized clinical trial of a group intervention for HIV positive men and women coping with AIDS-related loss and bereavement. *Death Studies, 28*(3), 187–209.

Singhal, A., & Rogers, E. M. (2003). *Combating AIDS: Communication strategies in action.* Thousand Oaks, CA: Sage.

Small, S. A., & Luster, T. (1994). Adolescent sexual activity: An ecological, risk-factor approach. *Journal of Marriage and the Family, 56,* 181–192.

Smith, S. R., Rublein, J. C., Marcus, C., Brock, T. P., & Chesney, M. A. (2003). A medication self-management program to improve adherence to HIV therapy regimes. *Patient Education and Counseling, 50*(2), 187–199.

Sonenstein, F. L., Pleck, J. H., & Ku, L. C. (1991). Levels of sexual activity among adolescent males in the United States. *Family Planning Perspectives, 23,* 162–167.

Spinola, S. M., Orazi, A., Arno, J. N., Fortney, K., Kotylo, P., Chen, C. Y., et al. (1996). Haemophilus ducreyi elicits a cutaneous infiltrate of CD4 cells during experimental human infection. *Journal of Infectious Diseases, 173,* 394–402.

Stanton, B., Li, X., Black, M., Ricardo, I., Galbraith, J., Kalijee, L., et al. (1994). Sexual practices and intentions among preadolescent and early adolescent low-income urban African-Americans. *Pediatrics, 93,* 966–973.

Stober, D. R., Schwartz, J. A. J., McDaniel, J. S., & Abrams, R. F. (1997). Depression and HIV disease: Prevalence, correlates and treatment. *Psychiatric Annals, 27*(5), 372–377.

Strunin, L., & Hingson, R. (1992). Alcohol, drugs, and adolescent sexual behaviors. *International Journal of the Addictions, 27,* 129–146.

Trickett, E. (2002). Context, culture, and collaboration in AIDS interventions: Ecological ideas for enhancing community impact. *Journal of Primary Prevention, 23,* 157–174.

Tubman, J. G., Windle, M., & Windle, R. C. (1996). Cumulative sexual intercourse patterns among middle adolescents: Problem behavior precursors and concurrent health risk behaviors. *Journal of Adolescent Health, 18,* 182–191.

Wasserheit, J. N. (1992). Epidemiological synergy: Interrelationships between human immunodeficiency virus infection and other sexually transmitted diseases. *Sexually Transmitted Diseases, 19,* 61–77.

Witte, K., Cameron, K. A., Lapinski, M. K., & Nzyuko, S. (1998). A theoretically based evaluation of HIV/AIDS prevention campaigns along the trans-Africa highway in Kenya. *Journal of Health Communication, 3*(4), 345–363.

Chapter 13

OBESITY

CYNTHIA J. STEIN AND GRAHAM A. COLDITZ

The United States is experiencing an epidemic of overweight and obesity. The prevalence of excess weight has rapidly increased across the country: close to 65% of the adult population is currently overweight or obese (Flegal, Carroll, Ogden, & Johnson, 2002). The prevalence of overweight (BMI $\geq$ 25 kg/m^2) has increased by 40% (from 46% to 64.5%) comparing the period 1976–1980 (Flegal, Carroll, Kuczmarski, & Johnson, 1998) to 1999–2000 (Flegal et al., 2002), and the prevalence of obesity (BMI $\geq$ 30 kg/m^2) has risen by 110% (from 14.5% to 30.5%).

We are also witnessing an alarming increase in weight among our youth. More than 10% of 2- to 5-year-olds and 15% of 6- to 12-year-olds are overweight (BMI $\geq$ 95th percentile for age and gender; Ogden, Flegal, Carroll, & Johnson, 2002). This represents a near doubling of overweight children and a near tripling of overweight adolescents over the past 3 decades (National Center for Health Statistics, 2001; U.S. Department of Health and Human Services, 2001). While some segments of the population are more likely to be overweight or obese than others, people of all ages, races, ethnicities, socioeconomic levels, and geographic areas are experiencing a substantial increase in weight (U.S. Department of Health and Human Services, 2001).

International data indicate that the epidemic is not isolated to the United States, but is a global health problem (Flegal et al., 1998; International Agency for Research on Cancer, 2002; Popkin, 1998). The prevalence of obesity is rising in other developed and affluent countries and is now spreading to less affluent countries (Popkin, 1998).

LIFESTYLE TRENDS

Overweight and obesity result from the interaction of many factors, including genetic, metabolic, behavioral, and environmental influences. The rapidity with which obesity is increasing suggests that behavioral and environmental influences, rather than biological changes, have fueled the epidemic. Increasing energy consumption, decreasing energy expenditure, or a combination of both has led to an energy imbalance and a marked increase in our society's weight.

Over time, we have changed our eating habits and activity levels, but the specific details of these complex behavior changes are not well understood. In evaluating caloric intake, the data from large national surveys have shown mixed results (Harnack, Jeffery, & Boutelle, 2000). For example, data from the National Health and Nutrition Examination Survey (NHANES) suggest that average energy intake increased between 1971 and 2000 (Centers for Disease Control and Prevention [CDC], 2004). However, Popkin, Siega-Riz, Haines, and Jahns (2001), analyzing data from the Nationwide Food Consumption Survey (1965 and 1977 to 1978) and the Continuing Survey of Food Intake by Individuals (1989 to 1991 and 1994 to 1996), did not find a large difference in caloric intake in 1994 to 1996 compared to 1965 (Popkin et al., 2001).

Aside from national surveys, ecological data seem to support the idea that energy intake has increased (Harnack et al., 2000). Despite the fact that there has been an increase in availability and consumption of low-fat food items over time, a number of trends could contribute to an increased energy imbalance and the observed rise in obesity: higher per capita energy availability (Frazao, 1999); increased percentage of food consumed outside the home, including fast food (Harnack et al., 2000; Nielsen, Siega-Riz, & Popkin, 2002); greater consumption of soft drinks (French, Lin, & Guthrie, 2003; Nielsen et al., 2002; Smiciklas-Wright, Mitchell, Mickle, Goldman, & Cook, 2003); and larger portion sizes (Harnack et al., 2000; Smiciklas-Wright et al., 2003).

The inconsistent data on energy intake suggest that the energy imbalance and rising levels of obesity may be more closely related to changes in energy expenditure. As with energy intake, competing influences exist. For example, the number of health clubs, recreational facilities, and homes with exercise equipment has grown (Jeffery & Utter, 2003). However, sedentary activities, such as television watching and videogame playing, have also increased. Of note, television viewing is associated with greater weight in children and adults (Gortmaker, Dietz, & Cheung, 1990), but it is unclear if this relationship is due more to a corresponding increase in food consumption or to a decrease in physical activity (Jeffery & Utter, 2003). Prospective data from the "Growing Up Today Study" of 16,000 adolescents indicate that television viewing is a strong and independent predictor of excess weight gain during adolescence (Berkey et al., 2000; Berkey, Rockett, Gillman, & Colditz, 2003).

Overall, it appears that levels of adult leisure-time activity have not changed significantly (CDC, 2001). What seems to have changed, however, is the level of activity required for work and daily living (Hill & Melanson, 1999), although this has not yet been well documented. Advances in technology have greatly reduced dependence on walking and cycling for transportation. Household physical activity has likely decreased due to labor-saving devices. The availability of mechanized labor aids has created a drop in occupational energy requirements, and in general, jobs have become more sedentary. Today 60% of the U.S. population do not participate in regular physical activity, and 25% are almost entirely sedentary (U.S. Department of Health and Human Services, 1996). In addition, physical activity in schools has declined, and almost half of young Americans between the ages of 12 and 21 are not vigorously active on a routine basis (U.S. Department of Health and Human Services, 1996).

Although the complexities of this relationship are not yet fully understood, the end result is quite clear: the imbalance of energy intake and energy expenditure has resulted in an epidemic of overweight and obesity across the United States.

MEASURING OVERWEIGHT AND OBESITY

As the prevalence of overweight and obesity continues to increase, efforts have been made to quantify this weight change in individuals and in the population. Because fat is stored throughout the body, it cannot be measured directly. Body weight itself can provide an indication of fat stores, but because body build and composition are extremely variable, there is no "ideal body weight." Instead, other measurements are often used to estimate body fat and better quantify health risk. These include body mass index (BMI), waist circumference (WC), waist-to-hip ratio (WHR), skin-fold thickness, and bioimpedence. These measurements cannot capture all the variables that impact risk, but they can be used as tools to estimate risk.

The measurement used most often to quantify body fat is BMI (see Table 13.1). It is relatively easy to calculate (weight in kilograms divided by the square of the height in meters); it has defined risk categories (overweight: BMI ≥ 25 kg/m^2; obesity: BMI ≥ 30 kg/m^2), and it is closely correlated with body fat in most people. It is not a perfect measure, however. BMI does not distinguish between fat mass and lean mass and therefore does not provide an accurate indication of body fat in extremely muscular individuals or in people who have lost significant muscle mass. In addition, BMI may not be a sensitive indicator of the

Table 13.1 Determining Body Mass Index (BMI) in Adults

$$BMI = \frac{\text{Weight (kilograms)}}{\text{Height}^2 \text{ (meters)}} = \frac{\text{Weight (pounds)} \times 703}{\text{Height}^2 \text{ (inches)}}$$

Height (feet and inches)	Weight (pounds)																
	100	110	120	130	140	150	160	170	180	190	200	210	220	230	240	250	260
4'10"	21	23	25	27	29	31	33	36	38	40	42	44	46	48	50	52	54
4'11"	20	22	24	26	28	30	32	34	36	38	40	42	44	46	49	51	53
5'0"	20	22	23	25	27	29	31	33	35	37	39	41	43	45	47	49	51
5'1"	19	21	23	25	26	28	30	32	34	36	38	40	42	44	45	47	49
5'2"	18	20	22	24	26	27	29	31	33	35	37	38	40	42	44	46	47
5'3"	18	20	21	23	25	27	28	30	32	34	35	37	39	41	43	44	46
5'4"	17	19	21	22	24	26	28	29	31	33	34	36	38	40	41	43	44
5'5"	17	18	20	22	23	25	27	28	30	32	33	35	37	38	40	42	43
5'6"	16	18	19	21	23	24	26	27	29	31	32	34	36	37	39	40	42
5'7"	16	17	19	20	22	24	25	27	28	30	31	33	35	36	38	39	41
5'8"	15	17	18	20	21	23	24	26	27	29	30	32	33	35	37	38	40
5'9"	15	16	18	19	21	22	24	25	27	28	30	31	33	34	35	37	38
5'10"	14	16	17	19	20	22	23	24	26	27	29	30	32	33	34	36	37
5'11"	14	15	17	18	20	21	22	24	25	27	28	29	31	32	34	35	36
6'0"	14	15	16	18	19	20	22	23	24	26	27	28	30	31	33	34	35
6'1"	13	15	16	17	19	20	21	22	24	25	26	28	29	30	32	33	34
6'2"	13	14	15	17	18	19	21	22	23	24	26	27	28	30	31	32	33
6'3"	13	14	15	16	18	19	20	21	23	24	25	26	28	29	30	31	33
6'4"	12	13	15	16	17	18	20	21	22	23	24	26	27	28	29	30	32
6'5"	12	13	14	15	17	18	19	20	21	23	24	25	26	27	29	30	31

☐ Underweight (BMI < 18.5)

☐ Healthy weight (BMI 18.5–24.9)

☐ Overweight (BMI 25–29.9)

☐ Obese (BMI 30+)

Note: For children and adolescents, overweight is defined as being at or above the 95th percentile of BMI, based on age- and sex-specific growth charts.
Source: BMI interpretation according to the National Heart, Lung, and Blood Institute.

health risks associated with moderate weight gain (10 to 20 pounds) in individuals that fall within the normal BMI range. Despite these limitations, BMI can be a reliable and valid measure for identifying adults at increased risk of overweight—and obesity-related morbidity and mortality (U.S. Preventive Services Task Force, 2003).

HEALTH CONSEQUENCES

Even small increases in weight across a population can have a devastating impact on public health. Close to 300,000 deaths each year in the United States may be attributable to obesity (Allison, Fontaine, Manson, Stevens, & VanItallie, 1999), making it the second leading cause of preventable death in this country (National Heart, Lung and Blood Institute, 1998). Excess weight increases the risk of multiple conditions, including cardiovascular disease, type 2 diabetes, cancer, and premature death (U.S. Department of Health and Human Services, 2001; see Table 13.2). The adverse health consequences do not occur only in those individuals classified as overweight and obese; disease risk starts to increase even for those at the upper end of the normal range (BMI of 22 to 24.9; Field et al., 2001).

Although there are a multitude of negative consequences associated with excess weight, many may be reversible with weight loss. For example, randomized trials have shown that weight loss leads to a reduction in blood pressure, better glucose tolerance, and an improved lipid profile (National Heart, Lung and Blood Institute, 1998). The U.S. Preventive Services Task Force (2003) has concluded that these improvements in intermediate outcomes provide indirect evidence of the health benefits achievable with modest weight reduction.

Heart Disease

A large variety of studies have linked obesity to an increased risk of heart disease, and it has been estimated that 20% to 30% of coronary heart disease (CHD) mortality may be attributable to excess body weight (Seidell, Verschuren, van Leer, & Kromhout, 1996). This is especially significant given that heart disease is the most common cause of death in the United States, killing over 700,000 Americans

Table 13.2   Risk Increase Associated with Obesity

Level of Evidence	None (RR 1–1.09)	Small (RR 1.1–1.34)	Moderate (RR 1.35–1.99)	Large (RR 2–4.9)	Very Large (RR 5+)
Convincing			Colon	Breast	Esophageal cancer
			CHD	Uterus	Type 2 diabetes
			Stroke	Kidney	Gallstones
				Osteoarthritis	
				Hypertension	
			High cholesterol		
Probable		Cataract	Prostate		

Relative Risk (RR) = Risk in obese population compared to risk in normal weight population.

each year (Anderson & Smith, 2003). Men and women who are overweight or obese may be two to three times more likely than their leaner peers to develop CVD (Harris, Ballard-Barbasch, Madans, Makue, & Feldman, 1993; Rimm et al., 1995), and they are also more likely to die from it (Seidell et al., 1996). Moreover, excess weight early in life is predictive of CHD mortality. Overweight adolescents may be more than twice as likely as their lean peers to die from CHD during adulthood (Must, Jacques, Dallal, Bajema, & Dietz, 1992).

Hypertension

Among men and women, hypertension is one of the most common conditions related to overweight and obesity (Must et al., 1999). The diagnosis and treatment of hypertension come with enormous personal and financial costs, and hypertension is associated with an increased risk of CVD, aortic dissection, renal damage, cerebrovascular disease, and dementia. In terms of its association with excess weight, there is a strong linear relation between BMI and blood pressure, and both weight (Ascherio et al., 1992; Folsom, Prineas, Kaye, & Soler, 1989; Witteman et al., 1989) and weight gain (Field et al., 1999; Yong, Kuller, Rutan, & Bunker, 1993) are positively associated with the development of hypertension. For example, compared to leaner women, overweight women may be almost three times more likely, and obese women nearly six times more likely, to develop hypertension (Witteman et al., 1989).

Diabetes

Over 18 million people in the United States have type 2 diabetes (CDC, 2002), which is the sixth leading cause of death in the United States (Anderson & Smith, 2003). Complications of diabetes include blindness, renal disease, heart disease, stroke, peripheral vascular disease, and neuropathy. Using data from the Nurses' Health Study (Hu et al., 2001), Hu estimated that as much as 80% of type 2 diabetes could be attributed to the combined effect of inactivity and overweight or obesity (F. B. Hu, personal communication, January 2001). There is a strong linear relationship between BMI and risk of type 2 diabetes mellitus (Chan, Rimm, Colditz, Stampfer, & Willet, 1994; Colditz et al., 1990; Colditz, Willet, Rotnitzky, & Manson, 1995; Lundgren, Bengtsson, Blohme, Lapidus, & Sjostrom, 1988); obese individuals have almost 10 times the risk of diabetes compared to their non-obese peers (Colditz et al., 1995). Independent of BMI, weight gain, WC, and WHR also strongly correlate with diabetes risk (Carey et al., 1997; Hartz, Rupley, Kalkhoff, & Rimm, 1983; Holbrook, Barrett-Connor, & Wingard, 1989; Lundgren, Bengtsson, Blohme, Lapidus, & Sjostrom, 1989; Ohlson et al., 1985).

Cancer

Excess weight has been linked to a variety of cancers. The International Agency for Research on Cancer (IARC, 2002) has estimated that overweight and obesity cause 9% of postmenopausal breast cancer, 11% of colon cancer, 25% of renal cancer, 37% of esophageal cancer, and 39% of endometrial cancer. Calle, Rodriguez, Walker-Thurmond, and Thun (2003) found that obesity was associated with a higher risk of death from 14 cancers, including cancer of the esophagus, colon and rectum, liver, gallbladder, pancreas, kidney, stomach, prostate, breast, uterus, cervix, and ovary, in addition to non-Hodgkin's lymphoma, and multiple myeloma. They estimated that overweight and obesity may account for 14% of all cancer deaths in men and 20% in women.

Cerebrovascular Disease

Stroke is the third leading cause of death in the United States (Anderson & Smith, 2003) and a leading cause of significant, long-term disability. Various measures of obesity have been associated with an increased risk of cerebrovascular disease in men and women. For example, Rexrode et al. (1997) reported that the risk of ischemic stroke increased with BMI, and obese women had approximately twice the risk as lean women. In men, associations between stroke and both BMI (Field et al., 2001) and WHR (Walker et al., 1996) have been reported.

Gallstones

Gallstones are fairly common, and though many are asymptomatic, they can cause pain and inflammation and often lead to treatment with laproscopic cholecystectomy. Although gallstones do form in lean adults, the relationship between weight and gallstone formation is very strong. Compared to women in the healthy weight range, overweight women have close to twice the risk of developing gallstones and obese women have 2.5 to 3 times the risk. Gallstones are more common in women; however, similar trends of increased risk with higher BMI have also been seen in men (Field et al., 2001).

Osteoarthritis

Over 20 million people in the United States have osteoarthritis (National Institute of Arthritis and Musculoskeletal and Skin Diseases, 1998). This condition, characterized by the degeneration of the joint cartilage, can cause severe pain and functional limitations. It is a leading cause of disability and also the most common reason for joint replacement surgery. Compared to their leaner peers, overweight adults are at increased risk of developing osteoarthritis of the knee (Cicuttini, Baker, & Spector, 1996) and hip (Cooper et al., 1998). Overweight and obesity are also associated with an increased risk of knee and hip replacement surgery (Wendelboe et al., 2003).

Additional Consequences

Overweight and obesity also increase the risk of a large variety of other conditions, including dyslipidemia, sleep apnea, asthma (U.S. Department of Health and Human Services, 2001), cataracts (Hiller et al., 1998; Schaumberg, Glynn, Christen, Hankinson, & Hennekens, 2000; Weintraub et al., 2002), benign prostatic hypertrophy (Giovannucci et al., 1994), menstrual irregularities, pregnancy complications, depression, and social discrimination (U.S. Department of Health and Human Services, 2001). Obesity also negatively affects physical functioning, vitality (Coakley et al., 1998), and general health-related quality of life (Fine et al., 1999).

ECONOMIC IMPACT

Excess weight not only causes widespread health effects, it also results in a tremendous economic burden. Assessing this economic cost is an additional method of summarizing the broad impact of the epidemic on society. It is estimated that obesity costs the United States $117 billion each year (U.S. Department of Health and Human Services, 2001). This estimate includes both direct costs (related to diagnosis and treatment of illness, including doctor visits, medications, hospitalizations, and nursing home stays) and indirect costs (resulting from lost wages and productivity due to illness or premature death; U.S. Department of Health and Human Services, 2001; Wolf, 1998).

The true cost of the current epidemic of overweight and obesity is likely much higher than the $117 billion estimate, which is based on the costs of obesity and does not fully address the costs related to individuals who are overweight but not obese. It also does not take into account other significant and costly conditions associated with obesity, such as reduced physical functioning, sleep apnea, pregnancy complications, and cataracts. Using a conservative approach, Thompson, Edelsberg, Colditz, Bird, and Oster (1999) estimated that the excess health care costs linked to obesity were nearly as high as those associated with smoking.

DEFINING OBESITY

Observed statistical associations between weight and mortality have driven recommendations. In setting the 1995 weight guidelines (U.S. Department of Agriculture & U.S. Department of Health and Human Services, 1995), the Dietary Guidelines Advisory Committee concluded that mortality risk increased significantly among persons with a BMI of 25 or higher (Lee & Paffenbarger, 1992; Rimm et al., 1995; Willet et al., 1995), whereas a linear increase in risk of diabetes, hypertension, and coronary heart disease is observed well below a BMI of 25 (Chan et al., 1994; Colditz et al., 1995; Willet et al., 1995). A two- to fourfold increase in risk is observed among those with a BMI of 24 to 25 compared to those with a BMI of 21. Because of the importance of total mortality as a summary measure of the public health impact of obesity, and because the designation of overweight at a point below a BMI of 25 would label over 50% of the adult U.S. population overweight, the committee concluded that a BMI of 25 represented a reasonable upper limit for healthy weight. Use of this cutpoint is consistent with that recommended by a steering committee of the American Institute of Nutrition (Kuller et al., 1993) and an expert committee of the World Health Organization (WHO; 1995). The International Obesity Task Force provided a more detailed breakdown of BMI categories. A BMI of 18.5 to 24.9 represents a healthy weight, 25 to 29.9 overweight, 30 to 34.9 class I obesity, 35 to 39.9 class II obesity, and 40+ class III obesity (WHO, 1998).

Body Mass Index

BMI is used in all these guidelines as a measure of adiposity, independent of height. Growing evidence suggests that BMI reflects adiposity well through middle age, but may be less clearly related to adiposity at older ages, when lean muscle mass may decrease and mass is redistributed to the abdomen. "Girth grow," or increasing WC with age, appears to predict risk of diabetes, heart disease, and stroke. Increasing abdominal girth has also been associated with benign prostatic hyperplasia (Giovannucci et al., 1994).

Waist Circumference and Waist-to-Hip Ratio

Debate continues regarding the possible use of WC or WHR as a measure of adiposity. Neither measurement is yet standard clinical practice. WC is a simple measurement that is easy to obtain and record. It correlates well with abdominal fat distribution and is associated with multiple disease risk factors (WHO, 1998) and quality of life (Lean, Han, & Seidell, 1998). Furthermore, it can indicate increased

Table 13.3   Disease Risk Based on Waist Circumference

Level of Risk	Women	Men
Increased risk	≥ 31 in. (80 cm)	≥ 37 in. (94 cm)
High risk	≥ 35 in. (88 cm)	≥ 40 in. (102 cm)

disease risk even among individuals of normal BMI (NITLBI, 1998). Table 13.3 suggests guidelines for estimating disease risk based on WC. Although the specific measurements that correspond to a given category may vary by population, a general guideline is that a waist that has reached or exceeded 31 inches for women or 37 inches for men may indicate an increased risk of disease (Lean, Han, & Morrison, 1995; WHO, 1998). WC should be measured at the midpoint between the lower edge of the rib cage and the iliac crest (WHO, 1998).

WHR has also been used to estimate intra-abdominal fat, and a WHR > 0.80 in women and > 0.95 in men has been associated with multiple disease risk factors (Lean et al., 1995). Both WC and WHR show a similar relationship to health outcomes, but WC may be preferable because it is easier to measure and may therefore be more clinically useful.

Weight Gain

Adult weight gain is observed in most countries with established market economies. Change in weight provides a single, readily interpretable number that is known, at least approximately, to most persons. As adult height is attained by approximately age 18, increase in weight after this point is almost exclusively through the addition of adipose tissue. Although it is possible to increase adiposity without changing weight, weight gain in adult life generally reflects an increase in adiposity. Many weight control guidelines recommend focusing first on the avoidance of weight gain before attempting weight loss. Because treatment of obesity has poor success and is often followed by regain of weight, preventing weight gain is a high priority and a necessary part of a public health approach.

DISPARITIES IN OBESITY

In the United States, the age-adjusted prevalence of obesity has increased tremendously over the past few decades (Kuczmarski, Flegal, Campbell, & Johnson, 1994). The proportion of the U.S. adult population over 20 exceeding the healthy weight ranges (i.e., the prevalence of BMI > 25) is high: 59.4% of men,

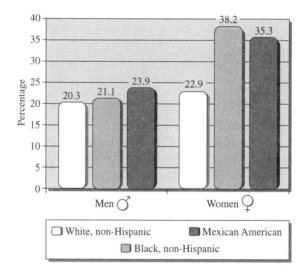

Figure 13.1   Prevalence of Obesity by Gender and Race/Ethnicity (Adults, Age 20 and Older). *Data source:* **NHANES III from "Prevalence and Trends in Obesity among U.S. Adults, 1999–2000," by K. M. Flegal, M. D. Carroll, C. L. Ogden, and C. L. Johnson, 2002,** *Journal of the American Medical Association, 288*(14), **pp. 1723–1727.**

50.7% of women, or 54.9% of the total U.S. population. Those who are obese (BMI ≥ 30) represent 24.8% of women and 20% of men, or, overall, 22.8% of the adult population (Flegal et al., 1998).

While the prevalence of overweight and obesity has increased across all racial and ethnic groups, certain trends have been observed (see Figure 13.1). For example, among non-Hispanic Black women and Mexican American women, the prevalence of obesity was markedly higher than among non-Hispanic White women in NHANES III (Flegal et al., 2002). Among men, the prevalence of obesity was comparable across ethnic groups, but overweight was more common among Mexican American men than among non-Hispanic White and non-Hispanic Black men (Flegal et al., 2002).

PREVENTION OF WEIGHT GAIN AND OBESITY

The prevention and treatment of excess weight is critical for both the health of individuals and the health of our society. When approaching issues such as weight control we should consider the factors necessary to bring about change: scientific knowledge about the disease and methods of reducing the disease burden, political will to allocate resources to address the problem, and social strategies to lower the hazards of weight gain and obesity (Atwood, Colditz, & Kawachi, 1997). In the category of social strategy we should address multiple reinforcing levels of intervention, including individual approaches (e.g., dietary adjustments, activity changes), health care system actions (e.g., screening, counseling), and policy actions (e.g., systemwide changes to promote weight control and physical activity). We address many of these intervention strategies next.

Individual Approaches

There are a number of effective strategies for managing weight. These include lifestyle change, behavior therapy, pharmacotherapy, and surgery (NHLBI, 1998).

Lifestyle Change

To achieve a healthy weight, it is important for people to set reasonable goals in terms of limiting caloric intake and increasing physical activity. Individuals should be encouraged to make small, sustainable changes in diet. For those who need to lose weight, reducing caloric intake by 500 to 1,000 calories per day will lead to a recommended weight loss of 1 to 2 pounds per week.

Increasing physical activity helps not only in losing weight but also in maintaining the weight loss over time. It's important to recognize that physical activity does not need to be strenuous to be beneficial. Many activities can be incorporated into daily routines, and even moderate exercise decreases health risk, burns calories, increases basal metabolic rate, and can reduce appetite.

Behavior Therapy

Behavior therapy has been shown to be helpful in weight control when used in combination with other weight-loss efforts, especially in the first year. Behavioral strategies include self-monitoring, stress management, problem solving, stimulus control, and social support. No single behavior therapy has been shown to be superior to others, but multidimentional therapies and those with the highest intensity appear to be the most successful.

Pharmacotherapy

Medications can help with weight loss when used as part of a comprehensive weight management program that includes diet, physical activity, and behavior therapy. If necessary, FDA-approved drugs (such as sibutramine and orlistat) can be used in combination with diet and activity modification in individuals who have the following risk profiles:

- BMI ≥ 27 with obesity-related risk factors and comorbidities, such as hypertension, abnormal lipid levels, heart disease, type 2 diabetes, and sleep apnea.
- BMI ≥ 30 even without any of the above-mentioned risk factors and comorbidities.

Because these medications can cause serious side effects, their use should be monitored closely for adverse effects and drug efficacy. The medications should not be combined and should not be prescribed without concomitant diet and exercise modification. For additional information on these medications, see the *Physicians' Desk Reference* (www.pdr.net).

Surgery

Gastrointestinal surgery is an option for those with severe obesity when used as part of a comprehensive program addressing diet, exercise, and social support. Surgery can be considered in individuals who have not been successful with medical treatment and who are severely obese:

- BMI ≥ 35 with comorbid conditions.
- BMI ≥ 40 with or without comorbidities.

Health Care Provider Strategies

Health care providers can play an important role in monitoring patients' weight and assisting with diet and physical activity counseling. The U.S. Preventive Services Task Force (2003) recommends that clinicians screen patients for obesity and offer intensive counseling and behavioral interventions. All patients should be encouraged to maintain a healthy weight by eating a nutritious diet and exercising regularly to balance energy intake and energy expenditure. Individuals who are overweight should be assisted in losing weight gradually, with a focus on long-term weight loss and maintenance. A variety of approaches can be effective in treating excess weight, and detailed guidelines have been created for providers to help patients with weight management (National Heart, Lung and Blood Institute, 1998).

The basis for treatment of overweight and obesity is to help patients improve their diets and increase their activity levels. It is important to determine weight status and monitor change in all patients. Measurements of height and weight should be recorded in every patient's chart at least once per year. BMI or WC should also be clearly recorded as an indication of disease risk.

Counseling Patients in the Normal Weight Range

Even a small amount of weight gain within the normal BMI or WC range can increase disease risk and should signal to the patient and provider that an imbalance exists between calorie intake and energy expenditure. Health care providers should talk to all patients about diet and exercise and should counsel patients to make small but sustainable changes. Indications that the patient may need counseling include:

- The patient's weight increases by 10 pounds or more.
- The patient's WC increases by 1 inch or more, even if weight remains stable.
- The patient is approaching the upper limit of normal in terms of BMI or WC.

It is important to intervene early and prevent the progression of weight gain before complications, such as diabetes and vascular disorders, develop. These complications may be irreversible and also may interfere with subsequent exercise and weight control efforts.

Counseling Overweight and Obese Patients

Patients should be counseled first to avoid additional weight gain by making diet and activity changes, then to strive for realistic weight reduction, and finally to maintain the weight loss over time (NHLBI, 1998). For individuals who are overweight or obese, the goal should not be to reach specific guideline end points because this may not be possible. Instead, smaller reductions of 5% to 10% of body weight should be recommended because they are more feasible and have been shown to bring significant improvements in disease risk factors, such as blood pressure, glucose tolerance, and lipid levels. After initial weight loss is achieved, additional weight loss can be attempted if necessary.

To counsel patients on weight control, dietary modification, and physical activity, the 5 As model for smoking cessation can be adapted and utilized:

Ask All Patients about Current Diet and Exercise
- Talk to patients about their food choices, activity levels, desired weight, and any history of weight change.
- Document this information clearly on the chart to help in setting goals and monitoring change.

Advise Patients about the Importance of Weight Control
- Help patients recognize the serious risks of excess weight and the health benefits of weight control.

- Emphasize that the only way to achieve and maintain a healthy weight is by balancing calorie intake and energy expenditure.

Assess **Patients' Attitudes toward Weight Control, Dietary Changes, and Exercise**

- Understanding the patient's readiness to change can help both the provider and the patient set realistic weight goals (see the Stages of Change box).

Stages of Change

All patients should be advised to achieve and maintain a healthy weight. However, this process takes time and effort. While assessing the patient's attitudes toward diet and exercise, it can be helpful to understand the patient's readiness to change. One learning theory used in studying behavior change is the transtheoretical model, which focuses on the stages of change through which individuals can move forward or back at varying rates. Even if patients are not yet ready to change their diet or activity pattern, health care providers may be able to help them move closer to the goal of maintaining a healthy weight.

- **Precontemplation:** The patient is not interested in changing his or her diet or physical activity level within the next 6 months.

  Stress the importance of weight control and offer information.

- **Contemplation:** The patient is not currently interested in weight control but intends to make changes in diet and/or exercise within the next 6 months.

  Provide motivational support, and help the patient become committed to changing diet and activity levels.

- **Preparation:** The patient plans to take steps in the next month to modify his or her diet and/or activity level.

  Work with the patient to identify personal goals and develop a plan of action.

- **Action:** The patient is taking steps to change his or her diet and/or activity level but has been making these changes for less than 6 months.

  Review the patient's goals and address barriers.

- **Maintenance:** The patient has been controlling his or her diet and exercise for 6 months or more.

  Continue to support the patient's activities, and reassess goals and barriers as needed.

Note: Based on Prochaska and DiClemente (1984), *The transtheoretical approach: Crossing traditional boundaries of therapy* (Homewood, Ill.: Dow-Jones/ Irwin).

- Discuss motivation to make changes, previous attempts to maintain or lose weight, and past barriers to change. Motivation is very important for successful weight loss.
- Those patients uninterested or not ready to make lifestyle changes may benefit from additional information on the health risks of overweight and obesity.
- Patients interested in making changes in diet and exercise should be encouraged and given assistance.
- For patients at a healthy, stable weight, provide positive reinforcement and encouragement to maintain a healthy weight.

Assist Patients Who Want to Maintain or Lose Weight

- Discuss realistic dietary changes to alter calorie intake. Focus on small calorie reductions that can be maintained over time.
- Help patients focus on physical activity levels to increase energy expenditure and maintain weight loss.
- Help patients set specific goals for changes in diet and activity.
- Suggest a diet and activity log to monitor progress and address challenges.
- Encourage patients to identify possible barriers and ways to overcome them.
- Discuss potential sources of support, such as friends and family members.

Arrange Follow-Up in 2 to 4 Weeks and Then Periodically as Needed

- Review the patient's diet and activity log.
- Support successful behavior change.
- Reinforce messages. Studies show that the number, type, and duration of reinforcements are central to the success of behavioral interventions.
- Examine barriers that persist or arise.
- Remind patients that successful weight control is an ongoing effort.

MESSAGES TO HELP PATIENTS CONTROL WEIGHT

To achieve and maintain a healthy weight, you must find a balance between the calories you take in from food and the calories you burn during physical activity. Eating more calories than you burn leads to weight gain; eating fewer calories or exercising more leads to weight loss.

To lose 1 pound of weight, you must burn 3,500 calories more than you take in. This is possible by combining healthy eating with increased activity. For example, eating 350 fewer calories and doing 30 minutes of moderate activity (burning 150 cal) leads to a 500-cal reduction per day. Over 7 days, this results in a 3,500-cal reduction and the loss of 1 pound. Even small changes can make a big difference: cutting out one soda (about 150 calories) or taking a 30-minute brisk walk (also about 150 calories) on most days can lead to a weight loss of more than 10 pounds over a year.

Tips on Diet and Weight

The best way to lose weight is to make small changes in diet and exercise that can be maintained over time:

- Set reasonable goals. First, avoid additional weight gain. If you are overweight or obese, aim to lose 10% of your body weight, which can bring significant health benefits.

- If you need to lose weight, do it gradually. Work to lose ½ to 2 pounds per week, and keep it off permanently.

- Motivation is key. You are more likely to succeed when you believe you can and are willing to take steps to control your weight.

- Avoid large, rapid changes in your diet. Your body may react by slowing its basal metabolic rate, making it harder to shed extra pounds. It is better to make small changes that can be maintained over time. Gradual weight loss can lead to decreased body fat, not just the temporary loss of water weight that can come with rapid weight change.

- Avoid fad diets that do not include a variety of nutritious foods or that promise quick and easy weight loss. Weight that is lost quickly is often regained quickly.

- Make healthy food choices. Focus on fruits, vegetables, and whole-grain foods. Many high-fiber foods provide nutrients and help you feel full.

- Know your eating patterns.

- Find ways to deal with stress other than by eating. Try exercising, joining a support group, meditating, or talking to friends.

- Eat a healthy breakfast, and don't skip meals. Try to eat small meals throughout the day to keep from feeling too hungry.

- Plan healthy snacks, and make them readily available. For example, have carrots and celery sticks or pretzels and popcorn around the house. Leave a bowl of fruit on the table. Bring healthy snacks to work.

- Drink water to keep yourself well hydrated, and avoid high-calorie sodas.
- Avoid alcohol, which can add a lot of calories without any nutritional benefit.
- Avoid snacking or eating meals in front of the television.
- Eat smaller portions, and use a smaller plate if you like seeing a plate full of food.
- Identify the barriers to healthy food choices and look for ways to overcome them.
- Mood can affect eating habits; if you feel that you may be depressed, speak to your health care provider about available treatment.

Tips on Exercise and Weight

Physical activity does not need to be strenuous to be healthy. Exercise not only burns calories but also raises the body's metabolic rate (how fast the body burns calories even when you're not exercising). Exercise also helps maintain weight loss over time, decrease appetite, reduce stress, and lower the risk of many chronic diseases.

- Start slowly and build up the amount of physical activity that you do each day.
- Even if your time is very limited, you can reach the recommended 30 minutes per day by doing just a few minutes of exercise several times per day.
- Decrease time spent doing sedentary activities such as watching TV.
- Plan family activities centered around fun and exercise.
- Pick activities you enjoy.
- Establish an exercise routine.
- Make exercise a priority.
- Find a friend to exercise with.
- If you start getting bored, make an exercise log to check your progress or consider adding other types of physical activity to keep up your interest.

Important Reminders

Weight control is a lifelong effort, so don't get discouraged by temporary setbacks. Losing weight can be very challenging. Work to keep yourself motivated.

- Make healthy food choices and stay active.
- Set short-term, realistic goals, and reward yourself for achieving them with nonfood items, such as a movie, a visit with a friend, or a new item of clothing.

- Keep a food diary and an exercise log to monitor your progress, identify barriers, and improve your efforts.
- Avoid weight gain over the holidays. If you do gain weight, take steps to lose it as soon as possible. Even a few pounds gained each year can add up to a large weight gain over time.
- Weight-loss diets should be lower in calories without compromising nutrition.
- Always think about healthy substitutions, such as having a baked potato instead of french fries, a bagel instead of a doughnut, fish instead of beef, pretzels instead of potato chips, or fruit instead of cookies.
- Don't deprive yourself. Instead, look for lower-calorie substitutes. If there is no acceptable substitution available, have a smaller portion or have it less frequently.

Ask for help if you need it: talk to family, friends, or your health care provider. Also, consider a weight-loss support group in your neighborhood or at a health club.

Community Intervention

Lifestyle interventions have proven effective in preventing and treating obesity (Gortmaker et al., 1999; National Heart, Lung and Blood Institute, 1998) and its health consequences (Knowler et al., 2002). However, to be most successful and to sustain positive change over time, individuals' efforts should be facilitated and supported by the larger physical environment. With this aim, a variety of resources have been developed to address the issues of overweight and obesity at the community and population levels (Task Force on Community Preventive Services, 2003; WHO Consultation on Obesity, 1998). Multilevel interventions are needed if we are to stem the epidemic and prevent the growing negative consequences of overweight and obesity.

PROGRAM AND POLICY OPTIONS

One essential part of effective program and policy planning is basing action on consistent messages. Yet, despite solid epidemiologic evidence that weight affects the risk of cancer and other chronic diseases—such as heart disease, diabetes, and hypertension—setting weight guidelines has long been problematic, and recommendations have evolved over time. In general, it is recommended that individuals eat a nutritious diet and exercise regularly to balance energy intake and energy expenditure. Those who are overweight should focus first on avoiding additional weight gain, and then strive to lose weight gradually with the goal of long-term weight loss and maintenance.

Koplan and Dietz (1999) note that lack of a national plan or focus has hindered the development and implementation of weight control strategies and obesity prevention programs. However, work has been done to coordinate efforts at the community level, and the CDC has set forth a range of recommendations (Task Force on Community Preventive Services, 2003; U.S. Department of Health and Human Services, Public Health Service, et al., 1999). These recommendations include understanding the problem and its causes, narrowing the focus of the intervention, targeting efforts, creating a supportive environment, establishing partnerships, setting objectives, and measuring success.

Policy messages must be accurate and consistent, but it is also important to tailor them to the current situation and the target population. Separate strategies should focus on different aspects of the obesity issue. For example, interventions may involve identifying opportunities to incorporate increased physical activity in daily life, providing access to safe areas for physical activity and recreation, or ensuring the availability of healthy food choices in neighborhoods, schools, and worksites.

Multidisciplinary teams can offer unique approaches to obesity prevention. For example, town planners and architects can be challenged to design ways to alter the physical environment to reintroduce physical activity into our modern lives. Parents and educators can create opportunities for increased physical activity in neighborhoods and schools. Employers can develop methods of encouraging weight control among employees. Town and county policy makers can reinforce these efforts by setting priorities and creating policy change. Fostering partnerships with schools, worksites, and local organizations not only helps develop well-targeted, effective programs, it also aids in building the social support and political will necessary for the intervention to succeed.

Reaching the populationwide goal of healthy weight maintenance and obesity prevention will require a concerted effort at many levels. Several proposed action steps can help organize these efforts:

- *Implement the consumer recommendation; balance the food you eat with physical activity to maintain or improve your weight:* This guideline, first recommended in 1995, focuses on the avoidance of weight gain rather than on weight loss (U.S. Department of Agriculture & U.S. Department of Health and Human Services, 1995). In the year 2000 guidelines, the recommendation was reworded slightly to encourage a focus on weight management (U.S. Department of Agriculture & U.S. Department of Health and Human Services, 2000). The principle remained the same, however: Those at a healthy weight should avoid weight gain, and individuals who are overweight should first prevent further weight gain and then aim to lose weight.

If this recommendation were successfully implemented, the increasing prevalence of obesity would be halted as the population maintained weight with increasing age. However, evidence suggests that the balance between energy intake and expenditure has not been readily achieved by the majority of the population. Implementing strategies to promote healthy weight control will require a shift in emphasis from a cosmetic ideal weight for height, to an acceptable weight for health (Koplan & Dietz, 1999).

- *Develop a national obesity prevention strategy:* A requirement for the response to the growing epidemic of obesity is a comprehensive national obesity prevention strategy that incorporates educational, behavioral, and environmental components. Efforts must be made to address obesity prevention across the life course.

- *Fund national obesity prevention and physical activity promotion strategies:* Ensuring that adequate funds are available to implement prevention strategies in a timely manner will be a major public health priority. Local implementation will be necessary, which will challenge our public health systems to communicate clearly the magnitude of the problem and the priority for primary prevention.

SUMMARY

Obesity is a complex problem with no single solution. Appropriate changes are necessary in individual behaviors, health care systems, community structures, and national policies. Multilevel interventions are required that deliver consistent messages on the risks and prevention of obesity across all stages of life. Reinforcement of individual efforts must come at the community, local, state, and national levels if we are to reverse the growing prevalence of obesity and the tremendous health and economic burden associated with it.

To learn more about ways to achieve a healthy weight, see the following resources:

- National Institutes of Health, National Heart, Lung, and Blood Institute (1998).

- Clinical guidelines on the identification, evaluation, and treatment of overweight and obesity in adults. U.S. Department of Health and Human Services, Public Health Service. Available online at www.nhlbi.nih.gov /guidelines/obesity/ob_home.htm.

- U.S. Department of Health and Human Services (2001). The Surgeon General's call to action to prevent and decrease overweight and obesity. U.S. Department of Health and Human Services, Public Health Service, Office of the Surgeon General. Available online at www.surgeongeneral.gov /topics/obesity/default.htm.

- National Institutes of Health, National Heart, Lung, and Blood Institute (2000). The practical guide: Identification, evaluation, and treatment of overweight and obesity in adults. National Institutes of Health. Available online at www.nhlbi.nih.gov/guidelines/obesity/practgde.htm.

- National Institutes of Health, National Institute of Diabetes & Digestive & Kidney Diseases. Weight loss and control. National Institutes of Health. Available online at www.niddk.nih.gov/health/nutrit/nutrit.htm.

For guidelines on communitywide preventive services, see:

- Community Preventive Services Task Force. Guide to community preventive services: Systematic reviews and evidence-based recommendations. Centers for Disease Control and Prevention. Available online at www.thecommunityguide.org.

REFERENCES

Allison, D. B., Fontaine, K. R., Manson, J. E., Stevens, J., & VanItallie, T. B. (1999). Annual deaths attributable to obesity in the United States. *Journal of the American Medical Association, 282*(16), 1530–1538.

Anderson, R. N., & Smith, B. L. (2003). Deaths: Leading causes for 2001. *National Vital Statistics Report, 52*(9), 1–85.

Ascherio, A., Rimm, E. B., Giovannucci, E. L., Colditz, G. A., Rosner, B., Willet, W. C., et al. (1992). A prospective study of nutritional factors and hypertension among U.S. men. *Circulation, 86*(5), 1475–1484.

Atwood, K., Colditz, G. A., & Kawachi, I. (1997). Implementing prevention policies: Relevance of the Richmond model to health policy judgments. *American Journal of Public Health, 87,* 1603–1606.

Berkey, C. S., Rockett, H. R., Field, A., Gillman, M., Frazier, A., Camargo, C., et al. (2000). Activity, dietary intake, and weight changes in a longitudinal study of preadolescent and adolescent boys and girls. *Pediatrics, 105,* E56.

Berkey, C. S., Rockett, H. R., Gillman, M. W., & Colditz, G. A. (2003). One-year changes in activity and in inactivity among 10- to 15-year-old boys and girls: Relationship to change in body mass index. *Pediatrics, 111*(4, Pt. 1), 836–843.

Blackburn, G. L., Dwyer, J., Flanders, W. D., Hill, J. D., Kuller, L. H., Pi-Sunyer, F. X., et al. (1994). Report of the American Institute of Nutrition (AIN) steering committee on healthy weight. *American Institute of Nutrition Journal on Nutrition, 124,* 2240–2243.

Calle, E. E., Rodriguez, C., Walker-Thurmond, K., & Thun, M. J. (2003). Overweight, obesity, and mortality from cancer in a prospectively studied cohort of U.S. adults. *New England Journal of Medicine, 348*(17), 1625–1638.

Carey, V. J., Walters, E. E., Colditz, G. A., Solomon, C. G., Willet, W. C., Rosner, B. A., et al. (1997). Body fat distribution and risk of non-insulin-dependent diabetes mellitus in women. The Nurses' Health Study. *American Journal of Epidemiology, 145*(7), 614–619.

Centers for Disease Control and Prevention. (2001). Physical activity trends: United States, 1990–1998. *Morbidity and Mortality Weekly Report, 50*(9), 166–169.

Centers for Disease Control and Prevention. (2002). Diabetes public health resource available from www.cdc.gov/diabetes/pubs/estimates.htm. Rockville, MD: U.S. Department of Health and Human Services.

Centers for Disease Control and Prevention. (2004). Trends in intake of energy and macronutrients: United States, 1971–2000. *Morbidity and Mortality Weekly Report, 53*(4), 80–82.

Chan, J. M., Rimm, E. B., Colditz, G. A., Stampfer, M. J., & Willet, W. C. (1994). Obesity, fat distribution, and weight gain as risk factors for clinical diabetes in men. *Diabetes Care, 17,* 961–969.

Cicuttini, F. M., Baker, J. R., & Spector, T. D. (1996). The association of obesity with osteoarthritis of the hand and knee in women: A twin study. *Journal of Rheumatology, 23*(7), 1221–1226.

Coakley, E. H., Kawachi, I., Manson, J. E., Speizer, F. E., Willet, W. C., & Colditz, G. A. (1998). Lower levels of physical functioning are associated with higher body weight among middle-aged and older women. *International Journal of Obesity and Related Metabolic Disorders, 22*(10), 958–965.

Colditz, G. A., Willet, W. C., Rotnitzky, A., & Manson, J. E. (1995). Weight gain as a risk factor for clinical diabetes mellitus in women. *Annals of Internal Medicine, 122*(7), 481–486.

Colditz, G. A., Willet, W. C., Stampfer, M. J., Manson, J. E., Hennekens, C. H., Arky, R. A., et al. (1990). Weight as a risk factor for clinical diabetes in women. *American Journal of Epidemiology, 132,* 501–513.

Cooper, C., Inskip, H., Croft, P., Campbell, L., Smith, G., McLaren, M., et al. (1998). Individual risk factors for hip osteoratheritis: Obesity, hip injury, and physical activity. *American Journal of Epidemiology, 147,* 516–522.

Field, A. E., Byers, T., Hunter, D. J., Laird, N. M., Manson, J. E., Williamson, D. F., et al. (1999). Weight cycling, weight gain, and risk of hypertension in women. *American Journal of Epidemiology, 150*(6), 573–579.

Field, A. E., Coakley, E. H., Must, A., Spadano, J. L., Laird, N., Dietz, W. H., et al. (2001). Impact of overweight on the risk of developing common chronic diseases during a 10-year period. *Archives of Internal Medicine, 161*(13), 1581–1586.

Fine, J. T., Colditz, G. A., Coakley, E. H., Moseley, G., Manson, J. E., Willet, W. C., et al. (1999). A prospective study of weight change and health-related quality of life in women. *Journal of the American Medical Association, 282*(22), 2136–2142.

Flegal, K. M., Carroll, M. D., Kuczmarski, R. J., & Johnson, C. L. (1998). Overweight and obesity in the United States: Prevalence and trends, 1960–1994. *International Journal of Obesity, 22,* 39–47.

Flegal, K. M., Carroll, M. D., Ogden, C. L., & Johnson, C. L. (2002). Prevalence and trends in obesity among U.S. adults, 1999–2000. *Journal of the American Medical Association, 288*(14), 1723–1727.

Folsom, A. R., Prineas, R. J., Kaye, S. A., & Soler, J. T. (1989). Body fat distribution and self-reported prevalence of hypertension, heart attack, and other heart disease in older women. *International Journal of Epidemiology, 18*(2), 361–367.

Frazao, E. (Ed.). (1999). *America's eating habits, changes and consequences.* Washington, DC: USDA, Economic Research Service.

French, S. A., Lin, B. H., & Guthrie, J. D. (2003). National trends in soft drink consumption among children and adolescents age 6 to 17 years: Prevalence, amounts, and sources, 1977/1978 to 1994/1998. *Journal of the American Dietetic Association, 103*(10), 1326–1331.

Giovannucci, E., Rimm, E. B., Chute, C. G., Kawachi, I., Colditz, G. A., Stampfer, M. J., et al. (1994). Obesity and benign prostatic hyperplasia. *American Journal of Epidemiology, 140*(11), 989–1002.

Gortmaker, S. L., Dietz, W. H., Jr., & Cheung, L. W. (1990). Inactivity, diet, and the fattening of America. *Journal of the American Dietetic Association, 90*(9), 1247–52, 1255.

Gortmaker, S. L., Peterson, K., Wiecha, J., Sobol, A., Dixit, S., Fox, M., et al. (1999). Reducing obesity via a school-based interdisciplinary intervention among youth: Planet Health. *Archives of Pediatrics and Adolescent Medicine, 153,* 409–418.

Harnack, L. J., Jeffery, R. W., & Boutelle, K. N. (2000). Temporal trends in energy intake in the United States: An ecologic perspective. *American Journal of Clinical Nutrition, 71*(6), 1478–1484.

Harris, T. B., Ballard-Barbasch, R., Madans, J., Makuc, D. M., & Feldman, J. J. (1993). Overweight, weight loss, and risk of coronary heart disease in older women. The NHANES I epidemiologic follow-up study. *American Journal of Epidemiology, 137*(12), 1318–1327.

Hartz, A. J., Rupley, D. C., Jr., Kalkhoff, R. D., & Rimm, A. A. (1983). Relationship of obesity to diabetes: Influence of obesity level and body fat distribution. *Preventive Medicine, 12*(2), 351–357.

Hill, J. O., & Melanson, E. L. (1999). Overview of the determinants of overweight and obesity: Current evidence and research issues. *Medicine and Science in Sports and Exercise, 31*(11, Suppl.), S515–521.

Hiller, R., Podgor, M. J., Sperduto, R. D., Nowroozi, L., Wilson, P. W., D'Agostino, R. B., et al. (1998). A longitudinal study of body mass index and lens opacities: The Framingham Studies. *Ophthalmology, 105*(7), 1244–1250.

Holbrook, T. L., Barrett-Connor, E., & Wingard, D. L. (1989). The association of life-time weight and weight control patterns with diabetes among men and women in an adult community. *International Journal of Obesity, 13*(5), 723–729.

Hu, F. B., Manson, J. E., Stampfer, M. J., Colditz, G., Liu, S., Solomon, C. G., et al. (2001). Diet, lifestyle, and the risk of type 2 diabetes mellitus in women. *New England Journal of Medicine, 345*(11), 790–797.

International Agency for Research on Cancer. (2002). *Weight control and physical activity*. Lyon, France: IARC Press.

Jeffery, R. W., & Utter, J. (2003). The changing environment and population obesity in the United States. *Obesity Research, 11*(Suppl.), 12S–22S.

Knowler, W. C., Barrett-Connor, E., Fowler, S. E., Hamman, R. F., Lachin, J. M., Walker, E. A., et al. (2002). Reduction in the incidence of type 2 diabetes with lifestyle intervention or metformin. *New England Journal of Medicine, 346*(6), 393–403.

Koplan, J., & Dietz, W. (1999). Caloric imbalance and public health policy. *Journal of the American Medical Association, 282*, 1579–1581.

Kuczmarski, R. J., Flegal, K. M., Campbell, S. M., & Johnson, C. L. (1994). Increasing prevalence of overweight among U.S. adults (The National Health and Nutrition Examination Surveys, 1960 to 1991). *Journal of the American Medical Association, 272*, 205–211.

Lean, M. E. J., Han, T. S., & Morrison, C. E. (1995). Waist circumference as a measure for indicating need for weight management. *British Medical Journal, 311*, 158:61.

Lean, M. E. J., Han, T. S., & Seidell, J. C. (1998). Impairment of health and quality of life in people with large waist circumference. *The Lancet, 351*, 853–856.

Lee, I. M., & Paffenbarger, R. S. (1992). Change in body weight and longevity. *Journal of the American Medical Association, 268*, 2045–2049.

Lundgren, H., Bengtsson, C., Blohme, G., Lapidus, L., & Sjostrom, L. (1988). Adiposity and adipose tissue distribution in relation to incidence of diabetes in women: Results from a prospective population study in Gothenburg, Sweden. *International Journal of Obesity, 13*, 413–423.

Lundgren, H., Bengtsson, C., Blohme, G., Lapidus, L., & Sjostrom, L. (1989). Adiposity and adipose tissue distribution in relation to incidence of diabetes in women: Results from a prospective population study in Gothenburg, Sweden. *International Journal of Obesity, 13*(4), 413–423.

Must, A., Jacques, P. F., Dallal, G. E., Bajema, C. J., & Dietz, W. H. (1992). Long-term morbidity and mortality of overweight adolescents: A follow-up of the Harvard Growth Study of 1922 to 1935. *New England Journal of Medicine, 327*(19), 1350–1355.

Must, A., Spadano, J., Coakley, E. H., Field, A. E., Colditz, G., & Dietz, W. H. (1999). The disease burden associated with overweight and obesity. *Journal of the American Medical Association, 282*(16), 1523–1529.

National Center for Health Statistics. (2001). *Prevalence of overweight among children and adolescents: United States, 1999–2000.* Hyattsville, MD: U.S. Department of Health and Human Services, Centers for Disease Control and Prevention.

National Heart, Lung and Blood Institute. (1998). Clinical guidelines on the identification, evaluation, and treatment of overweight and obesity in adults: The evidence report. *Obesity Research, 6*(Suppl. 2), 51S–209S.

National Institute of Arthritis and Musculoskeletal and Skin Diseases. (1998). *Arthritis prevalence rising as baby boomers grow older. Osteoarthritis second only to chronic heart disease in worksite disability.* Bethesda, MD: National Institutes of Health Department of Health and Human Services. (2004). Available from www.niams .nih.gov/ne/press/1998/05_05.htm.

Nielsen, S. J., Siega-Riz, A. M., & Popkin, B. M. (2002). Trends in energy intake in U.S. between 1977 and 1996: Similar shifts seen across age groups. *Obesity Research, 10*(5), 370–378.

Ogden, C. L., Flegal, K. M., Carroll, M. D., & Johnson, C. L. (2002). Prevalence and trends in overweight among U.S. children and adolescents, 1999–2000. *Journal of the American Medical Association, 288,* 1728–1732.

Ohlson, L. O., Larsson, B., Svardsudd, K., Welin, L., Eriksson, H., Wilhelmsen, L., et al. (1985). The influence of body fat distribution on the incidence of diabetes mellitus. 13.5 years of follow-up of the participants in the study of men born in 1913. *Diabetes, 34*(10), 1055–1058.

Popkin, B. M. (1998). The nutrition transition and its health implications in lower-income countries. *Public Health and Nutrition, 1*(1), 5–21.

Popkin, B. M., Siega-Riz, A. M., Haines, P. S., & Jahns, L. (2001). Where's the fat? Trends in U.S. diets 1965–1996. *Preventive Medicine, 32*(3), 245–254.

Prochaska, J., & DiClemente, C. (1984). *The transtheoretical approach: Crossing traditional boundaries of therapy.* Homewood, Il. Dow Jones-Irwin.

Rexrode, K. M., Hennekens, C. H., Willet, W. C., Colditz, G. A., Stampfer, M. J., Rich-Edwards, J. W., et al. (1997). A prospective study of body mass index, weight change, and risk of stroke in women. *Journal of the American Medical Association, 277*(19), 1539–1545.

Rimm, E. B., Stampfer, M. J., Giovannucci, E., Ascherio, A., Spiegelman, D., Colditz, G. A., et al. (1995). Body size and fat distribution as predictors of coronary heart disease among middle-aged and older U.S. men. *American Journal of Epidemiology, 141*(12), 1117–1127.

Schaumberg, D. A., Glynn, R. J., Christen, W. G., Hankinson, S. E., & Hennekens, C. H. (2000). Relations of body fat distribution and height with cataract in men. *American Journal of Clinical Nutrition, 72*(6), 1495–1502.

Seidell, J. C., Verschuren, W. M., van Leer, E. M., & Kromhout, D. (1996). Overweight, underweight, and mortality: A prospective study of 48,287 men and women. *Archives of Internal Medicine, 156*(9), 958–963.

Smiciklas-Wright, H., Mitchell, D. C., Mickle, S. J., Goldman, J. D., & Cook, A. (2003). Foods commonly eaten in the United States, 1989–1991 and 1994–1996: Are portion sizes changing? *Journal of the American Dietetic Association, 103*(1), 41–47.

Task Force on Community Preventive Services. (2003). *Guide to community preventive services: Systematic reviews and evidence-based recommendations.* Atlanta, GA: Centers for Disease Control and Prevention. 2004. Web address: www.thecommunityguide.org.

Thompson, D., Edelsberg, J., Colditz, G. A., Bird, A. P., & Oster, G. (1999). Lifetime health and economic consequences of obesity. *Archives of Internal Medicine, 159*(18), 2177–2183.

U.S. Department of Agriculture, & U.S. Department of Health and Human Services. (1995). *Nutrition and your health: Dietary guidelines for Americans* (4th ed.). Washington, DC: U.S. Government Printing Office.

U.S. Department of Agriculture, & U.S. Department of Health and Human Services. (2000). *Nutrition and your health: Dietary guidelines for Americans (5th ed).* Washington, DC: U.S. Government Printing Office.

U.S. Department of Health and Human Services. (1996). *Physical activity and health: A report of the Surgeon General.* Atlanta, GA: U.S. Department of Health and Human Services, Centers for Disease Control and Prevention, National Center for Chronic Disease Prevention and Health Promotion.

U.S. Department of Health and Human Services. (2001). *The Surgeon General's call to action to prevent and decrease overweight and obesity.* Rockville, MD: U.S. Department of Health and Human Services, Public Health Service, Office of the Surgeon General.

U.S. Department of Health and Human Services, Public Health Service, Centers for Disease Control and Prevention, National Center for Chronic Disease Prevention and Health Promotion, Division of Nutrition and Physical Activity. (1999). *Promoting physical activity: A guide for community action.* Champaign, IL: Human Kinetics.

U.S. Preventive Services Task Force. (2003). Screening for obesity in adults: Recommendations and rationale. *Annals of Internal Medicine, 139*(11), 930–932.

Walker, S. P., Rimm, E. B., Ascherio, A., Kawachi, I., Stampfer, M. J., & Willet, W. C. (1996). Body size and fat distribution as predictors of stroke among U.S. men. *American Journal of Epidemiology, 144*(12), 1143–1150.

Weintraub, J. M., Willet, W. C., Rosner, B., Colditz, G. A., Seddon, J. M., & Hankinson, S. E. (2002). A prospective study of the relationship between body mass index and cataract extraction among U.S. women and men. *International Journal of Obesity and Related Metabolic Disorders, 26*(12), 1588–1595.

Wendelboe, A. M., Hegmann, K. T., Briggs, J. J., Cox, C. M., Portmann, A. J., Gildea, J. H., et al. (2003). Relationships between body mass indices and surgical replacements of knee and hip joints. *American Journal of Preventive Medicine, 25*(4), 290–295.

Willett, W. C., Manson, J. E., Stampfer, M. J., Colditz, G. A., Rosner, B., Speizer, F. E., et al. (1995). Weight, weight change, and coronary heart disease in women:

Risk within the "normal" weight range. *Journal of the American Medical Association, 273,* 461–465.

Witteman, J. C., Willet, W. C., Stampfer, M. J., Colditz, G. A., Sacks, F. M., Speizer, F. E., et al. (1989). A prospective study of nutritional factors and hypertension among U.S. women. *Circulation, 80*(5), 1320–1327.

Wolf, A. M. (1998). What is the economic case for treating obesity? *Obesity Research, 6*(Suppl. 1), 2S–7S.

World Health Organization. (1995). *Physical status: The use and interpretation of anthropometry* (Report of a WHO Expert Committee, WHO Technical Report Series No. 854). Geneva, Switzerland: WHO.

World Health Organization. (1998). *Obesity: Preventing and managing the global epidemic* (Report of a WHO Consultation on Obesity, Geneva, 3–5 June 1997). Geneva, Switzerland: WHO.

Yong, L. C., Kuller, L. H., Rutan, G., & Bunker, C. (1993). Longitudinal study of blood pressure: Changes and determinants from adolescence to middle age. The Dormont High School follow-up study, 1957–1963 to 1989–1990. *American Journal of Epidemiology, 138*(11), 973–983.

Chapter 14

SLEEP DISTURBANCES

MARY ANN LEITZ

Sleep: For many, the word evokes thoughts of rest, slumber, and renewal. For others, the word is associated with anxiety, fatigue, and frustration. No matter one's attitude toward sleep, sleep is crucial for proper physical and psychological functioning. We spend approximately one-third of our entire lives sleeping (Hauri & Linde, 1996; Van Dongen, Maislin, Mullington, & Dinges, 2003). The amount and quality of sleep affects many areas of life: health, mood, energy level, emotional stability, professional functioning, and relationships (Hauri & Linde, 1996). Millions of Americans experience sleep disturbances at some time during their lives. A 1993 Harris poll indicated that approximately one-third of all adult Americans surveyed felt they were sleep-deprived (Hauri & Linde, 1996). Each year over 100 million Americans report sleep disturbances and as many as 10 million visit their doctor with a chief complaint of sleep problems (Hauri & Linde, 1996). Chokroverty (2000) studied sleep disturbance rates in 1,000 adults in the Los Angeles area. Results indicated that approximately 33% reported some type of sleep disturbance, marked by daytime sleepiness. Ban and Lee (2001) studied a sample of college students ($N = 1,414$) to determine the prevalence of sleep disturbances. Approximately 40% of the subjects reported having trouble sleeping; additionally, subjects reported daytime sleepiness, increased numbers of accidents, decreased productivity, more relationship problems, impaired concentration, and an inability to complete assignments. Sleep is so important that losing even one night of sleep temporarily decreases performance and learning (Dement & Vaughan, 1999). Heuer and Klien (2003) compared a group ($N = 12$) who were sleep-deprived for one night and a control group ($N = 6$). Findings indicated that subjects who were sleep-deprived exhibited decreased learning and motivation and were unwilling or unable to complete required tasks the next day.

NORMAL SLEEP NEEDS

Sleep was once believed to be a simple process of relaxing and letting go of daytime activities. We now know that sleep is a very dynamic and complex process in which the brain decreases some neurological activities while it increases others (Dement & Vaughan, 1999; Hauri & Linde, 1996; Siegel, 2002).

There is a constant interplay between chemical systems in the brain that affect levels of consciousness and motor activities (Hauri & Linde, 1996; Siegel, 2002). Sleep is a natural process in which the sleeping brain gradually isolates the conscious mind from the environment. For example, when one is in a light sleep, one is easily roused by external stimuli, such as loud noises and bright lights. However, once in a deep sleep, only an intense sensory stimulation will awaken one (Dement & Vaughan, 1999).

Sleep is essential for normal functioning and preventing serious physical and psychological disorders, but sleep needs vary among individuals. Sleep needs are determined by several factors, including heredity, physical activities, stress, and presence of physical or psychiatric disorders (Hauri & Linde, 1996). The amount of sleep needed varies among individuals. Sleep requirements for individuals remains relatively constant throughout their life, although sleep needs do decrease in old age (Hauri & Linde, 1996). Normal sleep needs usually range from 4 to 8 hours a night, with an average of 7 to 7½ hours. Six hours a night is considered the minimum number of hours of sleep for normal functioning (Dement & Vaughan, 1999; Hauri & Linde, 1996; Van Dongen et al., 2003). Less than 4 hours a night is considered unhealthy and will increase the risk of serious illness, such as coronary arterial disease and stroke (Chokroverty, 2000; Dement & Vaughan, 1999; Hauri & Linde, 1996).

Over the life span, sleep patterns and sleep needs change, with sleep needs decreasing with age. By middle age, individuals may be sleeping the same number of hours they always have, but more time is spent in the lighter stages of sleep and less in the deep sleep stages. As a result, they are more easily roused and disturbed while sleeping (Hauri & Linde, 1996). For the elderly, difficulties falling and staying asleep are frequent complaints. Due to physical and neurological degeneration, the elderly are more prone to physical conditions that disrupt sleep, including obstructive sleep apnea, sleep movement disorders, chronic pain, frequent urination, arthritis, inability to exercise, Alzheimer's disease, Parkinson's disease, and gastrointestinal problems (Dement & Vaughan, 1999). Complicating these conditions are increasingly sedentary lives and the elderly's tendency to nap, which decreases sleep needs (Dement & Vaughan, 1999). Older individuals also suffer from increased psychological and environmental stress that may interfere with sleep. Many are lonely due to the loss of social support and at the same time are experiencing stressful lifestyle changes. For example, they may suffer extreme stress related to being forced to support themselves with retirement funds and social security. Decreased finances may further indirectly cause stress by requiring seniors to reduce their standard of living (Barber et al., 2000; Dement & Vaughan, 1999; Piccone & Barth, 1983).

STAGES OF SLEEP

Sleep is composed of periods of core sleep and optimal sleep. Core sleep occurs in the first part of the night and is essential for normal functioning and for the brain to recover and heal from the effects of daily activities. Optimal sleep occurs in the later part of the night and is important for feeling energetic and refreshed during the day (Van Dongen et al., 2003). Sleep is further divided into stages through which we gradually cycle several times during a night (Hauri & Linde, 1996). There are two main stages of sleep: nonrapid eye movement sleep (NREM), which is further separated into four different stages (I, II, III, and IV), and rapid eye movement (REM) sleep (Chokroverty, 2000).

Stage I NREM marks the transition between wakefulness and sleep and accounts for approximately 8% of the entire night's sleep. During this stage, part of the brain is asleep and part remains active (Chokroverty, 2000). The body begins to slow down, decreasing heart rate, respiratory rate, and blood pressure (American Psychiatric Association, 2000; Chokroverty, 2000). Response to sensory stimulus is only slightly decreased and it is very easy to awaken someone during this stage (American Psychiatric Association, 2000; Chokroverty, 2000).

Stages II, III, and IV NREM account for approximately 42% of the night's sleep. As we cycle through each stage, we fall into deeper sleep (Van Dongen et al., 2003). Core sleep occurs during Stages III and IV (the deepest levels), when the body repairs itself from the damage caused by daily stress and activities (Hauri & Linde, 1996). Heart rate, respiration rate, and blood pressure are at the lowest of the night. This allows the cardiovascular system to rest, which helps to prevent cardiovascular diseases. In childhood and adolescence, growth hormones peak during these stages (American Psychiatric Association, 2000; Chokroverty, 2000; Siegel, 2003).

REM accounts for approximately 50% of all sleep. During this stage, we dream, and although the eyes are closed, they move rapidly in all directions as we dream. The movement under the lids is visible. When dreaming, the brain creates complicated and sometimes detailed scenarios and continues to send impulses to the body, telling it to move as if we were awake. However, during this stage, the body is temporarily paralyzed, except for muscles that control breathing and eye movements. Motor paralysis is caused by nerve cells in the brain stem that stimulate the muscles of the body, causing them to relax to such an extent that sleeping individuals cannot move during REM sleep, although there may be small muscle jerks and twitches. If the body were not paralyzed at this time, we would act out our dreams. REM sleep occurs approximately every 90 minutes throughout the night. The first REM period is very short, only about 5 minutes. REM sleep periods increase throughout the night until final REM periods last 30 to 60 minutes (Hauri & Linde, 1996; Lugaresi, 2003; Siegel, 2002). There are four to six complete sleep cycles lasting approximately 90 to 110 minutes during a normal night (Chokroverty, 2000).

REM sleep is necessary for mental and psychological recovery. While in REM sleep, individuals are only moderately responsive to the environment and very strong sensory stimulation is required to awaken them (Chokroverty, 2000; Hauri & Linde, 1996). Occasionally, REM sleep is suppressed due to illness, sleep deprivation, or medication. When REM sleep resumes, dreams are much longer, more bizarre, and more kinetic (Hauri & Linde, 1996). It appears that when deprived of dreaming for a period of time, the brain must make up for lost REM periods. Without dreams, individuals become increasingly irritable and emotionally unstable (Dement & Vaughan, 1999).

Sleep researchers have been unable to determine exactly how and why we sleep. However, it is known that our bodies function on a 24-hour biological clock, or circadian rhythm, that is regulated by chemical substances that partly determine sleep-wake cycles (Chokroverty, 2000; Green & Menaker, 2003). This cycle is also determined by external, environmental influences (Chokroverty, 2000; Dement & Vaughan, 1999). Circadian rhythms react to the amount of exposure to light and dark, which affects the secretion of hormones by the brain. When hormone levels are high, we are awake; conversely, when hormone levels are low, we become sleepy. Melatonin is the main sleep hormone secreted by the hypothalamus; it induces and controls sleep and feelings of sleepiness (Chokroverty, 2000; Dunlap, 1998; Green & Menaker, 2003). Melatonin decreases both body temperature and blood flow to the brain; it causes muscles to relax and become flaccid as individuals fall asleep. Melatonin is produced only in dark environments, such as darkened rooms, and is inhibited by light (Chokroverty, 2000; Dement & Vaughan, 1999; Dunlap, 1998; Green & Menaker, 2003).

Regular circadian rhythms with accompanying hormone secretions create good sleep-wake cycles and restful sleep. Ideally, we wake up in the morning feeling rested, with the most energy we will have for the entire day. As the day progresses, we become increasingly tired and accumulate sleep debt. Sleepiness increases throughout the day until the need to sleep becomes overwhelming (Van Dongen et al., 2003). Sleep debt is the amount of sleep the body needs to feel rested; the more tired we feel, the larger the sleep debt, which is resolved only by sleep (American Psychiatric Association, 2000; Dement & Vaughan, 1999). Sleep loss is cumulative and the amount of sleep needed is directly related to the amount of sleep lost (Dement & Vaughan, 1999; Van Dongen et al., 2003). Additionally, the negative effects of sleep loss are also cumulative and increase in direct relationship to the amount of sleep debt (Dement & Vaughan, 1999).

SLEEP DISTURBANCES

Sleep disturbances occur equally in both men and women and in all age groups; however, the elderly experience the highest rates of sleep disturbances (Piccone & Barth, 1983). There are several different types of sleep disturbances. Some are neurologically based, and others are the result of lifestyle choices. The number one symptom of sleep disturbance is daytime sleepiness (Chokroverty, 2000; Hauri & Linde, 1996).

Sleep is one of the strongest biological drives that exist. The sleep drive is so strong that at some point, it is beyond conscious control. Individuals will fall asleep even if they are actively trying to stay awake. The need to sleep can be so powerful that sleep-deprived individuals will experience frequent small microsleeps, in which they fall asleep for several seconds during the day. It may appear to others that these individuals have just stopped paying attention for a few seconds; the sleepers themselves are not even aware that they are sleeping.

Those who are sleep-deprived are frequently unaware that they are not functioning normally. Therefore, they do not realize that they must take extra care. Not only can sleep deprivation interfere with both social and professional functioning, but it is extremely dangerous for people engaged in activities such as driving (Piccone & Barth, 1983). Reaction times are reduced, and it is impossible to move and perform tasks quickly. Cognitive functioning is decreased, and the ability to code and remember new facts is impaired. For those engaging in safe, relaxed activities, this may not be a problem. However, it is very dangerous for those engaged in activities that require concentration and quick reactions. Additionally, sleep deprivation decreases the ability to successfully complete tasks that require creativity or abstract thought (Piccone & Barth, 1983).

CAUSES OF SLEEP DISTURBANCES

There are many causes of sleep disturbances, including poor sleep habits, alcohol and drug use, neurological, psychiatric, and physical disorders, chaotic schedules and irregular sleep-wake patterns, age, stress, sleep apnea, chronic pain, and lifestyle choices (Akerstedt, Fredlund, Gillberg, & Jannson, 2002; Akerstedt, Knutsson, et al., 2002; Piccone & Barth, 1983).

Lifestyle choices of diet, exercise, and stress directly affect quality of sleep. Unhealthy diets, especially those high in caffeine, negatively affect the quality of sleep. Caffeine is a stimulant and makes it much harder to relax and fall asleep. Additionally, poor diets reduce overall level of health, which makes the body more susceptible to illnesses and other disorders. Unhealthy diets are especially disruptive to sleep when combined with sedentary lives. Exercise is very important for proper sleep. Vigorous exercise in the morning or early afternoon dramatically improves sleep quality by decreasing stress and stimulating hormone secretion. However, vigorous exercise at night is arousing and will prevent or delay sound sleep (Chokroverty, 2000; Dement & Vaughan, 1999).

Medical and psychiatric conditions can also disrupt sleep patterns. Sleep disturbances are a symptom of many psychiatric disorders, including depression, schizophrenia, Bipolar Disorder, Anxiety Disorder, panic attacks, posttraumatic stress disorders, eating disorders, and Obsessive-Compulsive Disorder. Difficulty sleeping is reported by approximately 85% of those with a primary psychiatric diagnosis (Bender, 1990; Manber et al., 2003; Piccone & Barth, 1983). Because many of the medications used to treat these disorders are either stimulants or depressants, they can also cause sleep disturbances; in such cases, sleep disruption can be severe and prolonged (Chokroverty, 2000; Piccone & Barth, 1983). Among the many medical conditions known to cause sleep disturbances are Alzheimer's, Parkinson's, diabetes, heart disease, high or unstable blood pressure, chronic respiratory problems, gastrointestinal problems, fibromyalgia, arthritis, and renal problems (Chokroverty, 2000).

THE EFFECTS OF SLEEP DISTURBANCES

Sleep disturbances, especially if chronic, can have devastating effects on both physical and mental functioning. The effects of sleep disturbance are cumulative: The more sleep lost, the greater the negative effects in number and intensity (Van Dongen et al., 2003). Even short-term sleep disturbances will decrease overall levels of physical, emotional, and cognitive functioning (Van Dongen et al., 2003). Professional and social activities are negatively affected due to decreased energy and ability to focus on the task at hand (Chokroverty, 2000; Dement & Vaughan, 1999). Sleep disturbances and daytime sleepiness decrease mental focus, resulting in inattention, which can cause accidents and mistakes both at home and at work.

Jennings, Monk, and van der Molen (2003) studied college students ($n = 20$) who were sleep deprived for one night. Results indicated that subjects were unable to problem solve and complete difficult tasks. However, the effects of sleep deprivation were reversed once subjects were able to sleep (Jennings et al., 2003). Van Dongen et al. (2003) studied a group of healthy adults ($N = 48$) who were restricted to 8 hours, 6 hours, or 4 hours of sleep over a 14-day period and 0 hours of sleep for 3 days. Findings indicated that even a moderate sleep loss seriously impaired functioning, and subjects were unaware that they were functioning at a lower level. Additionally, effects were cumulative. When subjects slept 4 hours a night, they had more physical and cognitive problems than when they slept 6 hours. When completely sleep deprived, there was a sharp decline in performance (Van Dongen et al., 2003).

Mental health disorders frequently cause or result from sleep disturbances. An overwhelming number of individuals (90%) diagnosed with sleep disturbances also report concurrent physical or psychiatric problems (Edinger & Sampson, 2003; Piccone & Barth, 1983). Mood disturbances commonly co-occur with sleep disturbances and can be so severe that individuals may present with symptoms of psychiatric illness: sadness, loss of interest in life, blunted or exaggerated emotional responses, anxiety, and frustration (Edinger & Sampson, 2003; Piccone & Barth, 1983). As mentioned earlier, sleep disturbance is a symptom of several psychiatric illnesses, including depression, Bipolar Disorder, schizophrenia, and mood disturbances (Piccone & Barth, 1983).

Sleep problems also increase the risk for health problems such as cardiovascular diseases, high blood pressure, premature aging, gastrointestinal disorders, decreased immunity to infectious illnesses, and stroke. Sleep disturbances will also exacerbate existing medical conditions such as diabetes, respiratory ailments, sinus problems, and weight gain. Weight gain is caused by overeating because the brain interprets sleepiness as hunger. Leptin, a hormone secreted by the brain, signals the body that it is no longer hungry. When sleepy, the brain reduces the amount of leptin produced, resulting in sleep-deprived individuals feeling increased hunger (Chokroverty, 2000).

TYPES OF SLEEP DISTURBANCES

Individuals usually identify their specific sleep problem by their presenting symptoms, which may be difficulty falling asleep, daytime hypersomnolence (falling asleep during the day), daytime sleepiness, or sleeping at inappropriate times. Other common complaints are restless sleep, repeated leg and body jerks, frequent awakenings, fatigue, forgetfulness, sleepiness, and psychosomatic complaints (Chokroverty, 2000). There are two main categories of sleep disturbances: dyssomnias and parasomnias.

Dyssomnias

The more common group of sleep disorders, dyssomnias, involve difficulty either falling asleep or staying asleep.

Insomnia

Insomnia is defined as an inability to fall or stay asleep. Symptoms include inability to sleep at night, daytime sleepiness, difficulty waking in the morning, waking up too early in the morning, and sleep that is not refreshing (Piccone & Barth, 1983). Insomnia can be transient, lasting less than 1 week; short term, lasting 1 to 3 weeks; or chronic, persisting longer than 3 weeks (American Psychiatric Association, 2000; Chokroverty, 2000; Piccone & Barth, 1983). Most cases of insomnia are transient (Dement & Vaughan, 1999). Causes of insomnia include poor sleep hygiene, jet lag, shift work, stress, medication, acute illness, surgery, and diet (Chokroverty, 2000).

Insomnia can also be learned. For example, acutely stressful situations often result in problems falling asleep, causing feelings of frustration and increased anxiety, which further delays sleep. A cycle develops of escalating anxiety and frustration with decreasing ability to relax and fall asleep. A conditioned response of avoiding sleep develops. These individuals resist going to bed even when sleepy because they dread lying in bed waiting for sleep (Chokroverty, 2000). Insomnia then becomes a regular sleep pattern (Chokroverty, 2000).

Poor Sleep Hygiene

Good sleep hygiene involves activities that enhance sleep; poor sleep hygiene is caused by those that disrupt sleep routines. Poor sleep hygiene is the result of poor diet, use of alcohol, drugs, or tobacco, intense mental activity, vigorous exercise, an irregular sleep-wake schedule, an overstimulating bedroom environment, and irregular bedtime habits (Chokroverty, 2000). Thus, poor sleep hygiene is voluntary, a matter of lifestyle choices and habits (Chokroverty, 2000; Dement & Vaughan, 1999).

Restless Leg Syndrome

Restless leg syndrome is a sensorimotor disorder that results in an overwhelming desire to move the legs. It occurs when lying in bed and occasionally after sitting for long periods. Leg movements and discomfort can be severe enough to prevent sleep (American Psychiatric Association, 2000). Individuals with this disorder frequently describe feeling that insects and worms are crawling on the legs. Leg movements are conscious efforts to ease symptoms (Chokroverty, 2000).

This condition is more common in the elderly, but can occur at any age. Approximately 10% of the general population suffers from this condition, and it occurs equally in both men and women. It tends to run in families and is chronic and progressive. Aside from hereditary factors, causes of restless leg syndrome include physical conditions such as iron deficit anemia, decreased blood circulation in the lower legs, muscle disorders, kidney problems, alcoholism, vitamin and mineral deficiency, stopping or starting medications, caffeine, smoking, fatigue, and extreme temperatures (American Psychiatric Association, 2000; Chokroverty, 2000). The syndrome is worsened by anxiety, depression, illness, old age, sedentary lifestyle, and pregnancy (American Psychiatric Association, 2000; Chokroverty, 2000).

Periodic Limb Movement Disorder

This disorder is characterized by brief severe contractions of the limbs, usually legs, characterized by myoclunus (contract-release) movements and by an extension of toes and upward jerk of the leg. It can occur as frequently as every 30 seconds, usually during Stage II NREM (American Psychiatric Association, 2000; Chokroverty, 2000). Severity of symptoms is not consistent and can fluctuate from night to night (Chokroverty, 2000). Movements are unconscious and involuntary; if awakened by the movements, individuals frequently do not know why they have awakened.

The likelihood of periodic limb movement disorder increases with age. It occurs equally in both men and women. There is no known cause; it can occur alone or in combination with other medical and neurological disorders, such as narcolepsy and kidney problems (American Psychiatric Association, 2000; Chokroverty, 2000).

Circadian Rhythm Disorders

Circadian rhythm sleep disorders result from disruption of the sleep-wake cycle. The most common causes are jet lag, shift work, and delayed sleep phase syndrome. Jet lag results from traveling across several time zones, especially when traveling from east to west. Our body does not adjust to the different time zones as quickly as we travel through them; as a result, our body remains on the time schedule of the original time zone (Chokroverty, 2000).

Shift work sleep disorders affect as many as 5 million workers in the United States. Sleep disruption and chronic fatigue occur when job demands reverse natural waking and sleeping hours, so that individuals are awake at night and asleep during the day (Chokroverty, 2000).

Delayed sleep phase syndrome is a disorder of choice. The biological clocks of some people dictate that they stay up late at night and wake late in the morning. When these individuals must rise early in the morning to engage in their daily social and professional activities, chronic sleep loss results (Chokroverty, 2000).

Obstructive Sleep Apnea

Muscles usually relax and become flaccid during sleep. With obstructive sleep apnea, the tracheal muscles can become so relaxed that they collapse. Breathing stops (apnea literally means "absence of respiration"; Hauri & Linde, 1996, p. 201). After a few seconds, individuals begin to choke, which awakens them. Throat muscles become stimulated, contract, and become rigid again; the airway opens, and breathing resumes. Individuals fall asleep again and the cycle repeats, perhaps hundreds of times, continually throughout the night.

The symptoms of sleep apnea include very loud snoring, choking during sleep, cessation of breathing, frequent awakenings, frequent nighttime urination, daytime sleepiness, forgetfulness, morning headache, insomnia, night sweating, and gastrointestinal reflux (American Psychiatric Association, 2000; Chokroverty, 2000; Hauri & Linde, 1996; Piccone & Barth, 1983). Precipitating factors include nasotracheal abnormalities, overbite, large tongue, enlarged tonsils, tissue that blocks the airway, obesity, use of alcohol, medications, high blood pressure, menopause, old age, large neck size, and genetics (Chokroverty, 2000).

Sleep apnea causes insomnia, daytime sleepiness, impaired concentration, and fatigue (Piccone & Barth, 1983). More serious effects include life-threatening health conditions. Individuals with severe and long-term sleep apnea are more likely to suffer from high blood pressure and have an increased risk of stroke, myocardial infarction, and other cardiovascular problems (Chokroverty, 2000). Approximately 40% of the general population suffer from sleep apnea and approximately half of those cases are clinically significant (Dement & Vaughan, 1999).

Snoring

Individuals may snore without having sleep apnea. This type of snoring is caused by decreased muscle tone or some type of airway obstruction. There may be excessive tissue in the throat, sinus problems with swollen mucous membranes, large tonsils, or enlarged adenoids, which narrow air passages. Snoring is caused by air being forced through the narrowed passages. This condition is most common in men and postmenopausal women (Hauri & Linde, 1996).

Medical, Neurological, and Psychiatric Disorders

Sleep disturbances are frequently a symptom of medical and neurological conditions such as Alzheimer's, Parkinson's, cardiac difficulties, gastrointestinal disorders, pain, arthritis, brain tumors, strokes, and trauma (Chokroverty, 2000). Additionally, as mentioned earlier, sleep disturbances such as insomnia and oversleeping are frequently a major symptom of psychiatric disorders (Chokroverty, 2000).

Parasomnia Disorders

The second category of sleep disorder is parasomnia, which is characterized by abnormal muscle movements while asleep, including sleepwalking and sleep talking (Chokroverty, 2000). Parasomnia disorders are divided into four types: NREM disorders, REM disorders, sleep paralysis, and narcolepsy.

NREM Disorders

NREM sleep parasomnias include somnambulism (sleep walking) and sleep talking. These are most common in children between the ages of 5 and 12 years. It is rare for adults to experience these disorders. Sleep walking usually occurs in the first part of the night and may result in injury. Some precipitating factors include sleep deprivation, stress, illness, and medications (Buelow, Hebert, & Buelow, 2000; Chokroverty, 2000; Dement & Vaughan, 1999). Movements are involuntary and individuals are unaware of their activities (Chokroverty, 2000).

REM Disorder

REM sleep parasomnias include night terrors and nightmares, which also are more common in children. Although adults do experience nightmares, they become much less frequent with age (Chokroverty, 2000). However, there are rare episodes when muscles are not paralyzed during REM sleep and individuals may act out their dreams. This type of activity occurs more frequently in males over 60 years of age (Hauri & Linde, 1996).

Sleep Paralysis

Sleep paralysis occurs when falling asleep or waking up. When associated with falling asleep, it may be a symptom of narcolepsy. With this disorder, individuals are awake but unable to move any muscles except those needed for breathing and eye movement. This is a frightening disorder, but has no lasting negative effects (Chokroverty, 2000).

Narcolepsy

Narcolepsy is a chronic progressive neurological disorder that results in abnormal sleep patterns. It is defined as a sudden strong impulse to sleep (sleep attacks) at inappropriate times, usually during daytime activities. Sleep attacks last approximately 15 to 30 minutes and may be preceded by hallucinations. Narcolepsy develops in young adulthood, but is then a permanent condition that worsens with age. It is estimated that approximately 250,000 (0.18%) individuals in the United States suffer from narcolepsy. It occurs equally in both men and women and runs in families but is relatively rare (Chokroverty, 2000; Dement & Vaughen, 1999; Piccone & Barth, 1983).

Narcolepsy can be very mild and go unrecognized, or it may be so severe that professional and personal lives are completely disrupted (Piccone & Barth, 1983). It is often associated with other sleep disturbances, including restless leg syndrome, sleep apnea, and REM sleep disturbances. The nighttime sleep of narcoleptics stays mostly in the lighter sleep stages (Dement & Vaughan, 1999); as a result, even though they may sleep all night, their sleep is abnormally shallow. They are easily roused and experience an overall poor quality of sleep (Hauri & Linde, 1996). Cataplexy, a sudden, sometimes severe muscle weakness, usually accompanies narcolepsy. At times it can be so severe that there is a complete loss of all muscle tone and individuals collapse. Cataplexy is precipitated by strong emotions such as great happiness or deep sadness. It is estimated that approximately 70% of individuals with narcolepsy will develop cataplexy to some degree (Chokroverty, 2000).

PREVENTION OF SLEEP DISTURBANCES

Because of the potentially devastating consequences of sleep disturbances, it is important to prevent or at least minimize sleep problems. Gordon's model of prevention will be used to explain various preventive measures that are appropriate for different levels of risk. This model uses three different classifications of preventive measures. Universal measures of prevention are appropriate for the general public who do not have any risk factors for sleep disturbances. These measures are safe and can be used without medical supervision. Selective measures of prevention are slightly more specific; these are appropriate for individuals or groups who have identified high-risk factors for sleep disturbances. Indicated measures are the most specific measures and are appropriate for those who have already developed sleep disorders (Gordon, 1983).

Universal Measures of Prevention for Sleep Disturbances

Strategies that are useful in preventing sleep disturbances are assessing sleep needs, and practicing good sleep hygiene.

Sleep Assessments

Individuals should carefully assess their sleep habits to identify strengths and weaknesses. All activities should be evaluated, including lifestyle choices, drug and alcohol use, sleep hygiene, physical and psychiatric condition, and family history of sleep patterns (Chokroverty, 2000; Dement & Vaughan, 1999). In this way, individuals are able to analyze and identify habits before they lead to problems. A detailed sleep diary is a very useful tool for this process. All activities and feelings over a 24-hour period should be recorded: hours of sleep, quality of sleep, number of nighttime awakenings, day activities, feelings upon awakening, what is eaten and when, smoking, alcohol and drug use, when individuals feel tired, when they feel energetic, emotional responses and physical feelings (Chokroverty, 2000; Dement & Vaughan, 1999). The diary can then be used to determine personal sleep needs.

It is important to determine a personal range of sleep hours necessary for optimal health and functioning (Piccone & Barth, 1983). Then individuals know their exact sleep needs and can arrange their schedules so that they obtain at least the minimum amount of sleep needed (Chokroverty, 2000; Dement & Vaughan, 1999).

Sleep Hygiene

Good sleep hygiene is a combination of behaviors and environment that improve the quality of sleep. Engage in at least 2 hours of quiet time relaxing and slowing down before bed in order to get ready for sleep. Both mind and body relax slowly and time is required to transition from day to night (Hauri & Linde, 1996). Such techniques as progressive relaxation, listening to soft music, reading, gentle stretching, and meditation can enhance this process (Hauri & Linde, 1996). Develop a sleep ritual. This does not have to be an elaborate routine; simply do the same things at the same time and in the same order each night before going to bed. It is not important what is done as long as a routine and sequence is maintained. This signals both the body and the brain to get ready for sleep (Piccone & Barth, 1983). Do not bring work to bed (Chokroverty, 2000; Piccone & Barth, 1983).

Regular vigorous exercise in the morning or early afternoon improves sleep. However, exercise should be completed at least six hours before bedtime; exercise is a stimulant and will delay sleep if undertaken in the evening (Chokroverty, 2000; Hauri & Linde, 1996; Piccone & Barth, 1983). All evening activities should be calm and quiet (Piccone & Barth, 1983). Avoid naps except during illness because they decrease sleep needs and feelings of fatigue and disrupt sleep-wake cycles (Dement & Vaughan, 1999; Piccone & Barth, 1983).

During the early stages of sleep, there is a heightened state of sensory arousal; noises and lights that normally go unnoticed during the day will become so annoying that they may prevent or disrupt sleep. Therefore, it is important to reduce noise and light in the bedroom and create a relaxed environment (Dement & Vaughan, 1999). It is best to sleep in a dark room to reduce sensory input and stimulate the production of melatonin. The television should be turned off when ready for sleep because both the noise and the light can be disruptive (Dement & Vaughan, 1999; Piccone & Barth, 1983). Most people find it comfortable to sleep in a room that is a little cooler than what would be comfortable during the day (Piccone & Barth, 1983). The bedroom should be a pleasant room: clean, neat, and attractive. It is important to have a comfortable pillow, and the mattress should be supportive and have clean sheets and blankets. Consider moving the clock to a location that prevents clock watching during the night (Piccone & Barth, 1983).

Use the bed only for sleeping, sex, and illness. In this way, a connection between bed and sleep is made. Do not lie in bed when not sleeping. Get out of bed as soon as you wake up in the morning and go to bed only when you are ready for sleep (Chokroverty, 2000; Piccone & Barth, 1983). Trying to sleep when not sleepy creates anxiety and frustration, Sleep cannot be forced. If sleep does not come within 20 minutes, leave the bedroom and engage in some type of quiet activity such as reading, watching television, and playing quiet video games (Chokroverty, 2000; Dement & Vaughan, 1999). Even when not working, arising and sleeping times should be maintained to prevent disruption in sleep-wake routines (Chokroverty, 2000; Dement & Vaughan, 1999; Piccone & Barth, 1983).

A healthy diet is important for optimal functioning and good health. Caffeine and spicy foods should be limited and eaten early in the day; alcohol, drugs, and tobacco use should be restricted, especially in the evening. All of these substances are stimulants and it takes several hours for the body to metabolize them (Piccone & Barth, 1983). Taking vitamin and mineral supplements may be helpful because deficiencies in vitamin B complex, calcium, magnesium, and zinc are linked to insomnia. Tryptophan is a naturally occurring amino acid that induces sleep and is found in various foods, including milk. Melatonin (discussed previously) is a chemical released by the brain that controls the sleep-wake cycle. Both tryptophan and melatonin supplements are available at health food stores. However, high doses of vitamins and minerals can be toxic. Consult your physician to determine what supplements are needed and the appropriate dose (Hauri & Linde, 1996).

Selective Measures for the Prevention of Sleep Disturbances

Many individuals have risk factors that increase the likelihood that they will develop sleep disorders at some time during their lives. Therefore, preventive measures for this group must be more specific and aggressive. Those with family members who suffer from such conditions as sleep apnea, restless leg syndrome, periodic limb movement disorders, or narcolepsy are more likely to develop these disorders. Therefore, preventive strategies must be ongoing and intense.

Insomnia

When insomnia is the result of lifestyle choices, the suggestions described earlier should be instituted (Chokroverty, 2000; Dement & Vaughan, 1999; Hauri & Linde, 1996). Anxiety-induced insomnia may respond to strategies that reduce stress, such as relaxation techniques, biofeedback, meditation, acupuncture, and massage (Dement & Vaughan, 1999; Piccone & Barth, 1983). Sleeping pills should be avoided or taken for only a few days. They can disrupt the sleep-wake cycle, suppress REM sleep, and prevent the normal cycling between sleep stages. Tryptophan and melatonin will induce sleep without the negative side effects of sleeping pills (Hauri & Linde, 1996).

Sleep Apnea

Individuals who have family members with sleep apnea are more likely to develop this condition. By reducing risk factors, individuals may be able to avoid sleep apnea or at least minimize the problems associated with this condition. It is important to maintain normal weight to decrease the amount of tissue in the throat. Any sinus, throat, or respiratory problems should be treated to prevent airway obstructions. Occasionally, surgery is necessary to reshape the throat and remove obstructions. Tobacco, alcohol, and drugs should be avoided (Hauri & Linde, 1996).

Restless Leg Syndrome and Periodic Limb Disorders

Restless leg syndrome and periodic limb disorders run in families. Anyone who has family members with these disorders should be vigilant about maintaining preventive measures. A healthy diet and regular exercise are important to decrease leg cramps, maintain health, and relax muscles. Especially helpful is stretching the legs before bedtime to relax leg muscles and minimize or eliminate muscle cramping. Frequent breaks should be taken during the day to avoid sitting for long periods. Muscle spasms can be reduced by massage, warm baths, and heat or ice compresses (Hauri & Linde, 1996).

Medical and Psychiatric Conditions

Individuals who have precursors and risk factors for conditions with secondary symptoms of sleep disturbances should take precautions to prevent developing those conditions. Hereditary factors must be considered because many medical and psychiatric conditions run in families. Individuals who already have medical or psychiatric disorders that are known to interfere with sleep should aggressively try to prevent the development of secondary sleep disorders. Appropriate treatments for underlying medical problems may be the most effective way to prevent sleep disorders for this group (Chokroverty, 2000; Hauri & Linde, 1996).

Narcolepsy

Narcolepsy cannot be prevented. It is important for individuals who have family members with this disorder or who exhibit some of the signs of this disorder to be observant for other symptoms of narcolepsy. If daytime symptoms of narcolepsy occur, such as cataplexy and sleep attacks, individuals should seek medical care. Sleep attacks and cataplexy can result in accidents and embarrassing professional and personal situations (Chokroverty, 2000; Dement & Vaughan, 1999).

Indicated Measures of Prevention of Sleep Disturbances

Once sleep problems develop, treatment is more difficult but possible. Measures can be taken that are effective in eliminating or decreasing sleep disturbances. Several strategies to accomplish this goal are listed next.

Sleep Hygiene and Sleep Apnea

When poor sleep hygiene is the cause of sleep disturbances, the preventive measures listed earlier will be helpful. If sleep disturbances are caused by sleep apnea, there are several effective treatments. Weight loss reduces the amount of tissue in the throat that can narrow air passages and block air flow. Muscle relaxant medications should be avoided. Apnea is caused by an overrelaxation of throat muscles; muscle relaxants will increase this condition and worsen sleep apnea. Treat all respiratory ailments, sinus problems, allergies, asthma, problems with tonsils and adenoids promptly to prevent obstruction or interference with breathing. A mechanical device, CPAP, is an effective treatment for sleep apnea. CPAP is worn while sleeping; it forces air into the throat, holding it open and maintaining rigidity and thereby preventing tracheal collapse. CPAP is prescribed by a physician after sleep studies have been conducted and a definitive diagnosis of sleep apnea is obtained. A small amount of training is necessary to use the CPAP device correctly. Dental appliances that keep the throat open while sleeping will be effective in preventing some airflow obstructions. Surgery is sometimes recommended to remove and reshape tissues in the throat and mouth, including removing tonsils and adenoids to eliminate physical obstruction of air flow (Chokroverty, 2000; Dement & Vaughan, 1999).

Restless Leg Syndrome and Periodic Limb Disorder

To control these physical conditions it is necessary to control their symptoms. Stretching, walking, or otherwise moving the legs when cramped helps relax muscle contractions. Hot baths and gentle stretching before bed will help reduce muscle spasm when sleeping. Additional measures that relieve discomfort caused by these disorders are regular exercise, relaxation techniques, and applications of cold or heat compresses to the legs. Prescription medications ordered by physicians may be necessary to control symptoms and reduce discomfort (Hauri & Linde, 1996).

Narcolepsy

Any indication of narcolepsy should be noted and reported to a physician. There is no cure for narcolepsy, but it can be treated. Treatment requires physician-prescribed medications, usually stimulants. Additionally, the strategies listed earlier should be helpful (Hauri & Linde, 1996).

Circadian Rhythm Sleep Disorders

Circadian rhythm sleep disorders are treated by resetting the biological clock. Those with these disorders should stay awake in the daytime, even if tired, and sleep at night. Melatonin and tryptophan taken in the evening will encourage appropriate sleep-wake cycles (Hauri & Linde, 1996). While sleep disturbances caused by jet lag usually resolve naturally within a few days, there are some measures that can help. If possible, arrive at your destination a few days in advance to adjust to the new time zone. Set watches and clocks to the new time and try to schedule activities at hours appropriate to that time. Do not go to bed when you are tired; go to bed at the appropriate time in the new time zone (Chokroverty, 2000; Hauri & Linde, 1996).

Sleep Paralysis

Sleep paralysis is temporary muscle paralysis when falling asleep or waking up. In this condition, individuals cannot move any muscles except those that control eye movements and breathing. When individuals experience sleep paralysis, they should begin by moving the eyes, then gradually increase small body movements, starting with facial muscles and moving down the body until the paralysis disappears (Hauri & Linde, 1996).

PRACTICE AND POLICY IMPLICATIONS

Sleep disturbances are so prevalent that all practitioners will see clients who suffer from them. Therefore, practitioners and clinicians need to be educated about these frustrating and chronic problems so that they can work with clients to prevent and treat any sleep disorders and know when patients need a referral to a specialist in this field. Knowledge of sleep disorders is also important for accurate differential diagnosis. Sleep disturbances can mimic or obscure physical and mental conditions; determining the sleep problem and any associated medical or psychiatric conditions leads to appropriate treatment and the development of integrated treatment programs. Professionals can also be very supportive to their clients during this difficult period.

FUTURE DIRECTIONS

Sleep disturbances are dangerous, frustrating, and chronic conditions that negatively impact those who suffer from these disorders. Sleep problems rob sufferers of the chance to live healthy, active, and happy lives. It is crucial that they be identified and treated as soon as possible to prevent the development of long-term problems. Those that are neurological-motor-based such as restless leg syndrome, periodic limb movement, and narcolepsy are not usually preventable; however, they are treatable and the symptoms can be controlled. Sleep disturbances caused by stress and lifestyle choices can be prevented or reversed. Many of the measures contained in this chapter can be very effective, inexpensive, non-invasive, and even pleasant.

There is still much research to be done in the area of sleep disturbances. At this time, many sleep disorders cannot be prevented, cannot be cured, and can be only minimally controlled. Even with treatment, individuals with sleep disorders are often frustrated, stressed, and exhausted. Yet, exactly how and why we sleep is still a mystery. A thorough understanding of normal sleep is important to improve treatments and manage sleep disorders.

REFERENCES

Akerstedt, R., Fredlund, P., Gillberg, M., & Jannson, B. (2002). Sleep disturbance, work stress, and work hours: A cross-sectional study. *Journal of Psychosomatic Research, 53*(3), 741–748.

Akerstedt, R., Knutsson, A., Westerholm, P., Theorell, R., Alfredsson, L., & Kecklund, C. (2002). Work load and work hours in relation to sleep disturbance and fatigue in a large representative sample. *Journal of Psychosomatic Research, 53*(1), 585–588.

American Psychiatric Association. (2000). *Diagnostic and statistical manual of mental disorders* (4th ed., text rev.). Washington, DC: Author.

Ban, D. J., & Lee, T. J. (2001). Sleep duration, subjective sleep disturbances and associated factors among university students in Korea. *Journal of Korean Medical Science, 16*, 475–480.

Barbar, S. J., Enright, P. L., Boyle, P., Foley, D., Sharp, D. S., Petrovitch, H., et al. (2000). Sleep disturbance and their correlates in elderly Japanese-American males residing in Hawaii. *Journal of Gerontology: Series A, Biological Science and Medical Science, 55*(7), 406–411.

Bender, K. J. (1990). *Psychiatric medications: A guide for mental health professionals.* Newbury Park, CA: Sage.

Buelow, G., Hebert, S., & Buelow, S. (2000). *Psychotherapist's resource on psychiatric medication: Issues of treatment and referral.* Belmont, Ca: Brooks/Cole, Thomson Learning.

Chokroverty, S. (2000). *Clinical companion to sleep disorders medicine* (2nd ed.). Boston: Butterworth-Heinemann.

Dement, W. C., & Vaughan, C. (1999). *The promise of sleep: A pioneer in sleep medicine explores the vital connection between health, happiness, and a good night's sleep.* New York: Dell Trade Paperback.

Dunlap, J. (1998). An end in the beginning. *Science, 280,* 1548–1549.

Edinger, J. D., & Sampson, W. S. (2003). *Sleep, 26*(2), 177–182.

Gordon, R. S. (1983). An operational classification of disease prevention. *Public Health Reports, 98,* 107–109.

Green, C. B., & Menaker, M. (2003). Clocks on the brains. *Science, 301,* 319–320.

Hauri, P., & Linde, S. (1996). *No more sleepless nights* (2nd ed.). New York: Wiley.

Heuer, H., & Klien, W. (2003). One night of total sleep deprivation impairs implicit learning in the serial reaction task, but not the behavioral expression of knowledge. *Neuropsychology, 17*(3), 507–516.

Jennings, J. R., Monk, T. H., & van der Molen, M. W. (2003). Sleep deprivation influences some but not all processes of supervisory attention. *Psychological Science, 14*(5), 473–479.

Lugaresi, E. (2003). General introduction and historical review. In S. Chokroverty, W. A. Hening, & A. S. Walters (Eds.), *Sleep and movement disorders* (pp. 243–246). Philadelphia: Butterworth-Heinemann.

Manber, R., Rush, A. J., Thase, M. E., Arnow, B., Klein, D., Trivedi, M. H., et al. (2003). The effects of psychotherapy, Nefazodone, and their combination on subjective assessments of disturbed sleep in chronic depression. *Sleep, 26*(2), 130–136.

Piccone, P. M., & Barth, R. P. (1983). Sleep: An expanding field of practice and research. *Social Work, 24,* 228–233.

Siegel, J. (2002). *The neural control of sleep and waking.* New York: Springer.

Siegel, J. (2003). Neurobiology of the REM-non-REM sleep cycle. In S. Chokroverty, W. A. Hening, & A. S. Walters (Eds.), *Sleep and movement disorders (pp. 44–49).* Philadelphia: Butterworth-Heinemann.

Van Dongen, H. P. A., Maislin, G., Mullington, J. M., & Dinges, D. F. (2003). The cumulative cost of additional wakefulness: Dose-response effects on neurobehavioral functions and sleep physiology from chronic sleep restriction and total sleep deprivation. *Sleep, 26*(2), 117–126.

PART IV

Preventive Interventions for Adult Social Problems

Chapter 15

PROBLEM GAMBLING

THOMAS BROFFMAN

OVERVIEW

People have gambled since the beginning of recorded history. Over time, gambling activities have been understood from moral, mathematical, economic, social, psychological, cultural, and biological perspectives. During the early part of the twentieth century, most types of gambling were considered criminal and legal gambling was highly restricted. In the past decade, an unprecedented growth of legalized gambling occurred within a new and expanded public policy framework. The primary driving force behind this explosion of gambling in America has been the fiscal and economic needs of states and local governments. The United States has promoted leisure and recreational aspects of gambling.

Since the 1970s, legalized gambling has spread geographically and is now legal in all but two states, Utah and Hawaii. Moreover, according to the recently released National Gambling Impact Study Report (National Opinion Research Center [NORC], 1999), legalized gambling has become one of the fastest growing industries. Casinos now operate in 27 states. Legalized gambling has never been more available or socially acceptable. On the Las Vegas strip alone, there are 42 casinos, which earned $4.7 billion in 2002 (Atchison, 2003). Gambling on the Internet is also growing at a staggering rate, with 1,400 online wagering sites and over 400 sports betting sites, grossing over $1 billion annually compared to inconsequential revenues a few years ago (U.S. Senate, 1999). In 1999, Americans spent more on gambling ($50.9 billion) than on all other forms of recreation and leisure combined, including cruise ships, sporting events, music, movies, and amusement parks (NORC, 1999). Gambling varies by venue: casino gambling accounts for 40.3% of all U.S. gambling, lotteries 32.6%, tribal gambling 13.1%, parimutuel 7.5%, and charity gambling 6.5%. Amazingly, only 2.5% of bettors account for 15% of the wagering dollars in the United States (NORC, 1999).

It's fair to say that gambling is on a roll these days. In the past, there have been periods when gambling was viewed as sinful or as a vice associated with the underworld; that certainly has not been the case in recent years. Three primary forces appear to be motivating this growth: (1) the desire of governments to identify new sources of revenue without invoking new or higher taxes, (2) tourism entrepreneurs developing new destinations for entertainment and leisure, and (3) the rise of new technologies and forms of gambling (i.e., video lottery terminals, powerball mega-state lotteries, and computer offshore gambling on the Internet). Casino gambling, lotteries, and video slot machines at racetracks are not only tolerated by state and local governments, but actually supported and promoted because the states' share of the action is so substantial (it's the third leading source of revenue in several states). Gambling revenues are seen as a painless form of taxation, one that adults support freely and enjoyably.

The growth of the gambling industry throughout the United States has not been without consequence. As the availability of gambling options and venues has increased, so have the associated problems. The 1999 National Gambling Impact Study Commission Report illustrated a number of health and social costs associated with gambling. Problem gamblers and those at risk face higher rates of depression, stress, family and peer relationship problems, financial strain, alcohol dependence, and poor health (NORC, 1999). Gambling has not only become a high source of revenue for governments throughout the United States but also an important public health issue.

Gambling is one of the few activities that cuts across all barriers of race, gender, class, and culture. For the majority of people in the United States gambling is a form of recreation and entertainment; it provides an outlet for socialization and amusement at a reasonable price. One of the concerns relating to the increase in gambling opportunities is the potential rise in the number of problem gamblers. Associated with this phenomenon, there has been an increase in the prevalence of problem gambling (Korn & Shaffer, 1999). Gambling disorders arise from an interplay among many factors, including a person's biological or genetic predisposition, psychological constitution, and social environment and the nature of the activity itself.

A minority of gamblers have significant problems associated with gambling. Pathological gambling, as defined in the *Diagnostic and Statistical Manual of Mental Disorders* (*DSM-IV;* American Psychiatric Association, 1994), entails loss of control over one's gambling, a progression to more frequent and higher-stakes wagering, and gambling's becoming a life focus in spite of adverse consequences. Problem gambling implies a negative impact on one's life that falls short of pathological gambling. In evaluating the costs versus benefits of gambling to society, stories of ruined finances and destroyed relationships are balanced against individual freedom to enjoy a harmless activity that supplants tax increases. What has been rarely considered is the impact of a gambling culture on our society's values and measures to prevent the public from harm.

This chapter encourages the application of a public health perspective toward prevention of problem gambling. The classic public health model examines the interaction among host, agent, environment, and vector:

> For gambling the *host* is the individual who chooses to gamble and may be at risk for developing a gambling problem. The *agent* represents the specific gambling activity in which players engage (lotteries, slot machines, casino table games, bingo, scratch tickets, horse race betting). The *vector* is money, credit or something of value. The *environment* is both the micro-environment of the gambling venue, the family, the local community, and the socio-economic, cultural and political context within which gambling occurs. (Korn, Gibbons, & Azmier, 2000)

The public health model facilitates the incorporation of a range of prevention, harm reduction, and treatment strategies to address gambling disorders. Like all public health problems, there is a complex relationship among these factors that can produce a range of undesirable outcomes. A public health model also enables stakeholders to differentiate between potential costs and benefits of gambling and their impact on the community, including health and socioeconomic components.

HISTORY

There is nothing new about gambling or gambling problems. Archaeologists have identified gambling-related artifacts and records dating back as far as the ancient Babylonians in 3000 B.C. (Rosencrance, 1988). Both the Old and New Testaments make mention of the casting of lots, and Moses is instructed by God to divide the land west of the Jordan River by this means (Cox, Lesieur, Rosenthal, & Volberg, 1997). Gambling is also mentioned prominently in the literature and traditions of Eastern cultures (Rodgers, 1997). In Europe, organized lotteries date back to the Middle Ages. The first government-sponsored lottery was chartered by Queen Elizabeth I in 1566 (Rose, 1995).

Gambling is far from a new social issue, and over time a variety of perspectives has evolved. Apart from concerns about crime and protection of minors, gambling is a matter of individual freedom. It is both a recreational activity and a form of entertainment. It is a major source of public revenue, often referred to as a voluntary form of taxation. Gambling is touted as an important tool for economic development through increased tourism and employment. It is a ubiquitous cultural artifact that is more deeply embedded in some cultures than in others. Gambling is a way to escape the class restraints of American society, allowing winners to leap within a single bound into the ranks of the wealthy. Gambling addiction is an individual rather than a social pathology and therefore is treated with the medical model like other mental disorders.

Historically, gamblers were viewed by the psychiatric community as masochists or psychopaths rather than people with a disease or illness. The study of gambling-related health problems is a relatively new scientific field. In 1972, Dr. Robert Custer, a psychiatrist working at the Brecksville Veterans Administration Hospital in Ohio, proposed the medical syndrome "compulsive gambling" (Custer & Milt, 1985). He became an authority in the field of problem gambling and was first in identifying the progression of pathological gambling as including three phases: the winning phase, the losing phase, and the desperation or chasing phase (Custer & Milt, 1985). His efforts brought the problems associated with gambling into the health care arena. In 1980, the American Psychiatric Association included "pathological gambling" in its *Diagnostic and Statistical Manual of Mental Disorders* (*DSM*) categorizing it as an impulse control disorder. In the 1980s, Lesieur, Blume, and Zompa (1986) developed a clinical screening tool, the South Oaks Gambling Screen, to assist clinicians in identifying this disorder. The tool has become the main instrument used to study the prevalence of problem and pathological gambling.

The preponderance of gambling research has focused on the psychological consequences and the negative social impact on society. A range of social problems at the individual, familial, and community levels have been related directly or indirectly to gambling. These encompass crime, family dysfunction (domestic violence and child abuse), substance abuse, financial problems (bankruptcy and loss of employment), and comorbid psychiatric disorders (anxiety, depression, and Bipolar Disorder; NORC, 1999).

DEFINITIONS

The words *game, gamble, gambler,* and *gambling* are all derived from the Anglo-Saxon *gamen* (game) and *gameman* (to sport or play; Wykes, 1964). *Gambling* (used interchangeably with the terms *gaming* and *wagering*) is defined as placing something of value at risk in order to win a prize of value if a chance event (or an event in some part determined by chance) occurs (Korn & Shaffer, 1999). The chance events are usually determined by the outcomes of card or dice games, contests, or drawing of lots. The legal definition of gambling requires three elements: consideration, chance, and prize (Atchison,

2003). Gamblers Anonymous (1994) defines gambling as any betting or wagering, for self or others, if for money, no matter how slight or insignificant, where the outcome is uncertain or depends on chance or skill constitutes gambling. The casino industry prefers the term *gaming* as more acceptable than gambling. *Wagering* generally applies to betting on horse races, dog races, or pari-mutuel competitions such as jai alai.

Gambling occurs on a continuum from nonproblem (social or recreational gambling) to problem to compulsive or pathological gambling. A *social* or *recreational gambler* is a person who participates in gambling as a casual activity to fill time with friends or for excitement during leisure time (McGurrin, 1994). The player may expect to incur some losses, but these are seen as the cost of the entertainment experience. The losses are monies that the player can afford to spend on recreation. Social gamblers, unlike compulsive gamblers, can quit gambling at any time, win or lose: There is no self-esteem tied to winning or losing; other aspects of their lives are more important and rewarding; and they rarely have a big win (Blume, 1997).

In the mental health and addictions field, the most common terms used today are problem and pathological gambling. *Problem gambling* is defined as any pattern of gambling that compromises, disrupts, or damages personal, family, or vocational pursuits and leads to adverse consequences (Volberg, 2001). A problem gambler gambles excessively, usually more than he or she would like to, and losses exceed the amount of money the gambler can easily afford. The problem gambler maintains some control over his or her gambling activity, being able to stop and then avoid gambling activity; however, most pathological gamblers go through a stage of problem gambling. These gambling problems may be mild, moderate, or severe.

Problem gambling is not a well-defined concept. The *DSM-IV* (American Psychiatric Association, 1994) provides only a diagnosis of gambling problems at the pathological level. Currently, there is no diagnostic equivalent to substance abuse, such as gambling abuse or problem gambling. In the 16 states where prevalence studies have been conducted since 1986, the terms problem, compulsive, and pathological gambling have been used synonymously.

Pathological gambling is "persistent and recurrent maladaptive gambling behavior that disrupts personal, family or vocational pursuits" (American Psychiatric Association, 1994, p. 615; see Table 15.1). The pathological gambler has succumbed to a psychiatric impulse control disorder, evidenced by progression of gambling activity that cannot be controlled by the gambler, who becomes intolerant of losing and must keep betting to satisfy his or her inner drives. The gambling preoccupies the gambler's thinking to the point where the consequences of the gambling activity are completely disregarded. The gambler seems unable to stop;

Table 15.1 *DSM-IV* **Diagnostic Criteria for 312.31 Pathological Gambling**

A. Persistent and recurrent maladaptive gambling behavior as indicated by five (or more) of the following:

  1. Is preoccupied with gambling.
  2. Needs to gamble with increasing amounts of money in order to achieve the desired excitement.
  3. Has repeated unsuccessful efforts to control, cut back, or stop gambling.
  4. Is restless or irritable when attempting to cut down or stop gambling.
  5. Gambles as a way of escaping from problems or of relieving a dysphoric mood.
  6. After losing money gambling, often returns another day to get even.
  7. Lies to family members, therapist, or others to conceal the extent of involvement with gambling.
  8. Has committed illegal acts such as forgery, fraud, theft, or embezzlement to finance gambling.
  9. Has jeopardized or lost a significant relationship, job, or educational or career opportunity because of gambling.
  10. Relies on others to provide money to relieve a desperate financial situation caused by gambling.

B. The gambling episode is not better accounted for by a manic episode.

Source: From "Pathological Gambling," p. 615, by APA *DSM-IV* Task Force, in *Diagnostic and Statistical Manual of Mental Disorders,* fourth edition, 1994, in Washington, DC: Author.

he or she suffers from urges and cravings similar to those of other addictions. Eventually, gambling interferes with functioning in almost every aspect of life.

TRENDS AND INCIDENCE

Prevalence

While gambling is an entertaining and recreational pastime for the vast majority of players, it is evident that for a small minority, out-of-control gambling behavior causes problems for the individual, his or her family, and the community. The expansion of gambling arenas and methods over the past couple of decades has contributed to the public perception that gambling problems have exponentially increased.

The Harvard Medical School Division of Addiction meta-analysis of gambling addiction data published between 1977 and 1997 reviewed over 100 prevalence studies and estimated that there were 4.4 million adult and adolescent pathological gamblers and 11 million adult and adolescent problem gamblers (Shaffer, Hall, & Vander Bilt, 1997). In its national household phone survey conducted as part of the National Gambling Impact Study Commission to Congress, NORC (1999) estimated that there were 20.5 million pathological and problem gamblers. Even using the Harvard study's lower number of 15.4 million adult and adolescent problem and pathological gamblers and assuming five family members, friends, or coworkers are adversely affected by pathological and problem gamblers, there are approximately 70 million people indirectly impacted by gambling problems in the United States.

Gender Differences

Until the 1970s and 1980s, gambling in the United States was considered by the public to be largely a male pursuit. The traditional bastions of gambling, the racetrack, the casino, and card parlors, were male domains, and "ladies" were not seen at these venues (Goodman, 1995). However, in the 1990s, with the arrival of state-sponsored lotteries, modern-day casinos, high-stakes bingo parlors, and, most recently, video lottery, poker, and slots, more and more women are participating in all forms of gambling. With changes in traditional roles and lifestyles over the past decade, women have the time, money, and inclination to gamble. Women now constitute one of the fastest growing segments of casino and lottery gamblers (Moore & Carlson, 1998).

Since Freud's paper on compulsive gambling was published in 1914, there has been little systematic research into the female problem gambler (Lesieur, 1998). Historically, gambling and gambling problems have been considered male problems. Twenty-five years ago, 95% of gamblers were men (Rodgers, 1997). By 1997, 55% of gamblers were women (Shaffer, 1997). Men are more likely than women to develop gambling problems and men predominate among admissions to gambling treatment programs (Lesieur, 1998). About 33% of compulsive gamblers are female (Mark & Lesieur, 1992).

With few exceptions, until the recently published Harvard Medical School meta-analysis (Shaffer et al., 1997), gender comparisons were rare in gambling research (Hraba & Lee, 1996) because gambling was considered a disorder that primarily affected men. Researchers have contributed to this false perception by using either all-male or predominantly male samples in their investigations (Mark & Lesieur, 1992), with White males who served in the military being the most frequent subjects of research (Hraba & Lee, 1996). This set the stage for an inherent contradiction: Women's problem gambling was viewed as abnormal or different from men's, but women were studied as if their gambling problems were like those of men (Broffman & Scanlan, 1998). Inferring an understanding of gambling problems among women from studies on men creates many problems, particularly the "male-as-the-norm" bias (Wilke, 1994).

Gender differences among pathological gamblers have been hypothesized in stereotypical ways. For example, men are seen as "action" gamblers who tend to gamble for excitement or to prove themselves smarter than their opponents. Typically, the male uses his addiction to enhance his male image in a macho manner, by bragging and exaggerating about his behavior, winnings, and financial losses (Custer & Milt, 1985). Women are allegedly "escapist" gamblers, who tend to flock to the solitary pleasures of slot machines or video lottery slots to escape some problem in their personal life (Ohtsuka, Burton, DeLucs, & Borg, 1997).

The onset of gambling in women is often in adulthood rather than adolescence (Volberg, 1996), and in some cases much later in life as a result of developmental changes such as the empty nest, divorce, or widowhood (New Jersey Governor's Council on Alcoholism and Drug Abuse, 1996). Most males report winning a large sum of money early in their gambling experiences (Custer & Milt, 1985). Women report some winning episodes, but less often a tremendous win (Zebrowski, 1991). Females' enabling systems seem to be more limited to family and friends (Lesieur & Rosenthal, 1991). As with males, there is usually a history of addiction in either the nuclear or conjugal family (Lesieur, 1988).

While compulsive gambling affects both men and women, there are some differences worth noting. The addiction is progressive in women as it is in men, but with women it most often does not advance as far (Custer & Milt, 1985); social and economic factors seem to brake the descent earlier. Desperation for women comes when they cannot bear the guilt and shame any longer, and seems to come more from emotional exhaustion than from a lack of funds (Hunter, 1995).

Ethnic, Cultural, and Racial Factors

Information is beginning to emerge about the gambling habits of several special populations, although long-term consequences remain uncertain. Very few studies have focused on gambling problems among minority populations in the United States. Yet, the need for such research is critical, as gambling prevalence studies have found that pathological gambling is greater among people of color than among Caucasians (Murray, 1993; Volberg, 1996).

African American

The African American community is diverse in socioeconomic status, and its origins include people from the United States, Africa, and the Caribbean. Communal themes are race, oppression, discrimination, poverty, strengths, and survival. African Americans are not a monolithic group, though they do share a common cultural heritage rooted in slavery, the northern migration, urban living, the civil rights movement, and the continuing undercurrent of racism (Wright, 2001).

Gambling has been an indigenous part of American, African, and Caribbean cultures. For many African Americans, gambling has been used as an elixir for the emotional pain and stress of living in an oppressive environment. The numbers have long been a staple of the African American community, predating modern lotteries (Wykes, 1964). Gambling among African American males is normative, yet historically, gambling among women has been prohibited due to religious beliefs, role expectations, and family responsibilities. Economic frustration over not being able to get a job to fulfill their major financial responsibilities may be a factor among African American males (Goodman, 1995). Gambling is readily accessible and affordable, while providing escape from the unpleasant feelings and psychological pain of racism and discrimination. African American gambling is correlated with social pessimism and blossoms from a mood of despair, powerlessness, and hopelessness (Rodgers, 1997). It flourishes in communities where people no longer believe they can influence their present, much less their future.

To date, there have been limited studies of African American gamblers; equally distressing is the fact that few gambling studies address the race or ethnicity of participants. African Americans are underrepresented in both Gamblers Anonymous and problem gambling treatment (Lesieur, 1998). Many African Americans do not seek professional help for a variety of reasons. They instead use natural ecosystems to resolve problems, which include social supports and religious and spiritual networks (Wright, 2001). The issues that contribute to and perpetuate gambling problems in the African American community are as complex and diverse as the community itself. To decrease gambling problems among African Americans will require diverse strategies that are sensitive to the multiple racial and socioeconomic realities that challenge the African American community.

Asian American

Generally speaking, the Asian American community comprises people from Hong Kong, China, Taiwan, Korea, Vietnam, Cambodia, Laos, Thailand, the Philippines, and other Southeast Asian countries. When we talk about "Asians" or "Asian culture," we refer to a group that is far from homogeneous. People have come from different geographic areas, have come to the United States at different times and with different sociopolitical experiences and various lengths of stay in the United States. They have their own culture, language, and customs. Each subgroup has developed its own worldview and perceives and responds to situations differently.

Gambling has been part of the social life in Asian society for thousands of years; the first records of Chinese gambling appeared in 700 B.C. (Wykes, 1964). Historically, almost anything that involved chance and uncertainty was gambled on, including cock fights, dice, fish fights, cricket fights, mah-jongg, and horse racing. It was so widespread in China after the death of Chairman Mao, that it was considered a "social epidemic" (Chinese Family Life Services of Metro Toronto, 1996). The government has responded to this "social epidemic" by various attempts at prohibition and severe punishment.

In Asian culture, the line between gaming and gambling has never been well-defined. Some forms of gambling are socially acceptable and some are frowned upon. It seems some cultures condemn the consequences, not the activity. Some forms of gambling have become such an interwoven part of social life that they are highly acceptable and even considered to be healthy activities (Woo, 2003). A Chinese proverb says: "Small gambling is soothing and relaxing but heavy gambling can affect your mental health" (Wykes, 1964). Knowing how to gamble is also considered a sign of masculinity and manhood, even though heavy gambling is still not acceptable (Hwang & Lau, 2003).

Ethnicity and length of time in the United States are important factors in differentiating help-seeking behaviors of different groups in the Asian American community. The idea of social work or counseling is alien to most Asian Americans. In some subcultures, counselors or social workers are associated with government officials and treated with mistrust and suspicion. In traditional Asian culture, an individual's problems are often dealt with in the family system or among members of the extended family (Woo, 2003). Asian Americans will usually not reach out for help unless all resources in their private domain fail and the situation has escalated to a crisis. Seeking help in the public domain is considered rather shameful because it implies an admission that one is weak, feeble-minded, a burden to others, and a failure to the family (Hwang & Lau, 2003). When Asian Americans reach out to seek help, they usually look for tangible service and advice.

Hispanic/Latino American

According to the U.S. Census Bureau, the Hispanic population is the fastest growing and soon will be the largest minority group. It is a mosaic of many different people from Puerto Rico, Mexico, Cuba, and Central and South America. The impact of this shift in population may have a sizable impact on both gambling and intervention or prevention efforts. Research on Hispanic gambling behavior is largely nonexistent. The vast majority of individuals seeking help for gambling or already in treatment, including Gamblers Anonymous, are Anglo. The reasons for this discrepancy are not clear. Little research attention has been paid to possible cultural differences that exist between minority and Anglo gambling practices and beliefs that may influence persons seeking treatment for problem gambling or prevention efforts.

Hispanic cultural norms may present a barrier not only to seeking treatment, but to education and prevention activities. Spanish translations of existing Anglo-oriented materials are insufficient. Hispanics are often reluctant to use government or agency services perceived to be representative of the Anglo establishment. Machismo is a factor in highly permissive attitudes toward male drinking and gambling, making it difficult for men's gambling behavior to be labeled problematic (Cuadrado, 1999). For Hispanic women, *marianismo* requires them to be chaste, passive, submissive, and motherly. Gambling violates this image of a proper woman, although bingo is viewed as an acceptable type of gambling for women because it is commonly promoted by religious institutions as a fund-raising activity. Slot machines and video poker also offer limited social interaction and anonymity for Hispanic women.

Family problems are the most frequently stated reason both Anglos and Hispanics seek assistance for problem gambling. Cultural differences influence the definition of family problems. Linking gambling problems to addiction may be offensive to many Hispanics, who despise the stereotype of a "junkie" (Cuadrado, 1999).

RISK FACTORS

Co-Occurring Disorders

There is evidence that connects pathological gambling to other addictions. Studies demonstrate a large overlap among pathological gambling, alcoholism, and drug addiction (Lesieur, 1998). The potential role that casinos play in exacerbating alcohol-related disorders in pathological gamblers is significant because many of these facilities provide free alcohol to patrons. One of the rationales for this service may be related to alcohol's potential to impair judgment and therefore increase gambling activity. The substitution of one addiction for another has been reported by professionals in rehabilitation programs for both substance abuse disorders and pathological gambling, but research supporting this finding is limited (Spunt, Dupont, Lesieur, Liberty, & Hunt, 1998). Substance-dependent patients who are also problem gamblers have higher rates of stress-related diseases and serious psychiatric problems, including a suicide attempt rate six times higher than that of nongamblers (Ciarrocchi, 1987). The literature on simultaneous addictions and gambling disorders is still very much in its infancy. In treatment facilities for gamblers, approximately 30% to 70% of patients have an addiction to one or more substances (Ladouceur, Sylvain, Letarte, Giroux, & Jacques, 2002).

A variety of mental illnesses place people at greater risk for developing gambling problems. Similarly, problem gamblers have higher rates of psychiatric disorders than the general population. For example, the relationship between depression and gambling is complex and interactive. Depression increases the chance of developing a gambling problem, but it may also be a consequence of losses associated with gambling activity (Broffman, 2002). Problem gamblers have higher rates of depression than the general population. Among problem gamblers in treatment, rates of depression are three to five times higher than in the general population (Broffman, 2002).

Elders

Evidence suggests that problem gambling is rapidly increasing among seniors and may occur at higher rates than in the general adult population (NGISC, 1999). Convergent factors put elderly adults at higher risk: unresolved feelings associated with the multiple losses they experience in postretirement, increased longevity, isolation, increased free time, financial reserves, and decreased moral constraints (National Research Council, 1999). The data are scanty, but the underlying assumption is that seniors turn to gambling for comfort, friendship, dissociation to minimize depression, and pain reduction.

As legalized gambling, particularly casino and lottery gambling, has become increasingly available and accessible to those outside of Las Vegas and Atlantic City in the past 10 years, many older Americans (defined as persons age 65 and older) have discovered gambling as a new type of social activity. Though raised during the Great Depression, when gambling was a moral issue, considered either a sin or a vice, many seniors have embraced it as a new form of socially acceptable entertainment. Promotional programs such as inexpensive buffet meals, free transportation (especially during the first week of the month—"check week"), coupons, slot clubs, high-stakes bingo, dance clubs, and discount prescription offers are tailored to these older adults who remember their first WWII ration books. Such enticements encourage those who might not normally visit a casino or purchase a lottery ticket (McNeilly & Burke, 2000).

Though published studies on gambling and older adults are very limited, anecdotal reports abound on the potential public health problem of gambling among seniors. Those involved in treatment have described senior gamblers as escape gamblers, who gamble to relieve their negative dysphoric feelings of isolation, boredom, or depression, or to avoid difficult situations. At the same time, problem gambling treatment programs are reporting a telescoped period of time (1 to 3 years) for older adults to develop a gambling problem (National Research Council, 1999).

There is a great need for awareness of the impact of legalized gambling, particularly casino gambling, on seniors. Contrary to popular belief, the propensity for participating in gambling does not decline with age. Future research on gambling among older adults is important as a greater percentage of the population reaches retirement age at a time of unparalleled accessibility to legalized gambling as a form of mainstream entertainment (NORC, 1999).

EFFECTIVE UNIVERSAL PREVENTIVE INTERVENTIONS

Prevention can be defined as a process of fostering and creating conditions that promote the well-being of people (Substance Abuse and Mental Health Service Administration, Center for Substance Abuse Prevention, 2002). Prevention interventions provide individuals with the intentions and skills to act in a healthy manner, coupled with developing an environment that supports healthy behavior. The construction of nearly every prevention program begins with an understanding of factors that place people at risk for or that protect them from problem behavior. As gambling opportunities are likely to remain as they are, the question of who should be targeted for prevention efforts looms large. Preventing gambling problems is very complex because the loss of control for those with problems is just an exaggeration of the same set of emotions for those who gamble without problems. It is very difficult to effectively draw a line between the two groups.

A clear challenge for developing effective ways to prevent problem gambling is the lack of awareness of the dangers of excessive gambling. Placing a bet does not readily produce immediate adverse effects. Moreover, advertising by casinos and state lotteries suggest that gambling is a harmless form of recreation. Gambling advertising promotes the acceptance of gambling by portraying it as family entertainment or social recreation, emphasizing community needs for tax revenues generated, altering the norms surrounding the behavior, and publicizing successful gamblers (National Research Council, 1999).

Until the 1990s, public awareness of problem gambling was limited. Few prevention programs for problem gambling currently exist. Most of those that are available have no scientific basis, and even fewer have been empirically tested. The vast majority of programs have not delineated the risk or protective factors they were addressing. As well, most programs fail to explicitly state whether they use a harm-reduction or abstinence model. Prevention efforts in the field of problem gambling have included teaching gamblers about the odds of the games they play, providing helpline services, and developing public awareness campaigns about the potential risks associated with gambling (Derevensky, Gupta, Dickson, & Deguire, 2001). Nothing is known yet about the effectiveness of these efforts.

Universal prevention programs encompass efforts that target the general population, regardless of their relative risk. All members of a community, not just specific individuals or groups within the community, benefit from a universal prevention effort. Harm-reduction campaigns and programs that encourage individuals to use a decision-making process (maintaining and setting financial limits) are examples of universal initiatives (Derevensky et al., 2001).

The American Gaming Association (the trade group for commercial casinos) has developed a *Responsible Gambling Resource Guide* and sponsored an annual Responsible Gaming Education Week since 1996 held the second week in August at all participating properties. Founded in 1972, the National Council on Problem Gambling (NCPG) along with its 33 state affiliates attempts to increase public awareness of problem gambling, encourage research and prevention efforts, and ensure the availability of treatment. Initiated in 2003, the NCPG's mass media program, National Problem Gambling Awareness Week, is held during March to coincide with the NCAA National Basketball Championship ("March Madness"). Such universal prevention efforts need to be distinguished from more extensive mental health promotion efforts, which aim to help individuals more effectively cope with daily stresses and do not focus on gambling prevention per se.

In Canada, the provinicial governments of Ontario and Quebec have developed harm-reduction prevention initiatives for high school and college students. The programs are based on parallels to alcohol use and abuse: high prevalence, social acceptability, promoted in the home environment, continuum of harm, and adolescent experimentation. Student gambling is primarily motivated by an impulse for risk taking; harm-reduction prevention initiatives seek to identify both risk and protective factors for students. The key is to engage students: *Entering* into a supportive relationship, *nonblaming attitude, Gives* behavioral options, *Accepts* their choices, *Gains* awareness and *Educates* around potential harm (Derevensky et al., 2001). School-based programs focus on responsible gambling, including age-appropriate exposure to gambling information and strategies on how to gamble safely.

Another example of harm reduction is the curriculum developed at the Harvard University Project on Gambling and Health, *Facing the Odds: The Mathematics of Gambling and Other Risks,* which has been implemented in Massachusetts and Louisiana (Shaffer, Hall, Vander Bilt, & George, 2003). The curriculum teaches the mathematics of everyday life though games of chance. The purpose is to introduce and apply concepts of number sense, data, statistics, and probability through the use of gambling-related topics. Unlike traditional approaches that usually emphasize the health benefits associated with avoiding addictive behaviors or that attach particular values to behaviors (i.e., good versus bad drugs), this curriculum reveals the mathematical realities of various gambling activities and reinforces critical, statistical, and probability thinking. The goal is to delay the onset of gambling behavior, as the younger the age of initiation of gambling, the higher the correlation with the development of gambling-related problems (National Research Council, 1999).

As the legal age of gambling varies from 18 to 21 in various jurisdictions, it is important to intervene when young people are first legally able to gamble. According to the Harvard Meta-Analysis, people 18 to 24 have the highest rate of gambling participation and problem gambling, with surprisingly high rates among college and university students (Shaffer et al., 1997). One university prevention strategy has targeted these young adults, who have the highest rates of involvement with the most risky behaviors, including gambling. Several schools have modified their existing introductory course on probability and statistics to include lectures devoted to probabilities associated with gambling and gambling fallacies, and lab demonstrations of gambling. The goals are to decrease cognitive errors common in gambling, improve knowledge and ability to calculate gambling odds, change gambling attitudes, and modify gambling behavior (Shaffer et al., 2003).

EFFECTIVE SELECTIVE PREVENTIVE INTERVENTIONS

Selective preventive programs target those at higher-than-average risk for gambling problems. Targeted individuals are identified on the basis of the nature and number of risk factors for gambling problems to which they may be exposed. Selective strategies try to decrease risk factors or bolster protective factors (Derevensky et al., 2001). For example, a male with early initiation into gambling activities who struggles with depression displays several risk factors for problem gambling and would be a candidate for selective prevention programming. Other examples of selective strategies include harm-reduction problem gambling programs targeted to entire communities where the risk may be particularly high due to high crime rates, low socioeconomic status, and large number of single-parent households.

It is a selective intervention as college students are an "at risk" population, who engage in a variety of high risk, thrill seeking behaviors. In 1996, the Minnesota Institute of Public Health introduced the curriculum *Improving Your Odds* to help college students acquire the knowledge and skills necessary to make the right choices about gambling. The underlying premise was that responsible gambling was possible if the following guidelines were understood and respected:

1. The decision to gamble is a personal choice.
2. Gambling is not essential for having a good time.
3. Acceptable losses need to be established before starting to gamble.

4. Borrowing money to gamble should be avoided and discouraged.

5. There are times when people should not gamble.

6. Illegal gambling should be avoided and discouraged.

7. Use of alcohol and drugs when gambling is risky.

8. There are certain reasons for gambling that present a high risk for problems. (Svendsen & Griffin, 1996)

The curriculum was designed to teach students about the risks and benefits of gambling and to help them examine their perceptions about gambling and establish guidelines for low-risk gambling behaviors.

Another Minnesota program, *Gambling Away the Golden Years,* is a prevention program that targets senior citizens to address the onset of gambling problems during the retirement stage of life. This 15-minute video program and manual address senior problem gambling warning signs and where to seek help. The video stresses protective factors: learning a new skill, keeping busy with nongambling activities, and identifying activities that make one feel productive (North American Training Institute, 1997).

EFFECTIVE INDICATED PREVENTIVE INTERVENTIONS

Indicated prevention efforts encompass efforts aimed at individuals who possess noticeable signs (psychological or behavioral markers) of a problem or disorder even if they are not yet diagnosable. Screening is the primary strategy of indicated prevention. For example, screening for gambling problems in mental health care settings and community substance abuse treatment agencies is an important public health strategy to increase professional and public awareness of the potential for gambling-related harm and to provide indicated prevention through early identification and case finding.

Indicated preventive programs target those already gambling or engaging in other high-risk behaviors to prevent chronic or pathological gambling problems. Indicated interventions are aimed at individuals who may already display signs of gambling problems and are designed to prevent the onset of pathological gambling. There are three standard, common ways of dealing with the harm of gambling: harm reduction, harm minimization, and responsible gambling (Korn et al., 2000). Harm reduction supports strategies to reduce harmful negative consequences incurred through involvement in risky behaviors. For example, gambling might be limited to casinos or racetracks and prohibited at convenience stores. Harm minimization aims at lessening the harm of gambling to the lowest practical level. This approach implies that there is a known standard against which harm minimization measures can be judged. Presently, in Australia, these methods include efforts to program slot machines to warn players about the amount of money they have gambled or the time they have spent on the machine ("speed bumps"). Or machines may permit players to decide in advance how long they will play or what the speed of play may be.

Responsible gambling, by contrast, targets certain risk groups and attempts to move them to a lower level of risk through such methods as education and disclosure of gambling odds. Responsible gambling assumes that safe levels of gambling are possible. For those who do not gamble at all, of course, there is no risk of gambling addiction. Those who do gamble fall into one of three categories: moderate risk for a gambling disorder, severe risk, and pathological gambling. The last category implies that treatment, not prevention, is needed. Those in the moderate and severe risk categories are targeted for movement to a lower-risk category (Ladouceur et al., 2002).

An example of responsible gambling is the Connecticut Partnership for Responsible Gambling "Tips on Playing Responsibly," a statewide awareness program whose partners are the Connecticut Lottery Corporation, the Connecticut Council on Problem Gambling, and the State Department of Mental Health and Addiction Services. Responsible play reminders include:

1. Set a spending limit.
2. Once you reach your limit, stop playing.
3. Understand that winning and losing are both a part of gambling: If you expect to win, you should also be prepared to lose.
4. Understand that gambling is a recreational activity; it should not be used as an alternative to work or other activities.
5. Money for daily living expenses is just that; it should not be used for gambling.
6. Understand that all forms of gambling have the potential to be habit-forming.

The gambling industry has widely acknowledged the risks inherent in their products and as a result has an obligation to address gambling-related problems. The industry response to problem gambling is developing Responsible Gambling Programs in Australia, Canada, Europe, New Zealand, and the United States. Self-exclusion is a relatively new initiative by the casino industry: Individuals voluntarily have themselves barred from the premises of a casino or similar establishment. This nonintrusive intervention is an attractive self-control procedure for gamblers who have difficulty regulating their gambling activities but are not ready to seek professional help. Self-exclusion is a relatively new initiative by the casino industry. From a prevention point of view, self-exclusion programs have been advertised to reach people who are at risk of becoming pathological gamblers. Risky behaviors are described in signage and pamphlets to help gamblers decide whether such a step is appropriate for them. In the only published study of self-exclusion, which was conducted in Canada, researchers reported that self-excluded gamblers had a 30% success rate in avoiding all gambling activities, a powerful finding compared to statistics for other types of interventions (Ladouceur, Jacques, Giroux, Ferland, & LeBlond, 2000). Unfortunately, little documentation is available. No state or federal statutes mandate the inclusion of such programs. As well, questions have been raised as to the efficacy of enforcing such a program.

Other responsible gambling initiatives include strictly enforcing age limits, displaying information about treatment and a toll-free helpline number, and providing customers with information on the risks associated with gambling and guidelines for safer gambling. Most gambling establishments train staff to assist clientele who may have a problem. These actions are gradually becoming the general practice in the casino industry.

Several gaming providers and governments around the world are experimenting with new approaches that may prove useful in the future. Programs range from offering on-site counseling services to modifying electronic gaming machines to show users the time and money spent. Some are changing the gaming environment by removing bank (ATM) machines, installing clocks, or modifying lighting on their gaming floor. Some European countries have introduced more aggressive approaches, such as requiring gamblers to predetermine how much they will spend for each visit. Precommitment programs allow video poker machine players to precommit time and money expenditures.

PRACTICE AND POLICY IMPLICATIONS

With more people gambling, more people will have gambling problems and more social workers will counsel problem gamblers. Given this phenomenon, social workers need to understand the clinical manifestations of pathological gambling, as well as its effects on the family system.

Problem gambling is often a hidden disease: It is not discernible by merely looking at a person, breath or blood tests cannot detect it, nor does it leave needle marks. An old Gamblers Anonymous maxim advises, "You cannot smell cards on our breath." Pathological gamblers hide their gambling from their family, friends, and coworkers. A person with a gambling problem may seek assistance with either financial, relationship, or work problems, so gambling may be undetected as a primary problem.

Few social workers are adequately trained and prepared to deal with this newest addiction in our society. All should receive education and training in identification, assessment, and treatment of pathological gambling. Social workers require additional training in assessment and diagnosis of gambling problems. Gambling screening questions should routinely be included in all psychosocial assessments. In addition, social workers need assistance in identifying financial options to assist clients, because the costs of this addiction are enormous. A compulsive gambler can destroy a family system by undermining family finances, jeopardizing the physical and emotional health of family members, and destabilizing marital and parent-child relationships.

The research suggests that pathological gamblers can be found in psychiatric and substance abuse populations and are easily screened with existing instruments (Lesieur et al., 1986). An example is the Connecticut State Department of Mental Health and Addiction Services 4 Question Screen:

1. Have you ever borrowed money in order to gamble or cover money lost gambling?
2. Have you ever thought you might have a gambling problem, or been told that you might?
3. Have you ever been untruthful about the extent of your gambling, or hid it from others?
4. Have you ever tried to stop or cut back on how much or how often you gamble?

Substance abuse, use of illegal drugs, and gambling often occur concomitantly; knowing more about the interaction of gambling activity and other problem behaviors has significant implications for intervention (Spunt et al., 1998). In addition, social workers need to be aware of the social costs associated with gambling. The impact of pathological gambling goes well beyond the identified patient: Family and friends are pulled into the whirlpool of this deepening problem, and corporations are acutely affected, with the pathological gambler embezzling company funds to maintain the addiction. Social workers must be alert to avoid misdiagnosing or failing to identify the problem, particularly in the early stages, due to lack of familiarity or to the denial and mislabeling of the problem by clients and their significant others. In short, there is a real need to begin training social workers to assist problem gamblers and their families.

Policy Implications

Government has done with gambling what it has done, or is in the process of doing, with alcohol and tobacco. Under the guise of delimiting a vice, government itself has become the beneficiary of the vice. With alcohol and tobacco, government ostensibly keeps a respectable distance from the purveyors of the vice; however, with gambling, government has become a primary purveyor. Thus, we see the spectacle of government itself promoting and successfully increasing the number of persons involved with gambling. Politicians argue in favor of expanding legalized gambling to keep it out of the hands of organized crime and to keep revenues in their home states or out of the hands of Native Americans. All this despite knowledge that gambling ruins many lives.

Governments have the responsibility to create public policy in the public interest. The basic questions before state legislatures is whether to legalize additional forms of gambling (especially casinos and slot machines) and, in some cases, whether to abolish certain forms of gambling (e.g., Internet gambling). This means balancing gambling revenues with safeguards to prevent gambling-related problems and to help those who get into trouble. Governments have to ensure that gambling policies take into account both the benefits and the costs of gambling. They need to ensure that quality treatment and prevention and awareness programs are available. Because much is unknown about causes, treatment, and prevention in this field, ongoing research is important to increase understanding about what programs work best.

The public policy recommendations to address prevention of gambling problems are multifaceted and diverse. State and federal governments are urged to assess the impact of gambling expansion on the quality of life and balance the promotion of gambling with that of protecting the public from gambling-related harm. State governments have a dual role as purveyors and regulators of gambling. Public officials have an ethical, moral, legal, and fiduciary responsibility to protect the public safety from the direct and indirect impacts of gambling problems by educating the public about the possible dangers of gambling problems to allow individuals to make their own decisions. For a democracy to remain strong, people must be allowed to make their own choices. But for a society to prosper, these choices must be made in a responsible fashion (Yaffe & Brodsky, 1997).

FUTURE DIRECTIONS

As gambling has become more accessible, individuals, gambling providers, and the government have incurred the obligation to deal with gambling problems. Like most other social issues, there is no single cure for problem gambling. The programs that are in place or being put in place are essential, but not sufficient. There needs to be a better safety net in place to prevent gambling problems. Education must include basic statistics, teaching the laws of probability and the consequences of gamblers' fallacies. The gambling industry must take a responsible approach in their advertisements, akin to alcohol and tobacco warnings. Advertisements for gambling should include clear, visible warnings of the odds of losing and information on service centers, support groups, or helplines. Gambling advertisements should not be misleading, promoting gambling as the "ticket to happiness." Where there is an advertisement for gambling there should be a clear, visible warning of the odds of losing. There should be a clear, visible ad for service centers, support groups or helplines. The gambling industry rather than the taxpayer should be required to provide funds for prevention, treatment, and research on gambling problems. These funds could be obtained from a surtax on gambling industry profits; for example, the Ontario government commits 2% of revenues from slot machines and charity casinos to the treatment and prevention of gambling problems. The surtax should be a function of the rate of gambling problems revealed by biannual prevalence studies.

The public cares about problem gambling and problem gamblers. They also understand that the responsibility is shared between individuals, gambling providers, and the government. Like most other social issues there is no single cure for problem gambling. The programs that are in place or being put in place are essential, but not sufficient. There needs to be a better safety net in place to prevent gambling problems.

When we look to the experience of other sectors we see that improvements depend on many factors. If we learn one thing from experience in preventing or reducing other types of addictive disorders, it is that influencing individuals' behavior through education and awareness is essential. When we think about the reduction of motor vehicle injuries, drinking and driving, smoking, or any other public health interest issue, the informed consumer is the essential ingredient.

As noted, factors influencing the probability that a gambler will engage in preventive behaviors are varied and complex. No one strategy, approach, or perspective is likely to be effective by itself in achieving the level of risk factor change required to produce enduring public health effects in the prevention of gambling problems across subgroups of U.S. adults. Rather, combinations of approaches based on differing milieus and requiring the collaboration of a diversity of professional disciplines and interests, both public and private, are strongly indicated.

REFERENCES

American Psychiatric Associaton. (1994). *Diagnostic and statistical manual of mental disorders* (4th ed.). Washington, DC: Author.

Atchison, E. (2003). *Joe Gambel's hidden secrets: Behavioral control and psychosocial impact in Las Vegas.* Cheynne, WY: Pioneer Printing.

Blume, S. (1997). Pathological gambling. In N. Miller (Ed.), *The principles and practice of addictions in psychiatry* (pp. 422–432). Philadelphia: Saunders.

Broffman, T. (2002). *Gender differences in mental health and substance disorders as predictors of gambling disorders.* Unpublished doctoral dissertation, Boston College, Boston.

Broffman, T., & Scanlan, K. (1998, June). *Focus group research with female problem gamblers.* Paper presented at the National Conference on Problem Gambling Conference, Las Vegas, NV.

Chinese Family Life Services of Metro Toronto. (1996). *Working with gambling problems in the Chinese community.* Toronto, Ontario, Canada: Author.

Ciarrocchi, J. (1987). Severity of impairment in dually addicted gamblers. *Journal of Gambling Studies, 3*(1), 16–26.

Cox, S., Lesieur, H., Rosenthal, R., & Volberg, R. (1997). *Problem and pathological gambling in america: The national picture.* Columbia, MD: National Council on Problem Gambling.

Cuadrado, M. (1999). A comparison of Hispanic and Anglo calls to a gambling help hotline. *Journal of Gambling Studies, 15*(1), 71–81.

Custer, R., & Milt, H. (1985). *When luck runs out: Help for compulsive gamblers and their families.* New York: Facts on File.

Derevensky, J., Gupta, R., Dickson, L., & Deguire, A. (2001). *Prevention efforts toward minimizing gambling problems.* Toronto, Ontario, Canada: McGill University, International Centre for Youth Gambling Problems & High-Risk Behaviors.

Gamblers Anonymous. (1994). *Sharing recovery through gamblers anonymous.* Los Angeles, CA: Gamblers Anonymous.

Goodman, R. (1995). *The luck business.* New York: Free Press.

Hraba, J., & Lee, G. (1996). Gender, gambling, and problem gambling. *Journal of Gambling Studies, 12*(1), 83–102.

Hunter, R. (1995). Pathological gambling and its treatment. *The EAPA Exchange, 25*(2), 2–3.

Hwang, A., & Lau, L. (2003). *What's beyond: Cultural perspectives on problem gambling in the southeast Asian community.* St. Paul: Minnesota Department of Human Services.

Korn, D., Gibbons, R., & Azmier, J. (2000). Framing public policy towards a public health paradigm for gambling. *Journal of Gambling Studies, 19*(2), 235–256.

Korn, D., & Shaffer, H. (1999). Gambling and the health of the public: Adopting a public health perspective. *Journal of Gambling Studies, 15*(4), 289–365.

Ladouceur, R., Jacques, C., Giroux, I., Ferland, F., & LeBlond, J. (2000). Analysis of a casino's self-exclusion program. *Journal of Gambling Studies, 16*(4), 453–460.

Ladouceur, R., Sylvain, C., Letarte, H., Giroux, I., & Jacques, C. (2002). *Understanding and treating the pathological gambler.* Hoboken, NJ: Wiley.

Lesieur, H. (1988). Female pathological gamblers and crime. In W. R. Eadington & J. Cornelius (Ed.), *Gambling behavior and problem gambling* (pp. 495–515), Las Vegas: University of Nevada.

Lesieur, H. (1998). Costs and treatment of pathological gambling. *Annals of the American Academy of Political and Social Science, 556,* 153–171.

Lesieur, H., Blume, S., & Zoppa, R. (1986). Alcoholism, drug abuse, and gambling. *Alcoholism: Clinical and Experimental Research, 10,* 33–38.

Lesieur, H., & Rosenthal, R. (1991). Pathological gambling: A review of the literature. *Journal of Gambling Studies, 7*(1), 5–39.

Mark, M., & Lesieur, H. (1992). *Women who gamble too much.* New York: National Council on Problem Gambling.

McGurrin, M. (1994). *Pathological gambling: Conceptual, diagnostic, and treatment issues.* Sarasota, FL: Professional Resource Press.

McNeilly, D., & Burke, W. (2000). Later life gambling: The attitudes and behaviors of older adults. *Journal of Gambling Studies, 16*(4), 393–416.

Moore, T., & Carlson, M. (1998). Video poker and the new pathological gambler. *Counselor, 16*(5), 13–16.

Murray, J. (1993). A review of research on pathological gambling. *Psychological Reports, 72,* 791–810.

National Opinion Research Center. (1999). *Gambling impact and behavior study: Report to the National Gambling Impact Study Commission.* Chicago: University of Chicago, NORC.

National Research Council. (1999). *Pathological gambling: A critical review.* Washington, DC: National Academy Press.

New Jersey Governor's Council on Alcoholism and Drug Abuse. (1996). *Ad Hoc committee on women and addiction report: Women's addictions.* Trenton, NJ: Author.

North American Training Institute. (1997). *Gambling away the golden years.* Duluth, MN: Author.

Ohtsuka, K., Burton, E., DeLucs, L., & Borg, V. (1997). Sex differences in pathological gambling using gaming machines. *Psychological Reports, 80*(3), 1051–1057.

Rodgers, R. (1997). *Seducing America: Is gambling a good bet?* Grand Rapids, MI: Baker Book House.

Rose, I. (1995). Gambling and the law: Endless fields of dreams. In R. Tannenwald (Ed.), *Casino development: How would casinos affect New England's economy?* (pp. 18–46). Boston: Federal Reserve Bank of Boston Proceedings.

Rosecrance, J. (1988). *Gambling without guilt: The legitimation of an American pastime.* Belmont, CA: Brooks/Cole.

Shaffer, H. (1997). The most important unresolved issue in the addictions: The conceptual crisis. *Substance Use and Misuse, 32*(11), 1573–1580.

Shaffer, H., Hall, M., & Vander Bilt, J. (1997). *Estimating the prevalence of disordered gambling behavior in the United States and Canada: A meta-analysis of twenty years of gambling studies, 1977–1997.* Boston: Harvard Medical School, Division on Addictions.

Shaffer, H., Hall, M., Vander Bilt, J., & George, E. (2003). *Futures at Stake: Youth, gambling and society.* Reno: University of Nevada Press.

Spunt, B., Dupont, I., Lesieur, H., Liberty, J., & Hunt, D. (1998). Pathological gambling and substance misuse: A review of the literature. *Substance Use and Misuse, 33*(13), 2535–2560.

Substance Abuse and Mental Health Service Administration, Center for Substance Abuse Prevention. (2002). *Science-based prevention programs and principles.* Washington, DC: U.S. Government Printing Office.

Svendsen, R., & Griffin, T. (1996). *Improving your odds.* Anoka: Minnesota Institute of Public Health.

U.S. Senate, Committee on Indian Affairs. (1999). *National Gambling Impact Study Commission final report.* Washington, DC: U.S. Government Printing Office.

Volberg, R. (1996). Prevalence studies of problem gambling in the United States. *Journal of Gambling Studies, 12*(2), 111–128.

Volberg, R. (2001). *When the chips are down: Problem gambling in America.* New York: Century Foundation.

Wilke, D. (1994). Women and alcoholism: How a male-as-the-norm bias affects research, assessment and treatment. *Health and Social Work, 19*(1), 29–35.

Woo, K. (2003, April). The Chinese community problem gambling project. *Social Work Today,* 26–29.

Wright, E. (2001). Substance abuse in African American communities. In S. Lala Ashenberg Straussner (Ed.), *Ethnocultural factors in substance abuse treatment* (pp. 31–51). New York: Guilford Press.

Wykes, A. (1964). *Gambling.* London: Doubleday.

Yaffe, R., & Brodsky, V. (1997). Recommendations for research and public policy in gambling studies. *Journal of Gambling Studies, 13*(4), 309–316.

Zebrowski, M. (1991). *The significance of depression in the causality of the gambling phenomena in the female.* Unpublished doctoral dissertation. Cincinnatti, OH: Union Institute.

Chapter 16

INEFFECTIVE PARENTING

BARBARA THOMLISON AND SHELLEY CRAIG

Ineffective parenting significantly increases the risk of children's psychosocial problems, mental disorders, and adverse outcomes, whereas effective parenting during infancy and early childhood is a protective pathway for health, well-being, and competence of children and adolescents (Ehrensaft et al., 2003). There is now a substantial body of research literature affirming that when parents are competent, the risk that children and adolescents will develop mental health problems (internalizing and externalizing problems), delinquency, criminal behavior, and other problems is reduced, as are the factors that mediate these risks (Fraser, Kirby, & Smokowski, 2004; Kazdin & Weisz, 2003; Sanders, Turner, & Markie-Dadds, 2002; Saunders, Berliner, & Hanson, 2003; Shonkoff & Meisels, 2000).

Child, parent, and family characteristics influence parenting behavior therefore the prevention of ineffective parenting has a variety of origins but must focus on reducing risks and/or strengthening protection in these domains (Bavolek, 2002; Fraser, 2004; Kotchick & Forehand, 2002). Where the broad social and cultural environment supports positive parenting methods and skills, immediate outcomes include improved prenatal, perinatal, and early developmental outcomes for parent and child, as well as later outcomes such as improved education and employment, reduced risky behaviors and delinquency, and demonstrated competence for parenting (Fisher & Chamberlain, 2000; Olds, 2002; Osofsky & Thompson, 2000; Sanders et al., 2002).

Effective parenting programs are comprehensive in nature and utilize an ecological-developmental approach to understanding the parenting environment (Dishion & Kavanagh, 2003). Exemplary parenting programs are conceptualized as a *system* of parenting interventions and family supports to promote children's social competence and to manage developmental and behavioral problems (Sanders et al., 2002). Because of the substantial impact of parenting practices on the development of children, effective parenting programs target multilevel systems on a continuum, addressing the strengths in community, neighborhood, family, peer, and individual systems. For example, combining two or more effective programs, such as a home-based parenting approach and a school-based program, can be more effective than a single program in either system alone (Battistich, Solomon, Watson, & Schaps, 1997; Osofsky & Thompson, 2000).

Parental competence shapes the parenting environment, which primarily defines the quality of parenting that a child experiences. There is much to learn about the interrelationships of the factors that affect the quality of parenting, but research suggests that these factors include (1) a positive caring relationship with the child, (2) use of nonviolent problem-solving skills and communications between parent and child, (3) adequate contact between parents and members of their support network, and (4) the ability of parents to develop effective management and organization skills to monitor children and adolescents in their environments (Osofsky & Thompson, 2000). The parenting programs identified in this chapter focus on teaching adaptive parenting patterns, skills for nurturing, and nonviolent discipline approaches to child rearing where maladaptive or negative parenting conditions exist. They not only teach parenting skills, they address problems in the personal lives of parents, such as health care, stress, nutrition, and communication skills, and connect parents to community resources (Osofsky & Thompson, 2000; Sanders et al., 2002).

There are copious parenting programs available, and not all are equivalent. In fact, only a few have been subjected to rigorous evaluation or research. Popular parenting programs such as Parent Effectiveness Training (PET) and Systematic Training for Effective Parenting (STEP) lack evidence for their effectiveness, however, many parents have trained in these programs (Taylor & Biglan, 1998). Behavioral parenting training is the most widely evaluated and effective parenting intervention for child conduct disorders and other challenging parent-child problems. With all parenting programs, there is a great deal to learn about engaging parents, implementing the interventions, enhancing retention in programs particularly in diverse communities and populations, and the specific type of intervention that influences parents and the problems that challenge them (Kumpfer, Molgaard, & Spoth, 1996). Nevertheless, parents enroll in these programs every day, and agencies, courts, and practitioners refer many distressed parents and families for parenting skills, education, and support to improve their parenting abilities without knowing whether the program is based on well-defined theory with demonstrated evidence of a cause-and-effect relationship between an intervention and its benefits (Dunst, Trivette, & Cutspec, 2002). Some of these programs may unintentionally increase parenting problems and promote persistent parenting difficulties (Rutter, 1989).

Reflecting on the changing social trends, one realizes that serious parenting difficulties may be on the rise due to increasing changes in family structures, demands on parents, and the lack of sufficient resources, opportunities, and needs-based services. With our knowledge of preventive parenting interventions, there is now considerable opportunity for broadening the implementation of evidence-based parenting programs for greater public benefit. There are many challenging tasks, however, as program staff strive for program fidelity under different capacities and resources using proven parenting interventions.

In this chapter, parenting is viewed as a task concerned with rearing of children, and the provision of an interpersonal or environmental interaction between parent and child conducive to both cognitive and social development (Rutter, 1989). The parenting interventions summarized here are restricted to psychosocial interventions and focus on influencing affect, cognitions, and behaviors (the feelings, beliefs, and practices) of parents, and the services are designed to alleviate distress, reduce maladaptive behaviors, or enhance family structures for adaptive functioning of child and parent using systematic planned interventions. Exemplary universal, selective, and indicated preventive interventions to alleviate ineffective parenting practices and impact various parent-child problems in a positive way are reviewed. The chapter is organized as follows: first, the trends and incidence of parenting problems are presented, then the conceptual framework for parenting is defined; a summary of the risk and protective factors for prevention of ineffective parenting is presented, followed by descriptions of the universal, selective, and indicated parenting intervention programs. Finally, lessons from prevention research are suggested for policy and practice.

PARENTING TRENDS AND INCIDENCE

Social trends data reveal several shifts in parent-child relationships and family structures. Parenting is generally regarded now as a challenging endeavor. Many American adults (88%) believe that parenting is more difficult than it was for previous generations, and 86% of parents are unsure of the appropriate parenting practices to use with their children. They believe children have less moral and religious training (53%) and less supervision and discipline (56%) than children 10 years ago (National Commission on Children's National Survey, 1991).

More children are being raised in highly stressed environments by distressed parents. Children are living with violence in neighborhoods and homes, economic disadvantage, and community disorganization. There is a higher incidence of vulnerability to developmental problems among children living in poverty or living with a lone parent. More children are growing up in poverty, an experience that appears to be debilitating, although most children in these circumstances are not at risk. Other stressors on children identified in the trend data include (1) living with a parent who is distressed and at a distance from extended family assistance and support; (2) living with a parent who is depressed; (3) living in a family where the parents work extended hours, so that they are often unavailable to children; (4) living with a parent who provides inadequate linguistic or cognitive stimulation; and (5) living in a neighborhood where there are few community supports and resources (Fraser, 2004; Fraser et al., 2004; Sanders et al., 2002; Smith, 2000).

In addition, the increasing racial and ethnic diversity of the population contributes to the continuing effects of discrimination on development of children, whether caused by religious, ethnic, cultural, gender, or family background factors (Fraser et al., 2004). Stress of acculturation and discrimination and their impact on development remain understudied (Smith, 2000). Nevertheless, these structural factors tend to be correlated with family dysfunction and poor child developmental outcomes (Kumpfer et al., 1996). One in four young children live in poverty (Stormshak, Kaminski, & Goodman, 2002), and there is more homelessness, single-parent families, and exposure to street violence, illegal drugs, and life-threatening illnesses such as AIDS. Lack of affordable health services and child care are additional stresses. For example, poverty and other social and cultural risks may increase family stress, leading to inconsistent parenting and poor child-rearing practices, placing children at risk of social, emotional, behavioral, educational, and other developmental difficulties. Finally, parents of children with behavioral problems report child problematic behaviors as difficult to manage (Dishion & Kavanagh, 2003) and present greater amounts of parenting stress than parents of children without those behaviors. They also perceive that they have less parenting skill and less support than other parents to address these challenges (Eyberg, Boggs, & Rodriguez, 1992; Morgan, Robinson, & Aldridge, 2002).

Other noted trends identified in the child development literature indicate that for disadvantaged children, positive parent involvement in children's preschool education years is crucial to promoting social, emotional, and academic growth of children (Miedel & Reynolds, 2004) and therefore is the most critical time period to provide parenting interventions (Nixon, 2002; Olds, 2002). Research confirms that physical aggression and oppositional behavior (kicking and biting) is first observable at age 2 (Tremblay et al., 1999) and attributed to the social learning in preschool environments and ineffective parenting practices (Webster-Stratton, 2003). Physically aggressive behavior in 3-year-olds predicts development of violence, delinquency, substance abuse, depression, and school dropout (Webster-Stratton, 2003). Additionally, children whose level of aggression increases during school years have the single most important behavioral risk factor that is predictive of adolescent adjustment and problem behaviors (Smokowski, Mann, Reynolds, & Fraser, 2004; Webster-Stratton, 2000).

Early intervention for risk factors for aggressive behavior appears to have greater impact than later intervention by changing a child's developmental path away from problems to positive behaviors (Ialongo, Poduska, Werthamer, & Kellam, 2001; Offord, 2000). Approximately 7% to 20% of children meet the diagnosis of Oppositional Defiant Disorder and Conduct Disorder, and up to 35% of these children are from low-income families (Webster-Stratton & Hammond, 1998). Perhaps not surprisingly, externalizing behaviors are seen more frequently in boys than girls, with a rate of 2% to 9% in females and 6% to 10% in males (Offord, 2000). Fewer that 10% of school-age children in need of services for aggressive behavior actually receive them, and fewer than half of those get empirically supported interventions (Webster-Stratton & Taylor, 2001).

Parenting programs emerged during the 1960s, and the use of groups to train parents began in the 1970s. This trend has continued to grow, and group-based programs for parenting aggressive children and managing other child problems are now offered in a variety of settings. Research reviews of randomized controlled trials show that they are effective in improving behavior problems in young children (3 to 7 years; Barlow, Coren, & Stewart-Brown, 2002). In addition, it is thought that parenting programs have a role to play in improving maternal health and mental health, parenting attitudes and practices, and influence family dynamics (Barlow et al., 2002).

RISK AND PROTECTIVE FACTORS

Risk factors are characteristics or conditions that, if present for a given child, make it more likely that this child, rather than another child selected from the general population, will experience a specific problem. Protective factors are those factors that mediate or moderate the effect of the risk factors and result in reducing the risk that the problem will occur. Protective factors are the personal attributes and environmental conditions that lower the chances of poor developmental outcomes in the presence of risk (Fraser et al., 2004; Pollard, Hawkins, & Arthur, 1999; Thomlison, 2004a). The exact nature of the interactional processes among risk and protective factors is unclear. However, it is thought that in the absence of mediating factors, situational and predisposing contextual circumstances provide the opportunity for problems to emerge. Through a complex and dynamic set of processes, a range of individual, parent, family, and environmental risk and protective factors interact to have an effect on the onset, development, and maintenance of parenting problems (Hansen, Sedlar, & Warner-Rogers, 1999; Mrazek & Haggerty, 1994; Rutter, 2000).

Risk factors often occur together or cluster to produce heightened susceptibility for a parenting problem and, as the number of risk factors increases, the cumulation exerts an increasingly strong influence on parent and child (Dishion & Kavanagh, 2003; Fraser et al. 2004). Examples from research of common identified risk factors at the broad environmental level include few opportunities for education and employment, racial discrimination and injustice, and poverty. Risk factors at the family level include child maltreatment, family history of behavioral problems, family conflict and marital discord, poor parent mental health, poor parent-child relationship, poor supervision of the child, and harsh parenting (Fraser et al., 2004, p. 36; Thomlison, 2004a).

To be effective, interventions must identify and interrupt risk mechanisms at their first appearance, thereby increasing the chances that children at risk will have normal developmental outcomes. Thus, risk factors provide points of entry for the assessment process as well as focus to maximize treatment effectiveness. Not all risk conditions will be targeted at the same time; interventions target the most readily modifiable risk conditions while strengthening protective factors (Fraser & Galinsky, 2004).

Parent and Family Protective Factors

One consistent finding in the research on children is that positive parent-child interactions are the most influential factor in shaping individual behavior (Fraser et al., 2004). Positive parent-child relationships emerge among parents with high self-esteem and self-efficacy and who function within normal boundaries of behavior and social competence (Kinard, 1995; Rutter, 1987). Common parenting and family protective factors used by effective parents include (1) nonviolent methods of teaching and discipline with children; (2) high levels of warmth and acceptance and low levels of criticism; (3) low levels of stress and aggression in the family; (4) high levels of monitoring and supervision of children; (5) a positive and supportive parent-child relationship; (6) the presence of a supportive spouse or partner; (7) socioeconomic stability, success at work and school; and (8) sufficient social supports and positive adult role models in their life (Dishion & Kavanagh, 2003; Thomlison, 2004a). Research consistently emphasizes parenting skill and knowledge as giving comparatively greater protection against child problems than positive child characteristics such as easygoing temperament or other personal attributes (Guterman, 2001; Olds & Kitzman, 1993; Osofsky & Thompson, 2000; Veltman & Browne, 2001). Other common protective factors include access to adequate health, education, and employment for the benefit of their children (Fraser et al., 2004; Mrazek & Mrazek, 1987).

Children who are socially competent and prosocial in their behavior have parents who use exemplary parenting practices, such as offering regular amounts of praise, providing adequate supervision, maintaining a safe home environment, using nonviolent discipline techniques, and providing consistency through routines and supportive interactions with their children (Kazdin & Weisz, 2003; Thomlison, 2004a). Children of effective parents experience family cohesion, warmth, harmony, and the absence of neglect in their families (Ayoub, Jacewitz, Gold, & Milner, 1983; Thomlison, 2004a).

Parent and Family Risk Factors

Common parent and family risk factors for ineffective parenting include the following: (1) family conditions such as child maltreatment and family violence, interparental conflict, harsh or abusive parenting and child-rearing practices, and early negative childhood experiences of the parent; and (2) individual conditions such as child behavior problems, parental psychological distress, substance abuse, and poor or limited parent-child interactional skills and relationships. These situations are necessarily compounded when the risk factors occur in an environment with limited social contact and social network support.

Children who do not have positive parent-child interactions are twice as likely to have persistent behavioral problems as those who have positive interactions (Barlow et al., 2002; Dishion & Kavanagh, 2003; Garmezy & Tellegan, 1984). For example, poor parenting practices, such as inadequate supervision of children, inconsistent responses to children's behavior, and constant nagging, may increase the risk that a child will be noncompliant in home, school, and other settings (Patterson, 1974). With this in mind, professionals have an important role to play in promoting good parenting practices and in the development of family support and parenting skills management and the social and tangible resources (Barlow et al., 2002; Dishion & Kavanagh, 2003; Kazdin & Weisz, 2003).

Critical Factors of Ineffective Parenting Practices

A review of the literature indicates that there are two primary conditions contributing to ineffective parenting practices: family conditions and individual parent conditions.

Family Conditions

Four family conditions that lead to ineffective parenting are (1) child maltreatment and family violence, (2) interparental conflict, (3) harsh parenting and distorted child-rearing practices, and (4) limited social contact and social network support. Often, families may be experiencing several of these risk factors simultaneously, thereby compounding the developmental issues facing the child.

Child Maltreatment and Family Violence

Children exposed to any type of child maltreatment and family violence are more likely than children who have not been victimized to exhibit antisocial behavior, aggression, and delinquency and to engage in victimization behaviors with their peers (Fraser et al., 2004; Thomlison, 2004a). Risk factors that contribute to the development of these conditions are those situations when a parent perceives a child's behavior as difficult or stressful, such as poor eating and sleeping patterns and moodiness (Guterman & Embry, 2004). Learned patterns of abusive parenting and poor child-rearing practices are thought to be transmitted from parent to child and then repeated by the child when he or she is a parent (Bavolek, 2002; Dishion & Kavanagh, 2003). Children and adolescents exposed to maltreatment and violence tend to develop aggressive and violent coping styles in their interpersonal relationships and in their environment, thus placing them at risk for delinquency, criminal behavior, and school dropout (Thomlison, 2004a). Women who are exposed to intimate partner violence are less able to care for their children (Kumpfer et al., 1996).

Interparental Conflict

The presence of marital discord, threats of separation, poverty or lack of material resources, unemployment, and a conflictual social support network are associated with distress and ability to parent (Dishion & Kavanagh, 2003; Webster-Stratton & Taylor, 2001). Environments with high levels of conflict are associated with children's psychological difficulties (Hawkins, Catalano, & Miller, 1992; Hawkins, Catalano, Morrison, et al., 1992), and conflicts among family members may increase the risk for domestic violence and violence against others (Kumpfer et al., 1996). Children also learn aggression through observing aggression in their family. Single-parent households as compared with two-parent households often have higher levels of stress and are more likely to lack financial resources, which may be a barrier to effective parenting.

Harsh Parenting and Distorted Knowledge and Expectations

Rigid and unrealistic parental and child expectations about home, children, and self are common risk factors leading to ineffective parenting (Bavolek, 2002; Dishion & Kavanagh, 2003; Hawkins, Catalano, Morrison, et al., 1992; Olds, 2002; Sanders et al., 2002). Parents who are low on warmth and nurturing qualities and high on criticism are likely to use harsh or excessive physical punishment in their problem-solving responses to child-rearing situations (Bavolek, 2002; Hansen et al., 1999). Coercive parent-child interactions may emerge when children display aggressive and noncompliant behaviors toward a parent with distorted child-rearing knowledge (Dishion & Kavanagh, 2003; Hansen et al., 1999; Wolfe, 2001). Environmental stresses can exacerbate negative outcomes in the parent and thereby elevate distress or feelings of low sense of control, anger, and aggression (Webster-Stratton, 2003). Webster-Stratton and Taylor (2001) found that children who are more impulsive and quick to anger tend to overwhelm parents and raise the risk of negative parental responses such as those characterized by high arousal, anger, and harsh discipline—all risk factors for maltreatment and ineffective parenting.

Limited Social Contact and Social Support

Many ineffective parents have little or no personal or informal social support or resources to draw on for parenting assistance. Strengthening parental and family support networks is thought to reduce stress and isolation while increasing control over the environment and providing resources for dealing with children's behavior problems (Garbarino & Kostelny, 1992, 1994; Gaudin, Wodarski, Arkinson, & Avery, 1990–1991). As a result, these families are isolated from friends, family, and community networks.

Individual Parent Conditions

Parent conditions that lead to ineffective parenting are (1) children with behavioral and conduct problems, (2) nonnurturing parent-child relationships, and (3) parental psychological distress. These parent conditions or risk factors operate synergistically with the family conditions to create high-risk environments and processes that place children at risk.

Children with Behavioral and Conduct Problems

Over the long term, an ineffective parent is increasingly stressed if children display externalizing behaviors (Kazdin, 1995, 2001). Parents of children with disruptive or other difficult behaviors such as aggression and violent tendencies have described themselves as "under siege" (Webster-Stratton & Spitzer, 1996). Children with conduct disorders are more likely to live in families that have histories of criminal behavior and psychiatric dysfunction and child-rearing practices that contribute to the child's dysfunction (Kazdin & Weisz, 2003). High parent-child conflict, demonstrated as arguing, harsh physical punishment, and parent's overt dislike of the child, exacerbates behavioral problems (Ehrensaft et al., 2003). Several studies have confirmed that children's conduct can be influenced by positive and negative environmental reinforcement, including parent's attention or placation (Taylor & Biglan, 1998). It is also important to recognize factors thought to influence conduct behaviors, including coercive parent-child interaction, marital conflict, and parental depression (Sanders et al., 2002). Although not reviewed here, there is considerable literature on the risk factors for conduct disorders, and the reader is referred to Dishion and Kavanagh (2003) and Webster-Stratton and Spitzer for further information.

Nonnurturing Parent-Child Relationships

Attachment is an indicator of the quality of parent-child relations. Limited or inconsistent warmth, caring, and protection characterize nonnurturing parent-child relationships. Children who experience nonnurturing relationships show impairment in their ability to develop positive and reciprocal interpersonal relationships with others and are described by their parents as noncompliant compared with children who have strong bonds of attachment who develop a deep sense of belonging and security (Dishion & Kavanagh, 2003; Kolko, 1996). Parents who lack involvement with and spend little time with the child and who are unavailable to provide support in times of stress have maladaptive parent-child interactions and low levels of attachment to their children (Bavolek, 2002; Mrazek & Mrazek, 1987; Olds, 2002; Thomlison, 2004a, 2004b). A predictable, stable, and consistent parenting environment is central for attachments to develop.

Parental Psychological Distress

Psychopathology and psychological distress of the parent is a primary individual risk factor associated with ineffective parenting. Mental illness, psychosocial problems, criminality, and other personality problems interfere with the provision of child care and parenting (Thomlison, 2004a). Parent depression combined with external situational stress such as unemployment and reduced finances can lead to an increased rate of ineffective or dysfunctional parenting (Abidin, 1995, as cited in Morgan et al., 2002). Maternal depressive disorders, lack of involvement, and low emotional support have a direct and negative influence on parent-child transactions and the ability to provide a consistent and stimulating environment (Ehrensaft et al., 2003; Rutter, 2000). Mental illness can result in low monitoring or parental awareness of the child's friends and behavior, increasing behavior problems over time (Ehrensaft et al., 2003). Other psychological distress behaviors such as high anxiety levels, lack of impulse control under stress, and low social supports impact parenting directly (Mrazek & Haggerty, 1994; Olds, 2002; Osofsky & Thompson, 2000; Rutter, 2000). Parental problems such as alcoholism and antisocial behavior influence the quality of interactions and distort perceptions and other transactions in the parent-child environment (Dishion & Kavanagh, 2003; Thomlison, 2004a). Furthermore, research suggests that parents who have past or current substance abuse problems account for as many as 80% of child maltreatment cases (Dore, Doris, & Wright, 1995; Schinke, Brounstein, &

Gardner, 2002). Regardless of culture and source of distress, the risk for ineffective parenting increases when parents experience psychological distress, mental disorder, and a personal history of childhood maltreatment (English & Pecora, 1994, p. 465).

Approaches to Prevent Ineffective Parenting

Approaches to strengthening families through parenting intervention programs can be categorized as parent training, parent support, or parent education.

Parent Training

As the most empirically tested approach, parent training can be defined as a form of parent-child management training that teaches parents behavior guidance through the application of social learning principles (Nixon, 2002). Parent training programs teach parents of difficult children how to discipline more effectively and manage disruptive behaviors and conduct disorders. Parent training consists of four major components: initial assessment of parenting issues, teaching parents new skills, parent application (homework or out-of-session practice) of these new techniques with their children, and facilitator feedback (Taylor & Biglan, 1998).

Core elements of parent training programs include 8 to 14 weekly sessions for approximately two hours, following a treatment or intervention manual for session topics addressing information, skills, and strategies for managing child behaviors. Many of the parent training programs evolved from the model developed by Gerald Patterson (1974) of the Oregon Social Learning Center.

Parent Support

Parent support is an approach wherein parents are trained to become resources to one another. Social support is through formal and casual sources providing information and advice for parents trying to cope with the stress of child rearing (Dunst, 2000). An important characteristic of this intervention is the reliance on paraprofessionals rather than professionals, and groups in the neighborhood, church, and community. This is done through empowering peer partnerships and focused collaboration between families and practitioners to enhance family functioning, as opposed to extremely structured interventions (Dunst, 2000).

Parent Education

Parent education is based on the assumption that lack of knowledge about child development combined with insufficient skills contributes to poor parenting and child functioning (Cowen, 2001). This approach explains developmental principles such as normative stages as well as teaching skills of observation and interpretation of children's behaviors. Typically, teaching programs range from a single motivational lecture to a series of classes and use of experiential exercises. Often, programs teach parents about risk factors for specific problems, such as drug use. Programs use videotape aids and frequently tailor the program to high-risk and ethnic families (Kumpfer et al., 1996). This knowledge improves parental resources and overall coping skills and allows parents to learn different techniques from those they experienced as children (Cowen, 2001).

The intervention programs that follow are primarily examples of parent training, although some approaches use combinations of the previous parent programs.

PREVENTIVE INTERVENTION PROGRAMS FOR PARENTING

The parenting programs summarized here are organized by the guidelines proposed by the Institute of Medicine (Mrazek & Haggerty, 1994) and Gordon's (1983, 1987) operational definitions of prevention using three categories of classification, defined in the following sections.

Universal Preventive Interventions

Universal preventive intervention programs target the general public or an entire population of interest, such as schools (e.g., childhood immunizations, media-based parenting information campaign, first-time parents). A good example is the Don't Shake the Baby public awareness initiative targeting all professionals involved in the care of children (e.g., teachers, physicians, nurses, home visitors, parent educators) and parents to alert them to the dangers of shaking babies. These positive interventions are delivered independent of risk factors and thus minimize stigma and may reduce the incidence of poor parenting practices (Greenberg, Domitrovich, & Bumbarger, 2001; Offord, 2000). Healthy parenting practices, child safety skills, and protocols for preventing problems are part of these initiatives.

Selective Preventive Interventions

These intervention programs target subgroups of the general population who are at higher risk for developing a problem than other members of the broader population (e.g., information and advice for specific parenting of child behavior or development concerns, teen mothers). Interventions address risks specific to populations or parenting characteristics. For example, a selective program may be aimed at parents of all children with higher than average risk for school performance problems due to behavioral problems or aggression.

Indicated Preventive Interventions

These intervention programs target individuals who have detectable signs or symptoms of difficulty or who are engaging in high-risk behaviors or problems or have a clinical disorder (e.g., parent education and skills training for children with multiple behavior problems or aggressive behavior or learning delays, parenting programs for parents with substance abuse problems). Examples are training for parents of young children with behavior problems who do not meet guidelines for diagnosis (Greenberg et al., 2001; Offord, 2000) and a program for parents of delinquents to prevent chronic problems.

Selection Criteria for Programs

Parenting interventions selected for inclusion here met the following criteria: (1) interventions specifically focused on parents of children with challenging behaviors; (2) interventions were intended to decrease children's conduct and behavioral problems; (3) interventions were intended to improve parental competencies; and (4) interventions met the criteria for efficacious or possibly efficacious effects for treatment based on the categories outlined by Chambless and Hollon (1998). Some of the interventions address parenting at all three levels of the continuum, that is, universal, selective, and indicated intervention levels, such as the Nurse-Family Partnership Program (Olds, 2002) and The Incredible Years Program (Webster-Stratton, 2000). The included programs are conceptually sound, theory-based, ecodevelopmentally focused, and often have been adapted to be culturally sensitive for different ethnic groups. In most cases, an intervention or treatment manual is available. Research on the parenting programs presented here has produced enduring and replicated effects, and there is a need to support the implementation of parenting programs for greater public health impact.

UNIVERSAL PREVENTIVE INTERVENTIONS FOR PARENTING

Three universal interventions targeted to the general public and focused on parenting for prevention of child and adolescent problems are identified first. The programs combine multiple levels of intervention to address parenting skills and family support activities. All the programs have undergone randomized, controlled trials and have demonstrated success in reducing or curtailing parent-child prob-lem behaviors and enhancing parental social and emotional competencies and thereby lowered the risk for adverse mental health outcomes. Most parenting programs (selective and indicated) are not scaled to large populations as yet (Hawkins, Catalano, Morrison, et al., 1992; Mrazek & Haggerty, 1994; Olds, 2002; Spoth, Kavanagh, & Dishion, 2002). Although evidence-supported pro-grams are available, there are major challenges that make offering universal inter-ventions for parenting difficult to implement, particularly through the existing service systems and policies.

The three parenting programs summarized next are the Triple-P Positive Par-enting Program (Sanders et al., 2002), Fast Track (the Conduct Problems Pre-vention Research Group [CPPRG], 2002a, 2002b), and Project STAR: Steps to Achieving Resilience (Stormshak et al., 2002).

The Triple-P Positive Parenting Program

Category: Universal, selective, and indicated.

Program type: Parent training and parent support.

Target population: A multilevel intervention program targeting parents with children age 12 and under, with a range of common and severe developmental and behavioral problems, and with child problems and family dysfunction.

Cultural adaptation: The program has been used with different populations, including indigenous Australian families, using cultural reference groups, focus testing, and field trials (Sanders et al., 2002). The program is used in European and Asian countries such as Germany, Switzerland, Hong Kong, and Singapore.

Program summary: The Triple-P Positive Parenting Program incorporates five levels of behavioral family intervention for parents of preadolescent chil-dren from birth to 12 years. It is based on social learning models of parent-child interaction that highlight the reciprocal and bidirectional nature of parent-child interactions (Sanders et al., 2002). Based on the principle of suf-ficiency, the targeted risk factors include coercive parent-child interaction, marital conflict, and parental depression. This program is designed as a mul-tilevel system of parenting and family support with increasing levels of inten-sity, depending on the severity of the child's behavior and the sources of the child's problems (Sanders et al., 2002).

The primary goals of Triple-P are to encourage positive and healthy rela-tionships between parents and children and create effective parent manage-ment strategies. Activities teach information and skills address the way parents process information to modify parental cognitions such as attributions, expectancies, and beliefs as factors that contribute to parental self-efficacy, decision making, and behavioral intentions. The objective is to increase parents' sense of competence, improve communication, and reduce parenting stress (Sanders et al., 2002). The intervention levels progress from universal level 1 (promotional campaigns and videos) to level 2 (one to two two-session developmental stage education in primary health care setting) for children with mild behavior problems; selective level 3 (longer primary health contact), which targets children with mild to moderate behavior problems; indicated level 4 (intensive 8- to 10-hour parent training session) for children with severe behavioral problems; to indicated level 5 (5- to 11-session behavioral family intervention) that builds on level 4 to target support and coping skills (Sanders et al., 2002).

Evidence for the effects of treatment: Over 25 years, there have been numerous randomized controlled trials for the Triple-P intervention representing the progression of the evidence base from efficacy trials to effectiveness trials and finally to examining the dissemination of the program (Sanders et al., 2002, pp. 178–180). Parents report significantly decreased child behavior problems, greater parenting confidence, and less use of dysfunctional parenting techniques (Sanders et al., 2002). In addition, mothers reported more parenting confidence compared to controls. In a 1-year follow-up, children receiving self-directed behavioral modules showed additional improvements in behavior and continued decreased levels of disruptive behavior (Sanders et al., 2002). Overall, the Triple-P Positive Parenting Program provides a flexible and empirically sound intervention for reducing children's negative behaviors by enhancing parenting skills and family support.

FAST Track Program

Category: Universal and indicated.

Program type: Parent training.

Target population: First-grade children with impulsivity behavior, and families stressed with marital conflict and instability and living in low-income, high-crime communities. Children and their caregivers and teachers are the target populations.

Cultural adaptation: Rural and urban populations, diverse demographic characteristics, and cultural backgrounds.

Program summary: FAST Track is a comprehensive multifaceted intervention founded on developmental theory, which states that the interactions of a variety of influences assist in the growth of externalizing behaviors (CPPRG, 2000). Fast Track's primary objective is to prevent persistent conduct problems in high-risk children at school entrance (CPPRG, 2000; Webster-Stratton &

Taylor, 2001). Treatment goals include a reduction in the frequency and severity of externalizing behaviors of children, and helping parents understand the factors that influence successful school performance and family and community living (CPPRG, 2000). Fast Track extends through tenth grade. Social, academic, and behavioral gains in reducing aggressive behaviors occur, as does reduction in harsh discipline by parents.

Kindergarten students were identified by teachers as exhibiting externalizing behaviors and following random assignment by the school, they were put into a control or intervention group. The intervention included classroom management and tutoring, parent-child relationship therapies, cognitive and social skills training, home visits, and parent training (CPPRG, 2002b). Universally, all students were taught a version of the PATHS (Promoting Alternative Thinking Strategies; Kusche & Greenberg as cited in CPPRG, 2000) curriculum three times per week. This educational module focuses on self-control, awareness, peer social skills, and problem solving to increase competence.

At the standard indicated level, two-hour family groups that focused on communication skills and conflict negotiation were facilitated at the schools. Sessions occurred weekly for 22 weeks during first grade, biweekly for 14 sessions during second grade, and monthly for 8 sessions each year during grades 3 to 5. For each developmentally structured group, parents and children met separately for the first half and then participated in combined activities during the second half. Individualized indicated services included academic tutoring, home visits, and school peer pairing to increase children's levels of friendships and mentoring (Greenberg et al., 2001).

Evidence for the effects of treatment: Fast Track provided longitudinal evidence of decreasing externalizing behaviors for 891 children in grades 1 through 5 during a 6-year intervention (CPPRG, 2002a, 2002b). This randomized clinical trial involved 50 schools in four sites (Seattle, Washington; Durham, North Carolina; Nashville, Tennessee; and rural central Pennsylvania; Greenberg et al., 2001). The postintervention outcomes at 1 and 3 years showed significant reduction in conduct problems and consistent positive effects on children's social, emotional, and academic skills, peer interactions, and social status, and reductions in conduct problems and special education resource use (CPPRG, 2002a). Parents reported less use of physical discipline, increased warmth, higher comfort with parenting, and more engagement with school. At the end of the third year, 37% of the intervention group was without conduct problems as compared to 27% of the control group; very importantly, parent ratings agreed with that assessment (CPPRG, 2002a). Universally, intervention schools showed a lower overall level of aggression and higher ratings of the quality of the classroom atmosphere (CPPRG, 2002a).

Project STAR: Steps to Achieving Resilience

Category: Universal and selective.

Program type: Parent training, parent education, and parent support.

Target population: Early childhood populations, 4-year-old Head Start children and their families.

Cultural adaptation: Rural counties of Oregon with Caucasian and Hispanic populations.

Program summary: Based on a developmental-ecological model, this universal home-based intervention is implemented with Head Start families. Children in participating classrooms received 20 sessions focused on social competence, self-regulation, early literacy, and language development. Home visits and parent groups used the curriculum from The Incredible Years parenting curriculum for children ages 4 to 8 (Webster-Stratton, 1998).

Evidence for the effects of treatment: Results suggest that both parenting groups and home visiting interventions are effective at enhancing parenting skills, with more home visits leading to a higher participation rate both during the program and at follow-up. Parents who attended the parenting group showed gains in caregiver involvement over those who attended the home visiting program only (Stormshak et al., 2002). Parents who were more depressed required much more extensive intervention aimed at their child as well as contextual factors such as marital stress and substance use. The combined effect of a parenting group plus home visiting from a familiar staff person is the most effective set of interventions to increase caregiver involvement in children's life and school. Home visits need to be of sufficient frequency and duration to effect change, a finding similar to Olds (2002; Stormshak et al., 2002). Retaining families into kindergarten year and supporting families as they transition to school may have positive benefits for both children and families. Targeted interventions in universal strategies can be an effective means of engaging families in services to work more intensely on parenting problems and family-school relationships.

SELECTIVE PREVENTIVE INTERVENTIONS FOR PARENTING

The selective parenting programs identified here are directed at populations who face risks for developing serious problems although they may not have been identified as having specific difficulties. Two exemplary programs are the Nurse-Family Partnership (previously, NurseHome Visitor Program; Olds, 2002; Olds

& Kitzman, 1993; Olds et al., 1999) and the Incredible Years Training Series (Webster-Stratton, 2000; Webster-Stratton & Taylor, 2001).

The Nurse-Family Partnership

Category: Selective and indicated.

Program type: Parent education, parent support, and parent training.

Target population: Low-income first-time mothers (> 13 and unmarried).

Cultural adaptation: Spanish-speaking nurses assigned to monolingual Spanish-speaking clients. Mothers were of mixed ethnicity in all replication studies.

Program summary: The Nurse-Family Partnership is a comprehensive preventive intervention parenting program focused on maternal and child health and development through home visitation services provided by public health nurses. Interventions are grounded in theories of ecological-developmental theory, attachment, and self-sufficiency. The goal is to improve (1) pregnancy outcomes by reducing prenatal risks, (2) early childhood health and development by providing competent parental care, and (3) family economic self-sufficiency by helping parents' personal development and continued education. Professional nurses develop therapeutic relationships with the mothers following visit protocols that focus on health (physical and mental), home and neighborhood environment, family and friend supports, parental roles, and major life events such as education, pregnancy planning, employment, and substance abuse and other high-risk behaviors contributing to poor maternal and child outcomes. Visits begin prenatally and continue until the child's second birthday. The woman receives weekly visits during the first month of service enrollment and biweekly throughout the woman's pregnancy, then weekly for the first 6 weeks postpartum and every other week thereafter through the child's 21st month. In the final 3 months, nurses visit monthly until the child reaches age 2. Visits are 60 to 90 minutes in duration.

Evidence for the effects of treatment: Consistent outcomes from numerous randomized controlled trials have shown benefits to both mothers and children (Olds, 2002). Outcomes of a 15-year follow-up show the nurse-visited mothers had:

—A 43% reduction in subsequent pregnancies.

—A 44% reduction in maternal behavioral problems due to substance use.

—Fewer arrests (by 54%) and fewer convictions (by 69%) among the 15-year-olds.

—An 83% increase in the rate of labor force participation by the child's first birthday.

—Over 80% fewer verified cases of child abuse and neglect than their counterparts in the control groups through the child's second year.

The Incredible Years Training Series

Category: Selective and indicated.

Program type: Parent training and parent education.

Target population: The program targets parents and their children ages 2 to 12 who are exhibiting externalizing behaviors and at risk for developing Conduct Disorder and delinquency as well as academic problems. It is a prevention and intervention strategy, and the program components can be utilized simultaneously for children, parents, and teachers (Webster-Stratton, 2000).

Cultural adaptation: Replicated with African American, Asian, and Hispanic families, in urban, suburban, and rural communities.

Program summary: Incredible Years is a parent-training program whose theoretical foundation includes cognitive and social learning theories. Program goals for parents include increasing the level of involvement in children's school-related experience to reduce conduct problems and enhance social skills and academic competence as well as overall strengthening of parental competencies. Children's goals include reduced behavioral problems, increased engagement in school, and improved positive interactions with peers, teachers, and parents. Goals for teachers include enhanced competence and stronger home-school relationships.

Intervention activities target individual and familial risk factors, including children's aggressive behavior, critical parenting, harsh discipline, and poor parent-child attachment. In the school environment, the Incredible Years Series combats a negative and poorly managed classroom, child aggression toward others, and peer rejection and teaches positive reinforcement and classroom management techniques (Webster-Stratton, 2000; Webster-Stratton & Taylor, 2001).

The Incredible Years program series has three components that utilize discussion, coaching, and video clips in a group format to teach parenting techniques. The Early Childhood BASIC parent training program (ages 2 to 7) stresses positive play, nonviolent discipline, praise, incentives, limit setting, and correcting misbehavior (Webster-Stratton, 2000). The School Age BASIC parent training (ages 5 to 12) emphasizes the promotion of positive behaviors, problem solving with children and families, and consequences. ADVANCE (ages 4 to 10) tackles additional family risk factors such as depression, coping skills, and anger management by supplementing the BASIC program. EDUCATION is specifically designed to complement the BASIC program by increasing academic skills, encouraging good learning habits, and helping with homework (Webster-Stratton & Taylor, 2001). An additional teacher training program addresses classroom management concerns. This program also enhances communication skills and support by assigning participants a peer group member as a buddy (Webster-Stratton, 2000).

Evidence for the effects of treatment: Incredible Years shows positive outcomes in numerous randomized clinical trials. In one of the studies, parents of 114 children with externalizing behaviors were randomly assigned to one of four interventions: individual videotape modeling (self-administered), BASIC (video-based group therapy), group therapy only, or a wait-list control group. Few major differences were found between treatment groups, with a slight participant preference for the BASIC training, where two-thirds of the sample had statistically significant improvements in child behaviors and parenting skills. This study indicated that the improvements after treatment were maintained a year later (Webster-Stratton, Hollinsworth, & Kolpacoff, 1989).

Incredible Years has been field-tested in six randomized trials and in selective programs with Head Start (Webster-Stratton, 2000). Outcomes have included improved positive parenting skills; increased children's cognitive problem solving, use of conflict management skills, social competence, and school engagement; and reduced aggression. Overall decreased conduct problems at home and school have been noted in all studies (Webster-Stratton & Taylor, 2001).

INDICATED PREVENTIVE INTERVENTIONS FOR PARENTING

This section summarizes indicated interventions that have been successful in promoting positive family interactions and improving parenting skills. Three parenting programs are included: Multisystemic Therapy (Henggeler, Schoenwald, Borduin, Rowland, & Cunningham, 1998), the Nurturing Parenting Program (Bavolek, 2002), and Project 12 Ways (Gershater-Molko & Lutzker, 1999; Gershater-Molko, Lutzker, & Wesch, 2002; Lutzker, Bigelow, Doctor, & Kessler, 1998).

Multisystemic Therapy

Category: Indicated.

Program type: Parent training, parent education, and parent support.

Target population: Families with children 12 to 17 years with serious antisocial problems.

Cultural adaptation: Families in urban areas. Materials available in Norwegian.

Program summary: Multisystemic Therapy (MST) is a time-limited home- and family-centered program created for youth in difficulty with the juvenile justice system. Although this intervention addresses parenting, it essentially intervenes in school, peer, and community systems to effect change. This intervention is designed to impact all systems that influence a child's externalizing behaviors using methods that promote positive social behavior and decrease antisocial behavior. MST targets parental skills to improve their effectiveness by identifying strengths and developing support systems for parents. Parents collaborate with the therapist to use strategies such as setting rules and curfew and providing supervision to reduce child noncompliance utilizing cognitive and behavioral strategies for changes and promoting prosocial peer relationships for behavior maintenance (Brunk, Henggeler, & Whelan, 1987). Disengagement from harmful peers, stronger attachment to family and school, increased social competence, and improved family monitoring are encouraged simultaneously (Brunk, 2000). MST assumes that conduct problems are complex and addresses the stressing systems by using techniques of reframing, coaching, marital therapy, advocacy, and parent education (Brunk et al., 1987; Henggeler, Melton, Brondino, Scherer, & Hanley, 1997).

Evidence for the effects of treatment: MST has been proven efficacious for:
—Reducing adolescent substance use.
—Decreasing adolescent psychiatric symptoms.
—Reducing long-term rearrest rates by 25% to 70%.
—Reducing long-term out-of-home placement by 47% to 64%.
—Improving family relations and functioning.
—Increasing mainstream school attendance.
—Increasing parental monitoring (Alexander, Robbins, & Sexton, 2000; Brunk, 2000; Henggeler et al., 1997, 1998).

Eight randomized clinical trials have proven that MST enhances parenting skills and improves the familial environment. In a study with random assignment comparing MST group-based parent training with traditional parent training, MST achieved better outcomes in parental ability to control children's problem behaviors, increased parental positive responses to children, and improved child compliance (Brunk et al., 1987). However, parent training surpassed MST in the improvement of social problems, likely due to the group context of parent training. Both interventions show significant reductions in child externalizing behaviors, parenting stress, and family functioning (Brunk et al., 1987).

The Nurturing Parenting Program

Category: Indicated.

Program type: Parent training, parent education, and parent support.

Target population: Parents who have risk factors for maltreatment and a history of abuse and neglect.

Cultural adaptation: Various populations have received the program, including Hmong, Hispanic, and African American families.

Program summary: The Nurturing Parenting Program is a family-centered parenting initiative designed to address the generational cycle of violence in which parents rear children in the context of the violence they experienced as children. The intervention teaches parents how parenting patterns are learned and how acquiring nurturing parenting skills can lead to satisfaction in the parenting role. The intervention is developmentally focused on three categories of children: from birth to 5 years, from 5 to 11, and adolescents. Home-based approaches teaching parent-child activities and group sessions are conducted weekly for from 12 to 45 weeks. A program manual, videotapes, and handbooks guide the nurturing interactions between parent and child. The program is intensive, entailing six conceptual assumptions of how abusive parenting and child-rearing practice is learned through experience. Program objectives are to (1) stop intergenerational abuse by building nurturing parenting skills, (2) reduce the rate of recidivism in families receiving social services, (3) reduce the rate of juvenile delinquency among high-risk youth, (4) reduce the rate of alcoholism in high-risk families, and (5) lower the rate of multiple pregnancies among teenage girls.

Evidence for the effects of treatment: Replication has occurred in 13 separate sites across the United States, Canada, Mexico, Europe, South America, and Israel (Bavolek, 2002). Of the 121 adults who participated in the initial study, 95 (79%) completed the program. Of the 150 children who participated, 125 (83%) completed the program. Completers were rated by trainers as having successfully modified their abusive parent-child interactions. Seven adults (7%) who committed new acts of child abuse or did not achieve program goals were rated as having failed the program. Other changes included parents forming expectations more appropriate to the development of their children, an increased empathic awareness of child's needs, a decrease in the use of corporal punishment, and a decrease in parent-child role reversal. Children's attitudes about parenting practices improved, showing statistically significant increases. Evaluations of subsequently developed Nurturing Parenting Programs have yielded similar results, showing significant pretest and posttest change in parenting attitudes and child-rearing practices.

Project 12-Ways

Category: Indicated.

Program type: Parent training, parent education, and parent support.

Target population: Families at high risk for abuse and neglect of children.

Cultural adaptation: Spanish.

Program summary: Project 12-Ways (Lutzker et al., 1998) is based on the systems perspective and primarily strives to improve environments and support for families through the use of in-home interventions. The overall theory is that family problems can be minimized by dealing with family stressors and by teaching parenting skills. Delivered in home and community settings, the intervention targets child health, home safety, and parent-child interactions by using direct teaching methods to address the needs of individual families and children. The intervention occurs in 19 one- to two-hour sessions. An important component is planned activities training, which is utilized to teach parents the skills of structuring activities and child care. Paraprofessionals are integrated into the comprehensive process to address the issues of marital concerns, finances, and home health that impact levels of parenting stress. Targeted interventions include parent-child interactions, problem solving, daily routines, health maintenance, basic child development skills, stress reduction, self-control, social support, job training, substance abuse referrals, safety, and health information (Lutzer, Bigelow, Doctor, & Kessler, 1998).

Evidence for the effects of treatment: Although not empirically tested specifically for parents of children with externalizing behaviors, this program has proven to reduce parenting stress in child welfare populations (Thomlison, 2003, 2004b). In a quasi-experimental study with neglectful parents, wherein 352 families obtained Project 12 Ways treatment and 358 families received traditional services, those who received the Project 12 Ways intervention had fewer reports of child abuse 1 year later. The researchers reported a 21.3% recidivism rate for these participants, as compared to 28.5% for those families who received traditional service (Lutzker et al., 1998). Research that has been conducted on Project 12 Ways has been primarily single-subject designs with a few quasi-experimental studies (Lutzer et al., 2001), but the existence of evidence of effectiveness categorizes this program as promising.

PRACTICE AND POLICY IMPLICATIONS

The information in this chapter describes the risk and protective factors in the child, parent, and family environments contributing to ineffective parenting and the various preventive parenting and family support interventions that lead to positive outcomes for children. Indeed, there is a substantial amount of information about risk factors and their relationship to parenting competencies. And there are opportunities to improve clinical practice by implementing the interventions and thereby improving the mental health and adaptations of children and adolescents. Many programs incorporate a parenting component to address child or adolescent problems; however, the identified parenting interventions summarized here have a primary focus of early intervention for improving parenting skills, competencies, and supports for reducing behavioral and social problems and improving child and parent functioning.

Overall, there are limited exemplars of well-researched parenting programs. Those available share common characteristics such as combining parent training with other empirically supported strategies for enhancing effectiveness, for example, Fast Track (CPPRG, 1992). Other programs not included here but that are effective and designed specifically for parents of adolescents use group-based interventions and family interventions, for example, the Adolescent Transitions Program (Dishion & Kavanagh, 2003). Some effective family interventions have received considerable support from research findings, for example, Brief Strategic Family Therapy (Robbins et al., 2003), but this intervention focuses on delinquency and drug problems in the family. There continue to be many practice, dissemination, and policy concerns about the implementation of evidence-supported interventions.

Practice Concerns

There are multiple reasons that evidence-supported parenting programs are not implemented widely. Weisz and Kazdin (2003, p. 446) discuss five concerns that practitioners identify as reasons that manual-guided treatments are not relevant or appropriate for their clients: (1) manualized treatments limit therapist creativity, requiring them to use "cookie-cutter" procedures; (2) manualized treatments interfere with therapeutic relationship development and opportunities to individualize interventions; (3) evidence of interventions does not support work with the most severe client situations, but has been limited to work with simple cases and low levels of psychopathology; (4) treatments focus on single problems and not comorbid disorders; and (5) clients are unpredictable, and so predetermined session plans are unworkable. Not all of these concerns are valid, and it would be disappointing to dismiss many of the interventions as unworkable until they are perfect in development. Instead, it seems desirable to address the impediments to dissemination in practice settings and work more closely with practitioners and various settings to resolve differences in perspectives regarding the clinical and research gap to establish real-world practice acceptance and support.

Dissemination Concerns

Two dissemination concerns often voiced are training issues and lack of policies requiring use of empirically supported interventions. First, promoting the widespread use of parenting interventions will require training and consultation for many clinicians and settings. It is unrealistic to think that all staff will be able to deliver the interventions or to learn them. Nevertheless, adequate preparation is necessary. Most parenting programs impart behavioral knowledge and skills and commonly employ modeling and behavioral rehearsal skills, reinforcing techniques such as practicing skills at home, self-monitoring techniques to enhance awareness, and individualized strategies. Generic life skills or knowledge and skills related to parenting, child management, and substance abuse and maltreatment problems were usually part of the content. Support for developing this knowledge and skill in staff will need to be encouraged.

Second, it is important to make known to clinicians and practitioners those parenting interventions that are considered valuable. In addition, many of the interventions appear to be highly compatible with time-limited services, which should also make them appealing to policy makers. Helping agencies move toward evidence-based clinical practice is itself a process of change, and the idea of clinicians using empirically based interventions must be backed up with service provision policy support. One current policy of state agencies and insurance companies requires that identified clients be present at treatment, yet the evidence-supported interventions identified here suggest working with the parent when the child is the identified client for best outcomes, and the child's presence is not always necessary. Instead, it would make great sense for practitioners and policy makers to advocate for *use* of empirically supported treatment interventions for child behavior problems.

Cultural Sensitivity and Adaptation Concerns

Few parenting interventions have been adapted to be culturally sensitive to different ethnic groups. Changing the interventions to adapt to different ethnic groups has most often entailed changing the dosage or intensity or eliminating modules of core content. Kempner, Alvarado, Smith, and Bellamy (2002) report that reducing the amount of exposure to programs can increase retention by up to 40%, but this also reduces the positive outcomes. Clearly, there is considerable research needed in this area, and it would make great sense to involve consumers in designing and partnering with researchers and practitioners in developing culturally sensitive adaptations of evidence-supported interventions.

Policy Shifts

Research on changing health risk behaviors among the population suggests that information campaigns using print and electronic media are effective in raising awareness of parenting issues and normalizing participation in parenting programs. However, both policy and political support are required for responsive implementation. Such programs need to be embedded in policy and other service systems to raise awareness of resources and participation (Sanders et al., 2002). A public health policy perspective can extend our clinical knowledge about parenting and raising competent children.

Future Directions

Among the many issues in parenting interventions, it seems important that a focus on the prevention of challenging behaviors receive priority. Evidence-supported parenting intervention, using a comprehensive array of services from prevention to intensive intervention, can reduce the challenging behaviors of children. Parent training can be delivered at varying intensities or levels, and new interventions will emerge. Nevertheless, the best intentions must have a full complement of interventions that assist parents at all levels of children's development. Interventions must be understood in the context of what is necessary and sufficient for treatment benefits. Although the best interventions are parent-training approaches focused on increasing individual parental skills, this is not always sufficient; it is often necessary to provide assistance in other areas for parenting support and to use needs-based services. Highly stressed families need transportation, child care, services offered at convenient times and locations, and other supports to attend parenting programs.

Great strides have been made in identifying good practices, and researchers and practitioners need to be applauded for these gains. Yet, we must involve parents, policy makers, and politicians to enable more children to achieve their maximum potential. Others that influence family and parent functioning include the mass media, health care providers, schools, and religious organizations; increasing collaborations among these vested interests will benefit children and society. Translating research to service in community-based regular settings needs to be encouraged at the levels of policy and staff training, as well as collaboration with experts and interagency collaborations.

REFERENCES

Alexander, J., Robbins, M., & Sexton, T. (2000). Family-based interventions with older, at-risk youth: From promise to proof to practice. *Journal of Primary Prevention, 21*(2), 185–205.

Ayoub, C., Jacewitz, M., Gold, R., & Milner, J. (1983). Assessment of a program's effectiveness in selecting individuals "at risk" for problems in parenting. *Journal of Clinical Psychology, 39,* 334–339.

Barlow, J., Coren, E., & Stewart-Brown, S. (2002). Meta-analysis of the effectiveness of parenting programs in improving maternal psychosocial health. *British Journal of General Practice, 52*(476), 223–233.

Battistich, V., Solomon, D., Watson, M., & Schaps, E., Caring school communities. *Educational Psychologist, 32*(3), 137–151, 1997.

Bavolek, S. J. (2002). *Research and validation report of the Nurturing Parenting Programs.* Retrieved January 10, 2004, from www.ncjrs.org/pdffiles1/ojjdp/172848 .pdf and www.nurturingparenting.com.

Brunk, M. (2000). *Effective treatment of conduct disorder: Juvenile justice fact sheet.* Charlottesville: University of Virginia, Institute of Law, Psychiatry, and Public Policy.

Brunk, M., Henggeler, S., & Whelan, J. (1987). Comparison of multisystemic therapy and parent training in the brief treatment of child abuse and neglect. *Journal of Consulting and Clinical Psychology, 55*(2), 171–178.

Chambless, D., & Hollon, S. (1998). Defining empirically supported therapies. *Journal of Consulting and Clinical Psychology, 66*(1), 7–18.

Conduct Problems Prevention Research Group. (1992). A developmental and clinical model for the prevention of conduct disorder: The Fast Track Program. *Development and Psychopathology, 4,* 509–527.

Conduct Problems Prevention Research Group. (2000). Merging universal and indicated prevention programs: The Fast Track Model. *Addictive Behaviors, 25*(6), 913–927.

Conduct Problems Prevention Research Group. (2002a). Evaluation of the first 3 years of the Fast Track Prevention Trial with children at high risk for adolescent conduct problems. *Journal of Abnormal Child Psychology, 30*(1), 19–35.

Conduct Problems Prevention Research Group. (2002b). The implementation of the Fast Track Program: An example of a large-scale prevention science efficacy trial. *Journal of Abnormal Child Psychology, 30*(1), 1–17.

Cowen, P. (2001). Effectiveness of a parent education intervention for at-risk families. *Journal of the Society of Pediatric Nurses, 6*(2), 73–82.

Dishion, T. J., & Kavanagh, K. (2003). *Intervening in adolescent problem behavior: A family-centered approach.* New York: Guilford Press.

Dore, M. M., Doris, J. M., & Wright, P. (1995). Identifying substance abuse in maltreating families: A child welfare challenge. *Child Abuse and Neglect, 19,* 531–543.

Dunst, C. (2000, Summer). Revisiting "Rethinking Early Intervention." *Topics in Early Childhood Special Education,* 1–15.

Dunst, C., Trivette, C. M., & Cutspec, P. A. (2002). An evidence-based approach to documenting the characteristics and consequence of early intervention practices. *Centerscope.* 1(2). Available from Center for Evidence-Based Practices web site, http:www.puckett.org.

Ehrensaft, M. K., Wasserman, G. A., Verdelli, L., Greenwald, S., Miller, L. S., & Davies, M. (2003). Maternal antisocial behavior, parenting practices, and behavior problems in boys at risk for antisocial behavior. *Journal of Child and Family Studies, 12*(1), 27–40.

English, D., & Pecora, P. (1994). Risk assessment as a practice method in child protective services [Special issue]. *Child Welfare, 73,* 451–475.

Eyberg, S. M., Boggs, S. R., & Rodriguez, C. M. (1992). Relationships between maternal parenting stress and child disruptive behavior. *Child and Family Behavior Therapy, 14,* 1–9.

Fisher, P. A., & Chamberlain, P. (2000). Multidimensional treatment foster care: A program for intensive parenting, family support, and skill building. *Journal of Emotional and behavioral Disorders, 8*(3), 155–164.

Fraser, M. W. (Ed.). (2004). *Risk and resilience in childhood: An ecological perspective* (2nd ed.). Washington, DC: National Association of Social Workers Press.

Fraser, M. W., & Galinsky, M. J. (2004). Risk and resilience in childhood: Toward an evidence-based model of practice. In M. W. Fraser (Ed.), *Risk and resilience in childhood. An ecological perspective* (2nd ed., pp. 385–403). Washington, DC: National Association of Social Workers Press.

Fraser, M. W., Kirby, L., & Smokowski, P. R. (2004). Risk and resilience in childhood. In M. W. Fraser (Ed.), *Risk and resilience in childhood: An ecological perspective* (2nd ed., pp. 13–67). Washington, DC: National Association of Social Workers Press.

Garbarino, J., & Kostelny, K. (1992). Child maltreatment as a community problem. *Child Abuse and Neglect, 16,* 455–464.

Garbarino, J., & Kostelny, K. (1994). Neighborhood-based programs. In G. B. Melton & F. D. Barry (Eds.), *Protecting children from abuse and neglect: Foundations for a new national strategy* (pp. 304–353). New York: Guilford Press.

Garmezy, N., & Tellegan, A. (1984). Studies of stress-resistant children: Methods, variables, and preliminary findings. In F. J. Morrison, G. Lord, & D. P. Keating (Eds.), *Applied developmental psychology* (pp. 231–287). Orlando, FL: Academic Press.

Gaudin, J. M., Wodarski, J. S., Arkinson, M. K., & Avery, L. S. (1990–1991). Remedying child neglect: Effectiveness of social network interventions. *Journal of Applied Social Science, 15,* 97–123.

Gershater-Molko, R. M., & Lutzker, J. (1999). Child neglect. In R. T. Ammerman & M. Hersen (Eds.), Assessment of family violence. A clinical and legal sourcebook (2nd ed., pp. 157–183). New York: Wiley.

Gershater-Molko, R. M., Lutzker, J., & Sherman, J. (2002). Intervention in child neglect: An applied behavioral perspective. *Aggression and Violent Behavior, 7,* 103–124.

Gershater-Molko, R. M., Lutzker, J., & Wesch, D. (2002). Using recidivism data to evaluate Project Safecare: Teaching bonding, safety, and health care skills to parents. *Child Maltreatment, 7,* 277–285.

Gordon, R. (1983). An operational classification of disease prevention. *Public Health Reports, 98,* 107–109.

Gordon, R. (1987). An operational classification of disease prevention. In J. A. Steinberg & M. M. Silverman (Eds.), *Prevention mental disorders* (pp. 20–26). Rockville, MD: U.S. Department of Health and Human Services.

Greenberg, M., Domitrovich, C., & Bumbarger, B. (2001, March 30). The prevention of mental disorders in school aged children: Current state of the field (Article 0040001a). *Prevention and Treatment, 4*(1). Retrieved September 14, 2004 from http://journals.apa.org/prevention/volume4/pre0040001a.html.

Guterman, N. B. (2001). *Stopping child maltreatment before it starts: Emerging horizons in early home visitation services.* Thousand Oaks, CA: Sage.

Guterman, N. B., & Embry, R. A. (2004). Prevention and treatment strategies targeting physical child abuse and neglect. In P. Allen-Meares & M. W. Fraser (Eds.), *Intervention with children and adolescents: An interdisciplinary perspective* (pp. 130–158). Boston: Allyn & Bacon.

Hansen, D. J., Sedlar, G., & Warner-Rogers, J. E. (1999). Child physical abuse. In R. T. Ammerman & M. Hersen (Eds.), *Assessment of family violence: A clinical and legal sourcebook* (2nd ed., pp. 127–156). New York: Wiley.

Hawkins, J. D., Catalano, R. F., & Miller, J. Y. (1992). Risk and protective factors for alcohol and other drug problems in adolescence and early adulthood: Implications for substance abuse prevention. *Psychological Bulletin, 112*(1), 64–105.

Hawkins, J. D., Catalano, R. F., Morrison, D. M., O'Donnell, J., Abbott, R. D., & Day, L. E. (1992). The Seattle Social Development Project: Effects of the first four years on protective factors and problem behaviors. In J. McCord & R. Tremblay (Eds.), *Preventing antisocial behavior* (pp. 139–161). New York: Guilford Press.

Henggeler, S. W., Melton, G., Brondino, M., Scherer, D., & Hanley, J. (1997). Multisystemic therapy with violent and chronic juvenile offenders and their families: The role of treatment fidelity in successful dissemination. *Journal of Consulting and Clinical Psychology, 65,* 821–833.

Henggeler, S. W., Schoenwald, S. K., Borduin, C. M., Rowland, M. D., & Cunningham, P. B. (1998). *Multisystemic treatment of antisocial behavior in children and adolescents.* New York: Guilford Press.

Ialongo, N., Poduska, J., Werthamer, L., & Kellam, S. (2001). The distal impact of two first-grade preventive interventions on conduct problems and disorder in early adolescence. *Journal of Emotional and Behavioral Disorders, 9,* 146–160.

Kazdin, A. E. (1995). Child, parent, and family dysfunction as predictors of outcome in cognitive-behavioural treatment of antisocial children. *Behaviour Research and Therapy, 33,* 271–281.

Kazdin, A. E. (2001). *Behavior modification in applied settings* (6th ed.). Pacific Grove, CA: Wadsworth.

Kazdin, A. E., & Weisz, J. R. (2003). *Evidence-based psychotherapies for children and adolescents.* New York: Guilford Press.

Kempner, K. L., Alvarado, R., Smith, P., & Bellamy, N. (2002). Cultural sensitivity and adaptation in family-based preventive interventions. *Prevention Science, 3*(3), 241–246.

Kinard, E. M. (1995, July). *Assessing resilience in abused children.* Paper presented at the fourth international Family Violence Research Conference, Durham, NH.

Kolko, D. J. (1996). Individual cognitive behavioral therapy and family therapy for physically abused children and their offending parents: A comparison of clinical outcomes. *Child Maltreatment, 1,* 322–342.

Kotchick, B. A., & Forehand, R. (2002). Putting parenting in perspective: A discussion of the contextual factors that shape parenting practices. *Journal of Child and Family Studies, 11*(3), 255–269.

Kumpfer, K. L., Molgaard, V., & Spoth, R. (1996). The Strengthening Families Program for the prevention of delinquency and drug use. In R. D. Peters & R. J. McMahon (Eds.), *Preventing childhood disorders, substance abuse, and delinquency* (pp. 241–267). Thousand Oaks, CA: Sage.

Lutzker, J., Bigelow, K., Doctor, R., & Kessler, M. (1998). Safety, health care, and bonding, within an ecobehavioral approach to treating and preventing child abuse and neglect. *Journal of Family Violence, 13,* 163–185.

Miedel, W. T., & Reynolds, A. J. (2004). Parent involvement in early intervention for disadvantaged children: Does it matter? *Children and Youth Services Review, 26*(1), 39–62.

Morgan, J., Robinson, D., & Aldridge, J. (2002). Parenting stress and externalizing child behavior. *Child and Family Social Work, 7,* 219–225.

Mrazek, P. J., & Haggerty, R. J. (Eds.). (1994). *Reducing risks for mental disorders: Frontiers for preventive intervention research.* Washington, DC: National Academy Press.

Mrazek, P. J., & Mrazek, D. A. (1987). Resilience in child maltreatment victims: A conceptual exploration. *Child Abuse and Neglect, 11,* 357–366.

The National Commission on Children. (1991). *Speaking of Kids: A National Survey of Children and Parents* (ASI Publication No. 15528-2). Washington, DC: U.S. Government Printing Office.

Nixon, R. (2002). Treatment of behavior problems in preschoolers: A review of parent training programs. *Clinical Psychology Review, 22,* 525–546.

Offord, D. (2000). Selection of levels of prevention. *Addictive Behaviors, 25*(6), 833–842.

Olds, D. L. (2002). Prenatal and infancy home visiting by nurses: From randomized trials to community replication. *Prevention Science, 3*(3), 153–172.

Olds, D. L., Henderson, C. R., Kitzman, H. J., Eckenrode, J. J., Cole, R. E., & Tatelbaum, R. C. (1999). Prenatal and infancy home visitation by nurses: Recent findings. *Future of Children, 9,* 44–65.

Olds, D. L., & Kitzman, H. J. (1993). Review of research on home visits for pregnant women and parents of young children. *Future of Children, 3*(3), 53–92.

Osofsky, J. D., & Thompson, M. D. (2000). Adaptive and maladaptive parenting: Perspectives on risk and protective factors. In J. P. Shonkoff & S. J. Meisels (Eds.), *Handbook of early childhood intervention* (2nd ed., pp 54–76). New York: Cambridge University Press.

Patterson, G. (1974). Interventions for boys with conduct problems: Multiple settings, treatments, and criteria. *Journal of Consulting and Clinical Psychology, 42,* 471–481.

Pollard, J. A., Hawkins, J. D., & Arthur, M. W. (1999). Risk and protection: Are both necessary to understand diverse behavioral outcomes in adolescence? *Social Work Research, 23*(3), 145–158.

Robbins, M. S., Szapocznik, J., Santisteban, D. A., Hervis, O. E., Mitrani, V. B., & Schwartz, S. J. (2003). Brief strategic family therapy for Hispanic youth. In A. E. Kazdin & J. R. Weisz (Eds.), *Evidence-based psychotherapies for children and adolescents* (pp. 407–424). New York: Guilford Press.

Rutter, M. (1987). Psychosocial resilience and protective mechanism. *American Journal of Orthopsychiatry, 57,* 316–330.

Rutter, M. (1989). Intergenerational continuities and discontinuities on serious parenting difficulties. In D. Cicchetti & V. Carlson (Eds.), *Child maltreatment theory and research on the causes and consequences of child abuse and neglect* (pp. 317–348). New York: Cambridge University Press.

Rutter, M. (2000). Resilience reconsidered: Conceptual considerations, empirical findings, and policy implications. In J. P. Shonkoff & S. J. Meisels (Eds.), *Handbook of early childhood intervention* (2nd ed., pp. 651–683). New York: Cambridge University Press.

Sanders, M. R., Turner, K. M. T., & Markie-Dadds, C. (2002). The development and dissemination of the Triple-P Positive Parenting Program: A multilevel evidence-based system of parenting and family support. *Prevention Science, 3*(3), 173–189.

Saunders, B. E., Berliner, L., & Hanson, R. F. (Eds.). (2003). *Child physical and sexual abuse: Guidelines for treatment* [Final report: January 15, 2003]. Charleston, SC: National Crime Victims Research and Treatment Center.

Schinke, S., Brounstein, P., & Gardner, S. (2002). *Science-Based Prevention Programs and Principles 2002* (DHHS Publication No. SMA 03-3764). Rockville, MD: Center for Substance Abuse Prevention, Substance Abuse and Mental Health Services Administration.

Shonkoff, J. P., & Meisels, S. J. (Eds.). (2000). *Handbook of early childhood intervention* (2nd ed.). New York: Cambridge University Press.

Smith, C. (2000). *National extension parent education model of critical parenting practices.* Retrieved February 10, 2004, from www.cyfernet.org/parenting_practices /foundations.html.

Smokowski, P. R., Mann, E. A., Reynolds, A. J., & Fraser, M. W. (2004). Childhood risk and protective factors and late adolescent adjustment in inner city minority youth. *Children and Youth Services Review, 26*(1), 63–91.

Spoth, R. L., Kavanagh, K. A., & Dishion, T. J. (2002). Family-centered preventive intervention science: Toward benefits to larger populations of children, youth and families. *Prevention Science, 3*(3), 145–152.

Stormshak, E. A., Kaminski, R. A., & Goodman, M. R. (2002). Enhancing the parenting skills of Head Start Families during the transition to kindergarten. *Prevention Science, 3*(3), 223–234.

Taylor, T., & Biglan, A. (1998). Behavioral family interventions for improving childrearing: A review of the literature for clinicians and policy makers. *Clinical Child and Family Psychology Review, 1*(1), 41–60.

Thomlison, B. (2003). Characteristics of evidence-based child maltreatment interventions. *Child Welfare, 82*(5), 541–569.

Thomlison, B. (2004a). Child maltreatment: A risk and protective factor perspective. In M. W. Fraser (Ed.), *Risk and resilience in childhood: An ecological perspective* (2nd ed., pp. 89–133). Washington, DC: National Association of Social Workers Press.

Thomlison, B. (2004b). The prevention of child maltreatment. In L. Rapp-Paglicci, C. Dulmus, & J. Wodarski (Eds.), *Handbook of preventive interventions for children and adolescents* (pp. 381–415). Hoboken, NJ: Wiley.

Tremblay, R., Japel, C., Perusse, D., McDuff, P., Boivin, M., Zoccolillo, M., et al. (1999). The search for the age of "onset" of physical aggression: Rousseau and Bandura revisited. *Criminal Behavior and Mental Health, 9*(1), 8–23.

Veltman, M. W., & Browne, K. D. (2001). Three decades of child maltreatment research: Implications for the school years. *Trauma, Violence, and Abuse: A Review Journal, 2*, 215–240.

Webster-Stratton, C. (1998). Preventing conduct problems in Head Start children: Strengthening parenting competencies. *Journal of Consulting and Clinical Psychology, 66*, 715–730.

Webster-Stratton, C. (2000). *The Incredible Years Training Series: Juvenile Justice Bulletin.* Washington, DC: U.S. Department of Justice.

Webster-Stratton, C. (Ed.). (2003). Aggression in young children perspective: Services proven to be effective in reducing aggression. In R. Tremblay, R. Barr, & R. Peters (Eds.), *Encyclopedia on early childhood development.* Montreal, Ontario, Canada: Centre of Excellence for Early Childhood Development. Retrieved February, 1, 2004, from www.excellence-earlychildhood.ca/documents/Webster-StrattonANGxp.pdf.

Webster-Stratton, C., & Hammond, M. (1998). Conduct problems and level of social competence in Head Start children: Prevalence, pervasiveness and associated risk factors. *Clinical Child and Family Psychology Review, 1*(2), 101–124.

Webster-Stratton, C., Hollinsworth, T., & Kolpacoff, M. (1989). The long term effectiveness and clinical significance of three cost effective training programs for families with conduct-problems children. *Journal of Consulting and Clinical Psychology, 57*(4), 550–553.

Webster-Stratton, C., & Spitzer, A. (1996). Parenting a young child with conduct problems: New insights using qualitative methods. In T. Ollendick & R. Prinz (Eds.), *Advances in clinical child psychology* (pp. 1–62). New York: Plenum Press.

Webster-Stratton, C., & Taylor, T. (2001). Nipping risk factors in the bud: Preventing substance abuse, delinquency and violence in adolescence through interventions targeted at young children (0–8 years). *Prevention Science, 2*(3), 165–192.

Weisz, J. R., & Kazdin, A. E. (2003). Present and future of evidence-based psychotherapies for children and adolescents. In A. E. Kazdin & J. R. Weisz (Eds.), *Evidence-based psychotherapies for children and adolescents* (pp. 439–451). New York: Guilford Press.

Wolfe, D. A. (2001, July). *Interventions for physically abused children and adolescents.* Paper presented at the Second Biennial Niagara Conference on Evidence-Based Treatments for Childhood and Adolescent Mental Health Problems. Niagara-on-the-Lake, Canada.

Chapter 17 ———————————————————

PARTNER VIOLENCE

GRETCHEN ELY AND KAREN McGUFFEE

Intimate partner violence (IPV), also known as domestic violence, has been studied since the early 1970's feminist movement (Burke & Follingstad, 1999). It occurs in all societies, though it varies by culture (Sharma, 1997).

The psychological consequences for victims of IPV are numerous. Women who experience ongoing IPV report deteriorating physical and emotional health over time (Sutherland et al., cited in Arias et al., 2002). It has been conservatively estimated that nonlethal IPV results in financial losses of approximately $150 million per year (Greenfield et al., cited in Arias et al., 2002). Medical expenses accounted for approximately 40% of these costs, property loss another 44%, and lost pay consumes the remainder (Arias et al., 2002). Despite this, IPV is continually ignored, trivialized, and rationalized by professionals, institutions, and society, which inhibits prevention efforts (Sharma, 1997).

TRENDS AND INCIDENCE

Current estimates of the rate of IPV indicate that 1.5 million women are sexually or physically assaulted by an intimate partner each year in the United States (Tjaden & Thoennes, 1998). The highest rate of intimate partner violence occur among women ages 16 to 24: Almost 1 in every 50 women in this age group will be victimized (The 1998 National Crime Victimization Survey, cited in Waul, 2000). It is also reported that 834,700 men are physically assaulted or raped by intimate partners in the United States every year. However, not only is the victimization rate among men significantly lower than among women, but the differences between their rate of victimization become greater as the severity of assault increases (Tjaden & Thoennes, 1998). As an example, women were 2 to 3 times more likely than men to report that they had been pushed, shoved, or grabbed but were 7 to 14 times more likely to report that they had been beaten up, choked, threatened, actually assaulted with weapons, or almost drowned by intimate partners (Stets & Straus, cited in Arias, Dankwort, Douglas, Dutton, & Stein, 2002). As a consequence of severe IPV, women require more medical attention, take more time off from work, and spend more days in bed than men (Arias et al., 2002).

Accurate estimates of the rates of partner violence are difficult to discern due to methodological problems with intimate partner violence studies. Some studies have included both members of a dyad in their study samples, thus potentially doubling the data when respondents are asked about the presence of abuse in their relationships (Burke & Follingstad, 1999). Many studies do not separate out victims from perpetrators, which is necessary to accurately estimate the presence of abuse and to determine the use of force in self-defense (Burke & Follingstad, 1999).

Although a large body of literature related to heterosexual partner abuse has developed over the past 30 years, gay and lesbian partner abuse has remained an understudied issue (Burke & Follingstad, 1999). The relationship between homelessness and IPV is also understudied. Results from one study indicate that IPV in homeless adults is so prevalent that it seems a normative consequence of homelessness (Boris, Heller, Shepard, & Zeanah, 2002).

RISK FACTORS

U.S. societal norms and gender role expectations promote a cultural environment that perpetuates intimate partner violence (Mears, 2003). Factors such as stressful life events, family conflicts, cultural norms of male dominance, and families being socialized to violence have been found to contribute to involvement in IPV (Sharma, 1997; Straus & Gelles, 1990; Straus & Smith, 1990). Women in focus groups who had been free of partner violence for at least 6 months indicated that once partner violence began, it escalated over time (Short et al., 2000). Thus, prior involvement in IPV is a risk factor for future involvement.

Results from one study indicate that adolescents and pregnant women are at high risk for involvement in IPV and IPV ending in homicide (Shadigian & Bauer, in press) Depression, Posttraumatic Stress Disorder, and other mental disorders, physical injury, alcohol use, and suicide have been found to be associated with IPV (Mears, 2003; O'Leary, 2000; Thompson, Kaslow, & Kingree, 2002). Women in one study reported that problem gambling by the male partner was also associated with involvement in IPV (Mulleman, DenOtter, Wadman, Tran, & Anderson, 2002). Substance use has been associated with IPV, and individuals in substance abuse treatment have been found to be at high risk for involvement (Chermack, Fuller, & Blow, 2000). It is possible that batterer programs would be more effective if offered in conjunction with substance abuse programs (Stuart, Moore, Ramsey, & Kahler, 2003). Results from one study revealed that unsuccessful participants of a court-referred batterer program were more likely to be using alcohol at the time of arrest when compared to participants who successfully completed the program (Yarbrough & Blanton, 2000).

A recent survey conducted by the Commonwealth Fund found that women who were abused as children were more likely to experience violence as adults. Almost two-thirds (62%) of all women in this study reporting child abuse also experienced violence as an adult, as compared to 25% of adults with no history of child abuse (Waul, 2000).

EFFECTIVE UNIVERSAL PREVENTIVE INTERVENTIONS

A significant body of literature related to intimate partner violence is available. This literature suggests that IPV is prevalent in our culture but that efforts to prevent involvement in IPV before it occurs are virtually nonexistent, as very little research has been done on the subject (Wathen & MacMillan, 2003).

Universal preventive efforts are interventions that are targeted to the general public or a whole population group that has not been identified on the basis of individual risk for a particular disorder (Gordon, 1983, 1987). According to the current IPV literature, efforts to prevent initial involvement in IPV do not exist. However, there are prevention efforts that are universally directed toward individuals who have already become involved in IPV. Prevention efforts are targeted toward both victims and perpetrators. Many interventions take place in medical settings and in the court system.

Medical Screening

Because IPV often results in physical injury, medical professionals have a unique opportunity to intervene and prevent future involvement in IPV (Mears, 2003). Doctors and other medical professionals should do all they can to identify IPV and make referrals to social agencies where patients can get help (Rhodes & Levinson, 2003). Researchers propose that physicians should ask patients about abuse, provide validating messages when the abuse is revealed, acknowledge that IPV is wrong, confirm patients' self-worth, and document the symptoms and disclosures of abuse (Gerbert et al., 2002). Universal screening for IPV is recommended by medical professionals in both urban and rural health care settings (Bauer & Shadigian, 2002; Ulbrich & Stockdale, 2002).

In one study where IPV screening was implemented in a family planning clinic, 11.5% of the participants screened reported involvement (Shattuck, 2002). This screening gave the clinic staff an opportunity to intervene when such an opportunity had not been present before the implementation of the screening process. Results from an emergency room study of 4,641 women indicate that routine screening for IPV in emergency rooms increases the likelihood that women who are involved will get needed interventions (Glass, Dearwater, & Campbell, 2001). Results from another study recommend that using the Partner Violence Screen (PVS) during emergency room visits can help detect IPV 65% to 71% of the time (Feldhaus et al., 1997), thus giving professionals a chance to intervene and prevent many incidents of revictimization (Feldhaus et al., 1997).

IPV screenings for pregnant women should also be a part of routine medical screenings that assess for conditions such as hypertension, diabetes, and drug/alcohol use (Johnson, Haider, Ellis, Hay, & Lindow, 2003). Many studies indicate that IPV occurs in 3% to 13% of pregnant women (Campbell, 2002). Screenings should be conducted by a professional who is educated about the dynamics of IPV and who has been taught how to use the screening instrument (Shadigian & Bauer, 2003). Abuse screening may be the most effective intervention available for preventing IPV in pregnant women (McFarlane, Soeken, & Wiist, 2000).

Shelter, Counseling, and Other Community Services

In a meta-analysis that analyzed 22 studies on the topic of preventing IPV, researchers found evidence that women who spend at least one night in a shelter and receive counseling and other advocacy services do experience a decrease in rates of IPV (Wathen & MacMillan, 2003). In another study, counseling reduced the severity of involvement in IPV across time for a group of Hispanic women who were pregnant at the initial time of intervention (McFarlane et al., 2000). In a study of 81 women who received case management and counseling services at a domestic violence shelter, results indicate that after three contacts with the shelter services, victims reported that incidents of IPV had decreased (McNamara, Ertl, Marsh, & Walker, 1997).

In a study of a domestic violence program in an urban American Indian health center, intervention approaches that were successful at preventing further involvement in IPV were home visits and a domestic violence support group that incorporated values from the Native culture (Norton & Manson, 1997).

Orders of Protection

One of the first experiences domestic violence victims have with the legal system is when they come to the court requesting orders of protection. There is some controversy surrounding whether orders of protection are successful at preventing further incidents of IPV. If a defendant will abide by an order of protection, the victim can be provided safety and resources; however, if the defendant chooses to ignore the order, the only avenue for the victim is to have the defendant arrested for contempt and put back into the court system. Research suggests, however, that orders of protection do serve to reduce incidents of IPV in some cases (McFarlane et al., 2002). Thus, orders of protection as a universal prevention strategy are included in the analysis for this chapter.

According to research on protection order petitioners, women who sought court intervention had typically experienced severe abuse over an extended period of time and were seeking protection orders to interrupt the abuse (Waul, 2000). Researchers concluded that for most of the women in their studies, filing for a civil protection order was their desperate attempt to obtain help with an increasingly dangerous situation (Harrell et al.; Keilitz et al., cited in Waul, 2000). Based on this knowledge, many courts are offering extra assistance to those requesting orders of protection to increase the prevention of further incidents of IPV. Waul recently conducted a study of the Domestic Violence Intake Center in the District of Columbia to see if their method of obtaining orders of protection had any impact on the likelihood of a woman's returning to court to obtain a permanent protection order. The results of the study found some indication that a centralized case-processing system can help encourage women to continue involvement in the court process by providing direct assistance to petitioners (Waul, 2000). Thus, permanent orders of protection and continued involvement in the court system were considered successful interventions for preventing further involvement in IPV (Waul, 2000). Results from a study of immigrant women indicate that contact with the justice system to obtain an order of protection resulted in a significant reduction in levels of IPV, and these results were maintained at 6-month follow-up (McFarlane et al., 2002).

Domestic Violence Courts

Another universal prevention strategy employed in the court system is the use of domestic violence courts. A number of states have created these courts, which are separate systems from regular criminal courts. One of their distinguishing features is the assignment of cases to specialized judges and the use of personnel who typically have specialized training in issues related to handling IPV cases (Karan et al., cited in Weber, 2000). Some of these domestic violence courts use a "combined calendar" in which both civil and criminal IPV matters are heard (Weber, 2000). Screening court cases for domestic violence takes place by trained personnel. Some courts have specialized units staffed by personnel with experience working with victims and perpetrators to assist litigants in filling out forms, provide an orientation to the legal system, and escort parties through the courtroom process (Weber, 2000).

One common feature of domestic violence courts is the increased accessibility of social or community services for petitioners and respondents (Judicial Council of California, "Domestic Violence Courts: A Descriptive Study," cited in Weber, 2000). Some courts include frequent monitoring of offenders by the judicial officer. As a condition of probation, defendants are expected to appear at 30-, 60-, and 90-day intervals for meetings with the judicial officer assigned to hear the matter (Weber, 2000). Research indicates "a substantial increase in compliance" with batterers' program requirements when there is mandatory court monitoring (Gondolf, cited in Weber, 2000).

In Brooklyn, New York, there is a court dedicated to hearing domestic violence felonies. The court utilizes victim advocates to explain the court process, assist in safety planning, and provide social service referrals. Additionally, the court strictly monitors defendants' compliance with court orders. In the first 2 years of the court's operation, dismissal rates declined almost 60% and probation violation rates of defendants were nearly half the typical rates (Kaye & Knipps, 2000).

In Toronto, Canada, a domestic violence court operates through a coordinated and mandatory response involving the Crown attorney, the Victim/Witness Assistance Program, the police, the judiciary, court administration, probation services, and community groups offering intervention programs for offenders ("Domestic Violence Justice Strategy—The DVC Projects at Old City Hall and North York Courts," cited by Salvaggio, 2002). On July 9, 1999, the Women's Court Watch Project, a group monitoring judges' decisions and outcomes in domestic violence cases, released their results indicating that this innovative court program was better able to successfully prosecute domestic violence cases, had lower rates of withdrawals, dismissals, and peace bonds, higher and faster rates of guilty verdicts, and higher rates of victims attending courts than other courts surveyed. Overall, the number of spousal abuse cases reaching the courts had increased while the average time a case was completed from start to finish had decreased ("Violence at the Doorstep," *The Globe and Mail,* cited in Salvaggio, 2002).

Batterer Treatment Programs

In an attempt to reduce intimate partner violence, many batterers are ordered by the courts to participate in treatment programs. Researchers found that batterer intervention programs should include the following standards to increase their chances of effectiveness for preventing future incidents of IPV:

(a) promotion of a priority on victim safety and batterer accountability; (b) facilitation of a process by which those with varying interests and particular mandates can work together to end domestic violence; (c) promotion of consistency among programs and the existence of accountability to the community; (d) the existence of consumer education by virtue of publicizing the content of programs along with program limitations; (e) acknowledgement of expertise from victims' advocates; (f) encouragement of a coordinated community response to stopping domestic violence; (g) emphasis on the social dimensions of domestic violence; (h) exertion of influence for existing programs to develop new programs and facilitate the development of standards in other regions; and (i) legitimization of the need for specialized knowledge, training, and intervention approaches in relation to work with abusers. (Dankwort & Austin, cited in Arias et al., 2002)

Debate continues over whether court-referred batterer programs are effective at preventing perpetrators from becoming involved in future incidents of IPV (Rosenbaum, Gearan, & Ondovic, 2002). One study examined the relationship between referral sources, participant characteristics, treatment length, treatment completion, and recidivism in a sample of 326 men who had completed at least one section of a program designed to treat perpetrators of IPV (Rosenbaum et al., 2002). Study results revealed that court-referred men had significantly higher treatment completion rates than self-referred men. In this study, treatment completion was associated with significantly lower rates of recidivism for court-referred perpetrators when compared to self-referred perpetrators.

Domestic Violence Prosecutions

Central to the legal process is the prosecution of domestic violence cases. Without effective prosecution, victims of intimate partner violence will not receive legal assistance and their involvement in IPV will continue. In Quincy, Massachusetts, the Quincy Program has one of the most successful domestic violence programs in the country (Salzman, cited in Durham, 1998). This program stresses integration of the process and communication with the victims while implementing a strict, no-nonsense attitude toward abusers that domestic violence will not be tolerated (Salzman, cited in Durham, 1998). All participants in each stage of the legal process, from the police officer making the arrest to the judge hearing the case, are trained to take domestic violence charges seriously (Salzman, cited in Durham, 1998).

Comprehensive Legal and Community Services

Results from one study examined the relationship between women's receipt of counseling services, protective orders, partner's subsequent arrests, and police contacts (Weisz, Tolman, & Bennett, 1998). Results from this study indicate that when victims received battered women's counseling services or had a protective order, a completed court case was more likely and the number of perpetrator arrests rose, thus reducing continued victim involvement in IPV.

EFFECTIVE SELECTIVE AND INDICATED PREVENTIVE INTERVENTIONS

Selective prevention efforts are targeted toward individuals or a subgroup of the population who are at high risk for developing a particular disorder or problem at some point in their life (Gordon, 1983, 1987). Indicated prevention efforts are targeted toward high-risk individuals who do not presently meet the criteria for a certain problem or disorder, but who otherwise are identified as having minimal but detectable signs or symptoms of a disorder or who have a biological marker indicating predisposition for such (Gordon, 1983, 1987).

Upon examining the literature required for this chapter, it was determined that selective and indicated IPV prevention efforts are not taking place. Intervention efforts appear to be geared toward either universal prevention or treating IPV offenders and victims once the violence has already been initiated. Most studies related to interventions and IPV focus on treatment for men who are already batterers (i.e., Murphy, Morrel, Elliot, & Neavins, 2003) or women who are already victims (i.e., Sullivan & Bybee, 1999).

The lack of adult selective and indicated prevention efforts related to IPV is startling. Practitioners need to focus more of their efforts on preventing IPV before it begins. Women and men who have previously been in abusive relationships need to be targeted for selective preventive interventions to keep them from becoming involved in abusive relationships again in the future. Individuals who witnessed IPV as children also need to be targeted for selective preventive intervention efforts to decrease their chances of becoming involved in IPV in their own adult relationships, as research indicates that children exposed to IPV may be at risk for involvement in IPV as adults (Rosenbaum & Leisring, 2003; Williams, 2003). Results from one study revealed that individuals living in lower-income communities were five times more likely than individuals living in higher-income communities to be victims of IPV (Mears, Carlson, Holden, & Harris, 2001). Thus, medical clinics in lower-income neighborhoods could target patients for selective IPV preventive interventions. Further, because substance abuse is often linked to IPV (Easton & Sinha, 2002), individuals in substance abuse treatment could be targeted for selective preventive interventions related to IPV. Additionally, individuals involved in verbal abuse that has not yet turned physically violent need to be targeted for indicated preventive interventions before IPV leads to physical abuse and possibly death.

In the absence of selective and indicated preventive interventions for adults, it is important to consider recommendations from selective preventive efforts for young adult and youth populations that are intended for use before dating begins. Results from adolescent studies indicate that school- and community-based interventions targeted toward at-risk teens can help them develop healthier dating relationship behaviors (MacGowan, 1997; Wolfe, Wekerle, Straatman, Grasley, & Reitzel-Jaffe, 2003). Dating violence interventions aimed at at-risk youth may reduce incidents of physical and emotional abuse and symptoms of distress over time (Wolfe et al., 2003). School-based programs such as Safe Dates are designed to prevent violence and teach dating skills by challenging dating norms, addressing gender stereotyping, and improving conflict management skills, help-seeking skills, and cognitive factors that are associated with help-seeking (Foshee et al., 1998). Interventions like Safe Dates may affect IPV involvement in adulthood and thus could be considered preventive interventions for adult IPV.

PRACTICE IMPLICATIONS

Universal preventive interventions for adults are limited to individuals already involved in IPV and occur mostly through the medical and legal fields. Prevention efforts detailed in the literature examined for this chapter focus on preventing future involvement in IPV once it has already begun. Prevention efforts at the selective and indicated levels are virtually nonexistent. Professionals need to focus on developing interventions for adults that prevent initial involvement in IPV. Professionals could target individuals seeking other types of social service for IPV preventive interventions. Individuals who are involved in other types of violence could be targeted to participate in selective preventive intervention efforts to keep them from also becoming involved in IPV. Individuals who report a history of childhood maltreatment could be targeted for IPV prevention efforts to interrupt the cycle of violence in adulthood. Evidence from the literature suggests that there is not enough being done to prevent IPV in adults.

There is mounting evidence that men who commit IPV vary on many dimensions, such as severity of violence and personality traits (Saunders, 2002; Yarbrough & Blanton, 2000). Because of these differences, programs targeting those who commit IPV need to be designed to respond to their different levels of motivation and cultural differences via multiple forms of intervention (O'Leary, 2002; Saunders, 2002).

Research suggests that lesbians and gay men are just as likely to abuse their partners as are heterosexual men (Burke & Follingstad, 1999). The high prevalence rates of partner abuse in gay and lesbian populations needs to be recognized by providers of mental health services so that they can identify and provide interventions for both victims and perpetrators (Burke & Follingstad, 1999).

Culturally sensitive preventive interventions need to be developed. For example, researchers in one study suggest that when working with Native Americans, intervention efforts need to take into account the social histories of Native women and their families (Malcoe, Duran, & Ficek, 2002). Similarly, women of color require different considerations from White women. For White women and women of color, the experience of battering is similar, but when deciding whether to seek help or escape, women of color face many problems that White battered women generally do not (Fenton, cited in Martinson, 2001). They may consider the race's image as a whole, the position of African American men, the view of African American families, their economic situation, and the system's responsiveness if they decide to pursue legal avenues. Addressing these concerns while providing better domestic violence resources will help all domestic violence victims equally (Martinson, 2001).

One group of citizens participating in a Court Watch program in Bergen County, New Jersey, suggested the following to improve their court's response under the State of New Jersey Prevention of Domestic Violence Act: provide a drop-in child care center for those having court proceedings; provide information about the protection to which victims are entitled under the Prevention of Domestic Violence Act in written form (booklets, pamphlets) or in an alternate format such as video; increase awareness of victims' rights; form a coordinating committee to improve interaction and information sharing among all systems involved in domestic violence with the aim of developing collaborative procedures for handling cases and monitoring their consistent implementation, resolving problems as they arise; address issues of child support, risk assessment, counseling, and treatment services in the court process; and require judges to attend courses related to domestic violence (Bergen County Commission on the Status of Women, 1995).

POLICY IMPLICATIONS

Policies should be implemented that require medical professionals and court personnel, including judges, to be trained in screening for IPV in clients. Such training would improve professionals' ability to determine if clients are involved in IPV and allow such professionals to make referrals for those who are involved, so that further incidents of IPV may be prevented. In addition to screening techniques, court personnel should be taught the facts regarding domestic violence so their rulings will not consist simply of telling him to stop hitting or telling her to leave.

Substance abuse centers need to introduce policies that require worker training in assessment for domestic violence, as it seems that IPV prevention may be an appropriate complement to substance abuse interventions.

FUTURE DIRECTIONS

Despite a generous body of literature related to IPV, little attention is being paid to the need to prevent the problem. Much more research needs to be done to determine which interventions may be applied on the universal, selective, and indicated levels to prevent initial involvement in IPV.

Information about the real prevalence of partner violence in the general population is still unclear as there are no national data. The development of national data sets that can support more rigorous evaluations of IPV are necessary to improve information related to family violence policy and practice (Chalk, 2001). Information related to real prevalence rates is necessary if we are to develop screening protocols and intervention tools that will address the needs of this population (Tollestrup et al., 1999). Researchers need to conduct projects to follow people throughout their lifetime so that the effects of screening, health consequences, and death rates from IPV can be examined (Bauer & Shadigian, 2002).

Practice strategies need to be rigorously evaluated and intervention strategies that incorporate input from women of color need to be developed, as there is only limited information available related to IPV among various ethnic groups (Lee, Thompson, & Mechanic, 2002; Sharma, 1997).

There are many promising interventions available that are designed to address IPV once it begins (Mears, 2003). Yet, there are few, if any, adult interventions available to prevent violence in individuals who may be at increased risk for the problem. Thus, professionals must focus efforts on developing programs for adults that will prevent initial involvement in IPV.

Finally, more studies related to gay and lesbian IPV are needed. Researchers suggest that studies of gay and lesbian partners could be enhanced using national census data-gathering procedures rather than convenience sampling methods (Burke & Follingstad, 1999). Research related to other special populations such as immigrant groups, American Indians, and homeless individuals are also desperately needed.

REFERENCES

Arias, I., Dankwort, J., Douglas, U., Dutton, M., & Stein, K. (2002). Preventing injuries and abuse: Violence against women: The state of batterer prevention programs. *Journal of Law, Medicine, and Ethics, 30,* 157–164.

Bauer, S. T., & Shadigian, E. M. (2002). Screening for partner violence makes a difference and saves lives. *British Medical Journal, 325,* 1418–1420.

Bergen County Commission on the Status of Women. (1995). Community court watch: II. A study of the Bergen County family court system and the enforcement of the state of New Jersey Prevention of Domestic Violence Act. *Women's Rights Law Reporter, 17,* 79–92.

Boris, N. W., Heller, S. S., Shepard, T., & Zeanah, C. H. (2002). Partner violence among homeless young adults: Measurement issues and associations. *Journal of Adolescent Health, 30,* 355–363.

Burke, L. K., & Follingstad, D. R. (1999). Violence in lesbian and gay relationships: Theory, prevalence, and correlational factors. *Clinical Psychology Review, 19,* 487–512.

Campbell, J. C. (2002). Health consequences of intimate partner violence. *Lancet, 359*(9314), 1331–1336.

Chalk, R. (2001). Assessing family violence interventions: Linking programs to research-based strategies. *Journal of Aggression, Maltreatment and Trauma, 4,* 29–53.

Chermack, S. T., Fuller, B. E., & Blow, F. C. (2000). Predictors of expressed partner and non partner violence among patients in substance abuse treatment. *Drug and Alcohol Dependency, 58,* 43–54.

Durham, G. (1998). The domestic violence dilemma: How our ineffective and varied responses reflect our conflicted views of the problem. *Southern California Law Review, 71,* 641–665.

Easton, C., & Sinha, R. (2002). Treating the addicted male batterer: Promising directions for dual-focused programming. In C. Wekerle & A. Wall (Eds.), *The violence and addiction equation: Theoretical and clinical issues in substance abuse and relationship violence* (pp. 275–292). New York: Brunner/Routledge.

Feldhaus, K. M., Koziol-McLain, J., Amsbury, H. L., Norton, I. M., Lowenstein, S. R., & Abbott, J. T. (1997). Accuracy of 3 brief screening questions for detecting partner violence in the emergency department. *Journal of the American Medical Association, 277,* 1357–1361.

Foshee, V. A., Bauman, K. E., Arragia, X. B., Helms, R. W., Koch, G. G., & Linder, G. F. (1998). An evaluation of Safe Dates, an adolescent dating violence prevention program. *Journal of Public Health, 88,* 45–50.

Gerbert, B., Moe, J., Caspers, N., Salber, P., Feldman, M., Herzig, K., et al. (2002, February/March). Physicians' response to victims of domestic violence: Toward a model of care. *Women and Health,* 1–22.

Glass, N., Dearwater, S., & Campbell, J. (2001). Intimate partner violence screening and intervention: Data from eleven Pennsylvania and California community hospital emergency department. *Journal of Emergency Nursing, 27,* 141–149.

Gordon, R. (1983). An operational classification of disease prevention. *Public Health Reports, 98,* 107–109.

Gordon, R. (1987). An operational classification of disease prevention. In J. A. Steinberg & M. M. Silverman (Eds.), *Preventing mental disorders* (pp. 20–26). Rockville, MD: U.S. Department of Health and Human Services.

Johnson, J. K., Haider, F., Ellis, K., Hay, D. M., & Lindow, S. W. (2003). The prevalence of domestic violence in pregnant women. *British Journal of Obstetrics and Gynecology, 110,* 272–275.

Kaye, J. S., & Knipps, S. K. (2000). Judicial responses to domestic violence: The case for a problem solving approach. *Western State University Law Review, 27,* 1–13.

Lee, R. K., Thompson, V. L. S., & Mechanic, M. B. (2002). Intimate violence and women of color: A call for innovations. *American Journal of Public Health, 92,* 530–535.

MacGowan, M. J. (1997). An evaluation of a dating violence program for middle school students. *Violence and Victims, 12,* 223–235.

Malcoe, L. H., Duran, B. M., & Ficek, E. E. (2002). Social stressors in relation to intimate partner violence against Native American women. *Annals of Epidemiology, 12,* 525.

Martinson, L. (2001). An analysis of racism and resources for African-American female victims of domestic violence in Wisconsin. *Wisconsin Women's Law, 16,* 259–285.

McFarlane, J., Malecha, A., Gist, J., Watson, K., Batten, E., Hall, I., et al. (2002). Intimate partner violence against immigrant women: Measuring the effectiveness of protection orders. *American Journal of Family Law, 16,* 244–253.

McFarlane, J., Soeken, K., & Wiist, W. (2000). An evaluation of interventions to decrease intimate partner violence to pregnant women. *Public Health Nursing, 17,* 443–451.

McNamara, J. R., Ertl, M. A., Marsh, S., & Walker, S. (1997). Short-term response to counseling and case management intervention in a domestic violence shelter. *Psychological Reports, 81,* 1243–1251.

Mears, D. P. (2003). Research and interventions to reduce domestic violence revictimization. *Trauma, Violence, and Abuse, 4,* 127–147.

Mears, D. P., Carlson, M. J., Holden, G. W., & Harris, S. D. (2001). Reducing domestic violence revictimization: The effects of individual and contextual factors and type of legal intervention. *Journal of Interpersonal Violence, 16,* 1260–1283.

Mulleman, R. L., DenOtter, T., Wadman, M. C., Tran, T. P., & Anderson, J. (2002). Problem gambling in the partners of the emergency department patient as a risk factor for intimate partner violence. *Journal of Emergency Medicine, 23,* 307–312.

Murphy, C. M., Morrel, T. M., Elliot, J. D., & Neavins, T. M. (2003). A prognostic indicator scale for the treatment of partner abuse perpetrators. *Journal of Interpersonal Violence, 18,* 1087–1105.

Norton, I. M., & Manson, S. M. (1997). Domestic violence intervention in an urban Indian health center. *Community Mental Health Journal, 33,* 331–337.

O'Leary, K. D. (2000). Developmental and affective issues in assessing and treating partner aggression. *Clinical Psychology: Science and Practice, 6,* 400–414.

O'Leary, K. D. (2002). Conjoint therapy for partners who engage in physically aggressive behavior: Rationale and research. *Journal of Aggression, Maltreatment, and Trauma, 5,* 145–164.

Rhodes, K. V., & Levinson, W. (2003). Interventions for intimate partner violence against women: Clinical applications. *Journal of the American Medical Association, 289,* 601–606.

Rosenbaum, A., Gearan, P. J., & Ondovic, C. (2002). Completion and recidivism among court and self-referred batterers in a psychoeducational group treatment program: Implications for intervention and public policy. *Journal of Aggression, Maltreatment, and Trauma, 5,* 199–220.

Rosenbaum, A., & Leisring, P. A. (2003). Beyond power and control: Towards an understanding of partner abusive men. *Journal of Comparative Family Studies, 34,* 7–22.

Salvaggio, F. (2002). K-Court: The feminist pursuit of an interdisciplinary approach to domestic violence. *Appeal: Review of Current and Law Reform, 8,* 6–17.

Saunders, D. G. (2002). Developing guidelines for IPV offender programs: What can we learn from related fields and current research? *Journal of Aggression, Maltreatment, and Trauma, 5,* 235–248.

Shadigian, E. M., & Bauer, S. T. (in press). Screening for partner violence during pregnancy. *International Journal of Gynecology and Obstetrics.*

Sharma, S. (1997). Domestic violence against minority women: Interventions, preventions and health implications. *Equal Opportunities International, 16,* 1–14.

Shattuck, S. R. (2002). An IPV screening program in a public health department. *Journal of Community Health Nursing, 19,* 121–132.

Short, L. M., McMahon, P. M., Davis-Chervin, D., Shelley, G. A., Lezin, N., Sloop, K. S., et al. (2000). Survivors' identification of protective factors and early warning signs for intimate partner violence. *Violence Against Women, 6,* 272–285.

Straus, M. A., & Gelles, R. J. (1990). *Physical violence in American families: Risk factors and adaptation to violence in 8,415 families.* New Brunswick, NJ: Transaction.

Straus, M. A., & Smith, C. (1990). Violence in Hispanic families in the United States: Incidence rates and structural interpretation. In M. Straus & R. Gelles (Eds.), *Physical violence in American families: Risk factors and Adaptations to Violence in 8,145 Families* (pp. 341–363). New Brunswick, NJ: Transaction.

Stuart, G. L., Moore, T. M., Ramsey, S. E., & Kahler, C. W. (2003). Relationship aggression and substance use among women court referred to domestic violence intervention programs. *Addictive Behaviors, 28,* 1603–1610.

Sullivan, C. M., & Bybee, D. I. (1999). Reducing violence: Using community based advocacy for women with abusive relationships. *Journal of Consulting and Clinical Psychology, 67,* 43–53.

Thompson, M. P., Kaslow, N. J., & Kingree, J. B. (2002). Risk factors for suicide attempts among African American women experiencing recent intimate partner violence. *Violence and Victims, 17,* 283–295.

Tjaden, T., & Thoennes, N. (1998). *Prevalence, incidence and consequences of violence against women: Findings from the National Violence against Women Survey* (NCJ

172837). Washington, DC: National Institute of Justice and the Centers for Disease Control and Prevention.

Tollestrup, K., Sklar, D., Frost, F. J., Olson, L., Weybright, J., Sandvig, J., et al. (1999). Health indicators and intimate partner violence among women who are members of a managed care organization. *Preventive Medicine, 29,* 431–440.

Ulbrich, P. M., & Stockdale, J. (2002). Making family planning clinics an empowerment zone for rural battered women. *Women and Health, 35,* 83–100.

Wathen, C. N., & MacMillan, H. L. (2003). Interventions for violence against women: Scientific review. *Journal of the American Medical Association, 289,* 589–601.

Waul, M. (2000). Civil protection orders: An opportunity for intervention with domestic violence victims. *Georgetown Public Policy Review, 6,* 51–70.

Weber, J. (2000). Courts responding to communities: Domestic violence courts: Components and considerations. *Journal of the Center for Children and the Courts, 2,* 23–33.

Weisz, A. N., Tolman, R. M., & Bennett, L. (1998). An ecological study of nonresidential services for battered women within a comprehensive community protocol for domestic violence. *Journal of Family Violence, 13,* 395–397.

Williams, L. M. (2003). Understanding child abuse and violence against women: A life course perspective. *Journal of Interpersonal Violence, 18,* 441–452.

Wolfe, D. A., Wekerle, C., Straatman, A., Grasley, C., & Reitzel-Jaffe, D. (2003). Dating violence prevention with at risk youth: A controlled outcome study. *Journal of Consulting and Clinical Psychology, 71,* 279–291.

Yarbrough, D. N., & Blanton, P. W. (2000). Socio-demographic indicators of intervention program completion with the male court referred perpetrator of partner abuse. *Journal of Criminal Justice, 28,* 517–526.

Chapter 18

ELDER ABUSE AND NEGLECT

PATRICIA BROWNELL

Elder abuse and neglect, generally defined as harmful acts of commission or omission toward an older adult by a family member or significant other, is a relatively new social problem (Wolf, 1988). In its short history, it has been variously defined as a public health, legal/criminal justice, domestic violence, and social service problem (Nerenberg, 2000).

Early efforts to address this social problem focused on detection and crisis intervention. Prevention and early intervention models have begun to emerge relatively recently and reflect the orientations of the various disciplines that respond to problems involving older adults, their family members, and their care providers. However, the growing recognition among service providers that elder abuse is a multidisciplinary issue has stimulated the development of models of interdisciplinary practice that reflect prevention and early intervention strategies.

Models of prevention and early intervention in elder abuse are emerging as important strategies for several reasons. One is the recognition that elder abuse and neglect, estimated to affect approximately 5% of the older adult population at some point in the life span, will increase as the older adult population increases. In the United States, residents 65 years of age and older number 35 million and comprise 12.4% of the population (U.S. Census Bureau, 2002). The population of older Americans age 85 and above showed the highest population increase (an increase of 38%, from 3.1 million to 4.2 million 10 years ago), reflecting greater longevity of older adults than in the past. In contrast, the cohort age 65 to 69 years decreased by 11%, reflecting the relatively low birth rate in the United States during the years of the Great Depression in the late 1920s and early 1930s.

This trend is expected to change dramatically when the cohort born between 1946 and 1964, the so-called post-World War II baby boomers, begin to reach age 65 in 2011 (U.S. Census Bureau, 2002). This is a global phenomenon, as well. While developing countries are aging rapidly, developed countries like Japan, for example, are showing dramatic surges in longevity (Shibusawa, 2004). Preventive interventions may be cost-effective alternatives to large-scale social distress and expensive long-term interventions for seriously abused and neglected older adults.

Second, research, although primarily still at the exploratory and descriptive stages, has begun to identify risk factors for abuse and neglect and examine outcomes associated with interventions (Bonnie, 2003). While explanatory research in elder abuse is at a beginning stage of development, research findings and practice experience have begun to generate data on factors associated with vulnerability to abuse and neglect, as well as those associated with useful interventions (Reis, 2000). This is an important and positive step toward the development and institutionalizing of prevention and early intervention strategies to address this social problem.

TRENDS AND INCIDENCE

Elder abuse is defined as physical, financial, or psychological abuse, active or passive neglect or self-neglect (Wolf & Pillemer, 1984), or mistreatment (Hudson, 1989). Defining elder abuse and neglect has been controversial since it was first recognized as a social problem of significance in the 1970s. In addition to the definitional disputes, like all forms of family violence, elder abuse is difficult to quantify because it often occurs in the privacy of the home. All but four states in the United States have centralized reporting systems for elder abuse or mistreatment that occurs in the community; almost all of the state reporting systems are mandatory. All states have statutes mandating reporting of elder abuse in residential care settings.

In spite of the problems related to defining elder abuse and neglect, there have been efforts to estimate their prevalence in the United States. Estimates have ranged from 4% to 10%, depending on the definition used and the population studied (Pillemer & Finkelhor, 1988; Tatara, 1995; U.S. House of Representatives, 1990). Assuming a conservative estimate of 4%, over 1.3 million older adults 65 and older in the United States may be victims of abuse and neglect. The actual number is thought to be much higher. The National Elder Abuse Incidence Report, mandated by the Family Violence Prevention and Services Act of 1992 (Pub. L. No. 102-295), states that abuse and neglect of older adults living in the community have been largely ignored. However, increasing consciousness of elder abuse is likely to bring more cases to the attention of service providers and the public (Tatara & Thomas, 1998).

Quantification of elder abuse and neglect cases has been stymied for another reason. There are several primary service systems relevant to the prevention, early detection, and intervention of elder abuse that serve older adults and their families (Brownell, Welty, & Brennan, 2000). The conflicting definitions of elder abuse currently used in the United States are linked to the different systems in which this social problem is addressed. For the purpose of this discussion, these systems are defined as the social service system (area agencies on aging, not-for-profit agencies providing community-based services to older adults, and adult protective services programs mandated by state social service and mental hygiene laws); the health and mental health system; and the criminal justice system (police, district attorneys, and the attorneys general).

Each system generates its own remedies. For example, in the social services system, Adult Protective Service (APS) programs operate with state legislative mandates to exercise their role of parens patriae with impaired at-risk older adults (Somers, 2003) but have limited powers to protect older victims who are mentally or physically unimpaired and refuse services. Aging service programs funded through the Older Americans Act do not have the authority to provide services on an involuntary basis to victims of elder abuse and neglect. Health and mental health care systems provide medical and psychiatric care to impaired older adults, but may not be prepared to diagnose stress-related health problems or undernourishment among older patients related to psychological or financial abuse. The criminal justice system may generate legal remedies but be unprepared for or unaware of the social consequences of these remedies.

In addition to differing categories of elder abuse and different service systems, there are two primary settings in which abuse or neglect can occur, each with its own legislative and reporting mandates, remedies, and constraints. These are domestic or community settings and institutional settings. Older adults living in the community may receive informal (family) or formal (home health care) in-home services.

Elder Abuse in the Community

Older adults who are abused or mistreated by family members and significant others in the community represent a much more diverse population than those in nursing home settings. They may range from healthy and vigorous older adults, possibly with caregiving responsibilities for impaired spouses, partners, adult children, or grandchildren, to frail elders with severe cognitive and physical disabilities. All states have APS programs, which handle referrals of at-risk individuals who are a danger to themselves or others or who are unable to protect themselves from harm. In addition, most states have mandatory reporting statutes for older adults living in the community who may be victims of elder abuse or neglect.

Social service, health and mental health, and law enforcement systems provide protective and preventive services to older adult community residents who may be victims of abuse or neglect. Because these systems have different mandates to provide services to victims based on victim and perpetrator characteristics such as mental and physical capacity, level of risk, and nature of the abuse, they must work collaboratively to ensure optimal service responses.

Elder Abuse in Institutional Settings

All states have mandated reporting of elder abuse and mistreatment in nursing homes. The numbers of older adults entering nursing homes in most states have been stable over the past few years and may be expected to remain so with increasing home-based alternatives. However, the proportion of states' populations age 60 and older residing in nursing homes are among the most frail and vulnerable of older citizens.

Mandated reporters of elder abuse and neglect in nursing home settings usually must report suspected or actual incidents of mistreatment to the State Departments of Health, the states' licensing entities for nursing home facilities. Anyone, including family members, can report abuse or neglect of nursing home residents to state health departments, but employees of nursing homes are usually mandated reporters and can be sanctioned for failing to report known or suspected abuse or neglect of an older nursing home resident. Mandated reporters in nursing homes are required to report physical abuse, neglect, or mistreatment of nursing home residents. In addition, the Long Term Care Ombudsman Programs, which are part of state aging agencies, are mandated under the Older Americans Act to implement state Ombudsman Programs for residents living in long-term care facilities. The primary function of the Long Term Care Ombudsman is to receive, investigate, and resolve complaints from residents and family members regarding services and treatment by facility staff (Filinson, 2001).

MANDATED REPORTING OF ELDER ABUSE AND NEGLECT

Although it would appear that reports generated by mandated reporting statutes could provide substantial information on the incidence and prevalence of elder abuse, in fact this is far from the case. State mandatory reporting systems are modeled after child abuse and neglect reporting systems; they are based on the assumption that elder abuse is a form of domestic violence perpetrated on impaired and frail elders who are unable to protect themselves from harm. State legislation mandating reporting of domestic abuse of older adults living in the community does not always take into consideration the fact that most people 60 and older are physically and mentally vigorous. In addition, older adults, unlike children, are legally entitled to make decisions about their own lives—however unsound these decisions may appear to an outside observer—unless adjudicated as lacking capacity by a court of law.

Studies from states with mandatory reporting of elder abuse have found that mandated reporting systems are expensive and underfunded (Zorza, 1999). In addition, older adults at risk of abuse or neglect are entitled to refuse services if found able to understand the consequences of their decisions. Appropriate services are often lacking or inadequate even if the victim agrees to accept them. Finally, statutes defining elder abuse and neglect, as well as responsibility for reporting, are state-specific and vary accordingly. Federal leadership to date has not supported the subsidizing of state and local funding for APS staff salaries or professional development, nor has it supported the national standardizing of definitions and reporting procedures. This must happen before any meaningful prevalence data on elder abuse are generated. In the United States, there is no national definition of elder abuse and neglect that clearly defines and delineates what it is and how it is to be measured.

The lack of a common definition that transcends the cultural and institutional mandates and boundaries of agencies, institutions, counties, and states limits the ability of policy makers, advocates, gerontologists, and researchers in the United States to understand current trends in elder abuse and neglect. As a result, it is difficult to project future trends, recommend preventive measures, and plan for the kinds of services needed to reduce the prevalence of elder abuse and neglect. The national prevalence rate for elder abuse and neglect is really not known in the United States (Anonymous, 2002).

Although reliable national prevalence data are unavailable, data on reported elder abuse suggest that it is increasing. A national study by the National Center on Elder Abuse (NCEA) found that reported incidents increased 150% between 1986 and 1996 (Somers, 2003). The National Incidence Report estimates that five incidents of elder abuse go unreported for every one that is reported (Tatara & Thomas, 1998). Earlier studies suggest that the number of unreported incidents may be as high as 14 for each reported case (Pillemer & Finkelhor, 1988).

RISK FACTORS

Because elder abuse has only recently been identified as a significant social problem (Wolf, 1988), there is still a lot that is not known about its risk factors. Early studies (Lau & Kosberg, 1979) suggested that care-dependent older women age 75 and older were at greatest risk of abuse or neglect from daughter caregivers. Studies of specific cultural groups, such as Asians, identify the daughter-in-law as the most likely abuser of elderly care-dependent family members (Le, 1997).

However, other studies identify the typical abuse situation as one in which there is not adequate social support, the elder victim has experienced abuse at some earlier point in the life span, and the caregiver is troubled and has difficulty with interpersonal relationships (Reis, 2000). Other researchers have found that older adults caring for impaired adult children and even grandchildren may be at greater risk of abuse than care-dependent elders (Brownell, Berman, & Salamone, 1999; Pillemer & Finkelhor, 1989). Risk factors associated with financial abuse of older adults include victims' old age (over 70 years) and cognitive impairment (Choi, Kulick, & Mayer, 1999).

The extremely broad and sometimes contradictory range of risk profiles for elder abuse reflects the complexity of this social problem. It also suggests the need for multifaceted and interdisciplinary approaches to prevention and early intervention strategies. Most models of prevention, early detection, and intervention have emerged from a primary service response system, however. These include the social service, health and mental health, and criminal justice systems. The primacy of each system in generating remedies for elder abuse and neglect has depended on assumed causes of this problem, and each response strategy is not without controversy (Nerenberg, 2000).

GORDON'S MODEL OF PREVENTION

The system of social, health, mental health, and criminal justice services for older adults is complex and includes a range of interventions that could be identified as primary, secondary, and tertiary (Forgey, 2000). However, only recently has elder abuse prevention been of explicit interest to the field, including public education models (Bonnie, 2003). As a result of the crisis orientation of responses to elder abuse, prevention and early intervention models have been slow to develop. The model of prevention developed by Gordon (1983, 1987) is useful for understanding the distinctions among general prevention, targeted prevention, and early intervention to prevent escalation of elder abuse or neglect.

Gordon identifies three categories of preventive interventions:

- Universal preventive interventions targeted to the general public or a whole population group that has not been identified on the basis of individual risk for abuse or neglect.

- Selective preventive interventions targeted to individuals or subgroups of the population who are at high risk for experiencing abuse or neglect at some point in their lives.

- Indicated preventive interventions targeted to high-risk individuals who may not presently meet the criteria for elder abuse or neglect, but who are identified as having minimal but detectable signs or symptoms of abuse or neglect.

SYSTEMS OF ELDER ABUSE INTERVENTIONS: A HISTORY

Professionals working with elder abuse victims and their families are challenged to confront professional ethical mandates to respect the autonomy of their clients. The state is judicious in defining the circumstances in which and the extent to which it can intervene into the private lives of individuals and families. Two areas of intervention legislated to date are when a serious crime has been committed against one family member by another, and when victims lack the capacity to protect themselves from harm. Overriding the autonomy of unimpaired abuse victims because of their age alone is a matter of serious consideration for professionals and lawmakers. However, not to attempt to prevent or detect at an early stage suspected or known instances of abuse is also troubling, particularly for those in the helping professions. This has resulted in a system of elder abuse interventions that address the social problem after the fact and are more reactive than preventive.

This issue is especially critical in legislation proposed by the state legislatures. To date, most state elder abuse statutes have focused on reporting elder abuse and prosecuting abusers. This is in spite of studies that have suggested that community education is more effective in identifying and, more important, preventing elder abuse than mandatory reporting systems (Tatara, 1995). For the purpose of this discussion, these initiatives are presented in social service, health and mental health, and criminal justice frames.

Social Service Frame

Title I of the Social Security Act, legislated in 1935, represented one of the earliest attempts to develop a system of preventive services for older adults at risk for abuse or neglect. This title enacted the Old Age Assistance (OAA) program, a cash benefits program for the indigent elderly age 65 and older that included casework services carried out under the auspices of the county departments of social services (Burr, 1982). Responsibilities of the caseworkers included eligibility investigations and home visiting, ensuring the protection and well-being of their elderly clients, and assisting with social services as well as income support for food and housing (Burr, 1982).

In 1974, OAA, along with Aid to the Disabled (AD) and Aid to the Blind (AB), became consolidated through the earlier passage of Title 16 of the Social Security Act into a single cash benefits program, Supplemental Security Income (SSI), and federalized. At this time, Congress enacted Title XX of the Social Security Act, which provided funding for community-based social services to serve populations experiencing newly defined social problems like domestic violence, child care for the working poor, the community-bound elderly, chronic substance abuse, and deinstitutionalized psychiatric patients (Bonnie, 2003).

In the mid-1970s, with social service funding through Title XX, the deinstitutionalization of formerly hospitalized psychiatric patients into the community, and the federalizing of OAA, AD, and AB assistance, states began passing legislation to amend state social services and mental hygiene laws and create APS programs. The funding from Title XX (since 1981, the Social Services Block Grant) enabled states to expand APS to include anyone 18 years of age and older found in situations indicating neglect, abuse, or exploitation (Burr, 1982). APS programs provide services to at-risk adults that are intended to prevent abuse from escalating and to ensure the safety of the abuse victims. As an arm of state and local government, APS workers can intervene in family situations on an involuntary basis, if necessary, and provide services like financial management, guardianships, and heavy-duty cleaning to prevent further abuse, neglect, and exploitation (Susan B. Somers, personal communication, August 31, 2003).

The 1965 Older Americans Act funds a national system of state and local agencies that are responsible for establishing a system of community-based services to adults age 60 and older, including nutrition programs, transportation, case management, limited home care, information and referral, advocacy, and other services intended to empower older adults to remain living independently for as long as possible, whether in the community or in an institutional setting. While APS programs are intended to provide protective services to primarily mentally incapacitated adults 18 and older, services funded through the Older Americans Act are specifically targeted to adults 60 and older on a voluntary basis. Both APS and aging service programs have the mission to support independent living in the community as long as possible for the older adults they serve.

In 1992, the Older Americans Act was amended to address the need for advocacy to protect and enhance the rights and benefits of older adults. This included Prevention of Elder Abuse, Neglect and Exploitation Programs intended to "develop and strengthen activities to prevent and treat elder abuse, neglect, and exploitation . . . and coordinate with other State and local programs and services to protect vulnerable adults, particularly older individuals" (U.S. Administration on Aging, 2004, p. 2).

Health and Mental Health Frame

Elder abuse first came to the attention of the American public as a social issue of concern through a series of U.S. House of Representatives hearings on domestic violence in the late 1970s and early 1980s (U.S. House of Representatives, 1990). At that time, elder abuse was understood to include a frail, dependent elderly victim and an overwhelmed, inappropriate, or uncaring caregiver (Quinn & Tomita, 1997).

Prior to 1980, the health care system had developed protocols to identify domestic violence as it affected children and battered spouses (Wolf, 1988). It was something of a revelation to the American public as well as service providers that older adults were also being battered, neglected, and otherwise mistreated by family members in ways that seriously compromised their health. The medical profession, particularly physicians and nurses but also dentists, began to devise guidelines for the detection of elder abuse (Fulmer & O'Malley, 1987).

By the 1990s, concern about elder abuse prevention in the health care field prompted a number of initiatives, such as education of physicians and nurses on elder abuse and abuse prevention. The American Medical Association, the American Psychological Association, and the American Society of Nursing developed model protocols. Currently, the health and mental health care system is seeking to develop and implement prevention strategies as well as detection and intervention strategies to address elder abuse and neglect among patients.

Criminal Justice and Legal System Frame

The criminal justice and legal system took a long time to define elder abuse as an issue of concern to law enforcement. An early and important study on elder abuse and the police was undertaken by the Police Executive Research Forum and the American Association of Retired Persons (AARP; Plotkin, 1988). However, when law enforcement began to acknowledge elder abuse as a criminal justice issue, it modeled statutes after traditional domestic violence crimes, such as spousal assault, rape, stalking, and other criminal acts that are more likely to affect younger abuse victims.

Although the most prevalent crimes that constitute elder abuse are financial in nature, most law enforcement agencies do not identify financial crimes as forms of domestic violence. However, the district attorney and attorney general offices have moved aggressively against financial abuse of the elderly in the form of scams, financial exploitation by strangers, and related crimes. These include fraudulent mail solicitations targeting the elderly, where the U.S. Postal Service has collaborated with law enforcement to identify and prosecute con artists who prey on the elderly.

EFFECTIVE PREVENTIVE INTERVENTIONS

In spite of the difficulties in establishing a nationally uniform response system to address elder abuse and neglect as a significant social problem, a number of states, localities, professional organizations, agencies, and grassroots groups, including older adults themselves, have developed innovative elder abuse prevention programs and initiatives. These include prevention strategies that have been developed in the social services, health and mental health, and criminal justice frames.

While prevention is a relatively new concept in the field of elder abuse and neglect, preventive interventions have been developed and piloted that reflect universal, selective, and indicated preventive interventions. Outcome research is only beginning in the elder abuse field, however, and effectiveness has not been determined on an empirical basis for most initiatives (Bonnie, 2003).

Universal Preventive Interventions

Universal preventive interventions targeted to the general public or a whole population group that has been identified on the basis of age but not individual risk for elder abuse include the following.

Universal Preventive Social Service Programs
- Coalitions and consortiums of agencies serving older adults are supported by the area agencies on aging. An example is the East Bay Consortium for Elder Abuse Prevention, a California-based coalition established in 1984, which includes more than 150 public and private agencies and individuals in Alameda and Contra Costa counties. The mission is to coordinate, improve, and develop services that prevent and resolve problems of elder abuse and promote greater cooperation within the service system. It also provides training and technical assistance, multidisciplinary consultation, and information and referral.

- Public education campaigns, including subway poster campaigns, define elder abuse and neglect and explain how older adults can protect themselves from abuse and neglect.

- Pamphlets written for older adults give instructions on prevention of elder abuse and neglect from family members and in the community. The AARP provides fact sheets explaining the definition of elder abuse and identifying ways to prevent it.

- Education is provided for consumers, family members, and professionals. The Colorado State University Cooperative Extension provides educational seminars in preventing elder abuse and neglect. Many schools of social work include content on elder abuse in their educational curriculum.

- Speakers bureaus, such as one from Senior Services of Northern Kentucky, advertise the availability of abuse prevention speakers on the Internet.

- Elder abuse prevention services for immigrant populations are developed and publicized in native languages. Examples of this approach include the Asian Elder Abuse Prevention Project, serving the Asian and Pacific Islander community, and Mosaic, a multiservice program for older refugees in Phoenix, Arizona.

Universal Preventive Health Care Programs

- Medical societies educate their members on speaking to older adult patients about elder abuse and neglect as a preventive measure. The State Medical Society of Wisconsin has defined elder abuse for its members and provided guidelines on how to discuss this problem with older patients as a form of prevention.

- Coalitions of health care providers have formed to address the issue of elder abuse prevention. The Nutritional Screening Initiative led by the American Academy of Family Physicians and the American Dietetic Association, along with other health care provider organizations, is a project of a long-term care task force convened to address the problem of elder abuse and neglect as reflected in poor nutrition and to issue alerts to its members.

- The American Nursing Association has been active in developing protocols for discussing the prevention of elder abuse and neglect with older patients and their families.

- Both national and local advocacy groups have initiated nursing home abuse prevention through education of consumers and family members. The Bauman and Rasor Group, Inc., maintains a web site with information on choosing a nursing home, federal and state laws, remedies, and ensuring care is provided (www.nursinghomeabuse.com).

• States have passed laws encouraging the use of advance directives and health care proxies to enable older adults to retain control of their health care decision making even if faced with a mentally incapacitating condition like Alzheimer's, dementia, or stroke.

Universal Preventive Criminal Justice Programs

• Professional law enforcement organizations have developed and issued handbooks that include information on elder abuse prevention. An example is the National Sheriffs' Association, which prepared and disseminated a handbook that includes crime prevention tips for older adults.

• State attorneys general have become active in fraud and abuse prevention. The Consumer Protection Division of the Office of the Attorney General of Texas has focused efforts on the advertising and sale of insurance and retirement-oriented investments, financial planning services, estate planning, and legal services directed at older Texans; the advertising and sale of home improvements, medical devices, and other services and products that target seniors; and telemarketing and mail fraud aimed at senior citizens.

• Certified public accountants have initiated a campaign to educate themselves on elder financial abuse and issued guidelines for being proactive in financial abuse prevention with older clients.

• State bar associations are educating members on topics like financial abuse of older adults.

• Seminars are given to older adults in senior centers, retirement associations, religious settings, and other places where older adults may congregate, by law enforcement and other groups like bank tellers and officers, on how to recognize and avoid financial exploitation.

Selective Preventive Interventions

Selective Preventive Social Service Programs

• Multidisciplinary teams prevent elder abuse from occurring or escalating. An example is the L.A. Metro Multi-Disciplinary Team for Consultation on Elders at Risk. This program is funded through the Los Angeles adult protective services program.

• Caregivers' support programs and groups funded through the Older Americans Act and organizations like the Alzheimer's Foundation are intended to educate and provide emotional support to caregivers of older adults and prevent abuse and neglect.

- Respite care enables caregivers to get a break from the pressure of caregiving, particularly if the older adult being cared for is an Alzheimer's patient.

- Counseling is offered to family members who may have unresolved conflicts with older adult family members and are at risk for becoming abusive.

Selective Preventive Health Care Programs

- Health care institutions can also provide information and support for caregivers of family members with dementia and other forms of severe cognitive impairment. Counseling protocols, such as those developed at the New York University School of Medicine's Alzheimer's Disease Center, reflect a selective preventive intervention strategy (Mittelman, Epstein, & Pierzchala, 2003).

- Substance abuse screening conducted at hospital and clinic settings can identify substance abuse among older adult patients (Fink, Tsai, Hays, Moore, Morton, et al., 2002). While substance abuse by the elderly is not a cause of elder abuse, it can cause would-be victims to be more vulnerable to abuse by a family member or predatory significant other.

Selective Preventive Criminal Justice Programs

- Community policing initiatives have been developed that target prevention of elder abuse that rises to the level of a crime. One of the most promising community policing movements on a national level is TRIAD, a cooperative initiative of the National Sheriffs' Association, the International Association of Chiefs of Police, and the AARP. On the local level, TRIAD unites seniors with police and sheriffs' departments (www.oag.statetx.us/elder/elder.htm).

- State legislation has been passed to strengthen state-based elder abuse prevention efforts. In California, Assembly Bill 1819 was signed into law in 2000, requiring peace officers to be better trained to recognize and report elder abuse and help with prosecution of individuals who attempt to manipulate older adults into handing over their assets. This law has also stimulated county-based elder abuse public awareness campaigns (http://democrats .assembly.ca.gov/members/a12/press/p122000021.htm).

Indicated Preventive Interventions: Early Detection of Elder Abuse

Once elder abuse and neglect was framed as a social issue of concern through a series of hearings held by the U.S. House of Representatives in the late 1970s and early 1980s, professionals and groups representing older adult constituents, such as the AARP, began to develop and issue guidelines for the detection and intervention of elder abuse. Initially, the focus was on the frail elderly, and social service agencies were active in forming coalitions, sponsoring conferences, and training staff.

Physicians and nurses in the health care system were also beginning to recognize serious cases of elder abuse and neglect, particularly among the frail elderly, and developed assessment and intervention models (Fulmer & O'Malley, 1987). Social workers developed training for professionals in the social service, health, and mental health care systems on detection and intervention of elder abuse (Breckman & Adelman, 1988). Private and public sector APS lawyers called attention to the plight of the mentally incapacitated elder abuse victim and worked to change restrictive state mental hygiene laws related to conservatorships and guardianships. Law enforcement also developed and implemented training protocols on elder abuse (Plotkin, 1988).

Most of the systems that respond to the problem of elder abuse and neglect, once identified, are able to do so only when the abuse or neglect becomes serious enough to rise to the level of a housing crisis, health emergency, or crime. Interest in prevention has followed once some sense of the etiology of elder abuse and neglect became known and remedies developed. However, only recently has interest and attention been focused on early detection of elder abuse and neglect. This is a critical part of the continuum of responses to this issue.

It is also probably the most problematic. One reason is that remedies tend to come into play only when the abuse or neglect has reached a serious level, so early detection may not lead to any immediate possibility of intervention, frustrating professionals, family members, neighbors, and victims alike. A second reason is that early signs of elder abuse and neglect may be ambiguous, and calling attention to them may upset the victims and their family members and raise concerns among professionals, friends, and neighbors about undue intrusiveness. However, efforts targeting early detection have begun, linking scrutiny to known risk factors and the notion, based on what has been learned in the field of domestic violence, that abuse escalates over time. The early detection initiatives in elder abuse are analogous to Gordon's indicated preventive intervention category.

Indicated Preventive Intervention in Social Service Systems

- Senior centers and in-home meals programs serve as part of an early detection system for elder abuse or neglect. Center directors who notice that a member has suddenly stopped coming and may be a victim of civil confinement and home-bound meals providers who suddenly lose access to an older adult's household or hear shouting by other family members are the first line of defense against emergent abuse or neglect.

- Community-based agencies may notice a change in the cognitive functioning of an older adult that coincides with the relocation of an adult child or grandchild to the older adult's household. Some studies have indicated that two risk factors for abuse and neglect are a past history of abuse for the victim, something a social service agency that does psychosocial assessments may know, and characteristics of the abuser like substance abuse, mental illness, or criminal history. Cognitive impairment of the victim is not in itself a causative factor in elder abuse and neglect, but may render older adults less able to protect themselves if it occurs.

Indicated Preventive Interventions in Health and Mental Health Systems

- The American Society of Geriatric Dentistry uses professional journals to inform members on how to identify dental problems that may be suggestive of elder abuse or maltreatment, including nutritional deprivation.

- Nursing home advocates monitor staffing and salary levels of nursing home personnel, training, and staff-to-resident ratio and use these indicators as a flag for early detection of abuse or neglect. In Florida, an initiative called Operation Spot Check inspects nursing homes and adult living facilities. This represents collaboration among the Florida state attorney general's office, the Long Term Care Ombudsman's Council, and the Florida Area of Health Care Administration.

- Medical societies educate their members about red flags for elder abuse or neglect, including weight loss, anxiety and insomnia, pressure sores, absent devices such as hearing aids, dentures, or eyeglasses, scratches, and subtherapeutic levels of prescribed drugs. Although these may be indicators of other conditions, the possibility of abuse or neglect can be explored and ruled out.

Indicated Preventive Intervention in Criminal Justice/Legal Systems

- Local community policing programs, which have a crime prevention agenda, are also useful for the early detection of elder abuse and neglect. Community police are assigned to a specific neighborhood, where they get to know building superintendents, mail personnel, community residents, local bank managers, social service providers, and community activists. An adult protective services program may not accept referrals of suspected low-level or emergent abuse or neglect, but community police can respond to information from residents and workers about red flags such as older residents who withdraw money in the company of others, unclaimed mail, unsanitary living conditions, and family disputes loud enough to be heard by neighbors. These can be checked by community police and concerns referred to community-based social service agencies or senior centers for follow-up.

• Bank personnel and court personnel may be able to detect efforts to exploit older adults financially by con artists or guardians at an early stage and refer the information to local district attorneys for follow-up.

GAPS IN PREVENTIVE SERVICE SYSTEMS: PRACTICE AND POLICY IMPLICATIONS

The service needs of elder abuse victims extend beyond the traditional aging service network. Practice experience and studies have both demonstrated that older adults at risk of family abuse will not accept services for themselves if services are not also offered to their abusers (Dundorf & Brownell, 1995). Primary interventions for impaired family members can serve as elder abuse preventive service strategies. Intensive case management, substance abuse, mental health, housing, and counseling services must be expanded and earmarked for impaired family members who, without services, could become abusers. With younger spouse/partner abuse, traditionally there has been serious opposition to spending service dollars on abusers instead of victims. This has not been found to be an appropriate strategy for addressing elder abuse.

Continuation and support of interdisciplinary programs and coalitions are essential for ensuring that representatives of the many disciplines and service sectors coming into contact with older adults continue an ongoing dialogue. This should include the review and drafting of legislation that relates to elder abuse. This effort should not be targeted only to those bills that relate specifically to elder abuse. It should also target those that address the needs of impaired family members. One example is the New York State law, named Kendra's Law, that permits assisted outpatient treatment and involuntary medication of selected mentally ill patients who, as an unintended consequence of deinstitutionalization, may present a danger to others unless medicated (Somers, 2003). This is especially pertinent to elder abuse, as almost half of all mentally ill adults in New York State live with elderly parents after discharge from hospitals or prisons, according to Joy Braun, New York City National Alliance for the Mentally Ill (NAMI; personal communication, June 15, 1999). Legislation should be preventive as well as protective and should preserve the autonomy of elder abuse victims as much as possible.

The gaps in service identified here illustrate the limitations of taking a single-focus approach to elder abuse and neglect prevention. Criminal penalties for potential abusers may serve as part of a preventive strategy, but they are not always appropriate. Other policy areas have an impact on this problem as well. In fact, most existing policy and legislative remedies to date are at best bandages. Many service interventions used to address elder abuse are after the fact; not enough is done as a preventive measure. If prevention is a goal, the target of services must be extended beyond older people to include the larger network and community. Education and outreach and engaging other types of community organizations such as churches, synagogues, and mosques, as well as tribal leaders and libraries, are essential. Legislation such as the law passed in August 1999 giving New York State courts new authority to order former mental patients to comply with treatment is controversial, but at least attempts to take a proactive approach to violence prevention. This is important not only for the general public but for families of the mentally ill as well.

FUTURE DIRECTIONS

There have been many achievements in the past 30 years in framing elder abuse as a significant social problem in the United States. The challenges are threefold. First, the U.S. government should develop a national definition of elder abuse and neglect that transcends agency, service system, county, and state boundaries. Second, the search must continue for new and effective ways to address the current fragmentation among all the existing criminal justice, social service, and health and mental health care systems that assist elder abuse victims and their abusers. This fragmentation is reflected in uncoordinated legislation, social policies, and programs for abuse victims in the United States today. Third, providers, advocates, legislators, and older adults and their families are challenged to develop and implement a comprehensive approach to elder abuse and neglect, drawing on models of synthesis to develop common ground among service providers, legislators, and the aging advocacy community. The United States should also expand the efforts already under way to take a more proactive response to elder abuse and neglect, emphasizing prevention and early detection over crisis intervention, which is the primary method of addressing elder abuse and neglect today. With this foundation, the United States will be ready to move forward and address more effectively the problems of elder abuse and neglect in the new millennium.

A promising start has been made by the National Center for Elder Abuse (NCEA) with funding from the Administration on Aging and the Department of Justice's Office for Victims of Crime. NCEA sponsored the First National Policy Summit in Washington, DC, in December 2001. Over 80 distinguished experts from multiple disciplines and all parts of the country came together and prioritized recommendations that became an action agenda for elder abuse in the United States in the twenty-first century. Key among them are recommendations to enact a national elder abuse act and develop and sustain a public education campaign.

The Elder Justice Act was introduced in the U.S. Congress with broad bipartisan support in beginning in September 2002, and has been reintroduced in September 2004. If enacted into law, this act will focus federal attention on the issue of elder abuse and exploitation for the first time in the history of the United States. It will also provide funding to develop and test new models of prevention and early intervention services to older adults who may be at risk of mistreatment, both in the community and in institutional settings. This represents an important first step in recognizing the issue of elder abuse and neglect at the national level (Blancado, 2002; Breaux, 2002).

REFERENCES

Anonymous. (2002). Protecting older Americans: A history of federal action on elder abuse, neglect, and exploitation. *Journal of Elder Abuse and Neglect, 14*(2/3), 9–31.

Blancado, R. B. (2002). The elder justice act: A landmark policy initiative. *Journal of Elder Abuse and Neglect, 14*(2/3), 181–183.

Bonnie, R. J. (2003). Risk factors for elder abuse. In R. J. Bonnie & R. B. Wallace (Eds.), *Elder mistreatment: Abuse, neglect, and exploitation in an aging America* (pp. 88–103). Washington, DC: National Academy of Sciences.

Breaux, J. (2002). To promote elder justice and for other purposes (§ 333 IS, 109th Cong., 1st Sess.). *Journal of Elder Abuse and Neglect, 14*(2/3), 87–178.

Breckman, R., & Adelman, R. (1988). *Strategies for helping victims of elder mistreatment.* Thousand Oaks, CA: Sage.

Brownell, P., Berman, J., & Salamone, A. (1999). Mental health and criminal justice issues among perpetrators of elder abuse. *Journal of Elder Abuse and Neglect, 11*(4), 81–94.

Brownell, P., Welty, A., & Brennan, M. (2000). *Project 2015: The future of aging in New York State.* Albany: New York State Office for the Aging.

Burr, J. J. (1982). *Protective services for adults.* Washington, DC: Administration on Aging, Office of Human Development Series.

Choi, N. G., Kulick, D. B., & Mayer, J. (1999). Financial exploitation of elders: Analysis of risk factors based on county adult protective services data. *Journal of Elder Abuse and Neglect, 10*(3/4), 39–62.

Dundorf, K., & Brownell, P. (1995). Elder abuse: What is it; what can be done about it? *Family Advocate, 17*(3), 81–84.

Filinson, R. (2001). Evaluation of the impact of a volunteer ombudsman program: The Rhode Island experience. *Journal of Elder Abuse and Neglect, 13*(4), 1–19.

Fink, A., Tsai, M., Hays, R., Moore, A. A., Morton, S. C., Spritzer, K., et al. (2002). Comparing the alcohol-related problems survey (ARPS) to traditional alcohol screening measure in elderly outpatients. *Archives of Gerontology and Geriatrics, 34,* 55–78.

Forgey, M. (2000). Capitalizing on strengths: A resiliency enhancement model for at-risk youths. In E. Norman (Ed.), *Resiliency enhancement: Putting the strengths perspective into social work practice* (pp. 213–226). New York: Columbia University Press.

Fulmer, T., & O'Malley, T. (1987). *Inadequate care of the elderly: A health care perspective on abuse and neglect.* New York: Springer.

Gordon, R. (1983). An operational classification of disease prevention. *Public Health Reports, 98,* 107–109.

Gordon, R. (1987). An operational classification of disease prevention. In J. A. Steinberg & M. M. Silverman (Eds.), *Preventing mental disorders* (pp. 20–26). Rockville, MD: U.S. Department of Health and Human Services.

Hudson, T. (1989). An analysis of the concepts of elder mistreatment, abuse and neglect. *Journal of Elder Abuse and Neglect, 1,* 5–25.

Lau, E. A., & Kosberg, J. I. (1979, September/October). Abuse of the elderly by informal care providers. *Aging,* 10–15.

Le, Q. K. (1997). Mistreatment of Vietnamese elderly by their families in the United States. *Journal of Elder Abuse and Neglect, 9*(2), 51–62.

Mittelman, M., Epstein, C., & Pierzchala, A. (2003). *Counseling the Alzheimer's caregiver: A resource for health care professionals.* Chicago: American Medical Association (AMA) Press.

Nerenberg, L. (2000). Developing a service response to elder abuse. *Generations, 24*(11), 86–94.

Pillemer, K., & Finkelhor, D. (1988). The prevalence of elder abuse: A random sample survey. *Gerontologist, 28*(1), 51–57.

Pillemer, K., & Finkelhor, D. (1989). Causes of elder abuse: Caregiver stress versus problem relatives. *American Orthopsychiatric Association, 59*(2), 51–57.

Plotkin, M. (1988). *A time for dignity: Police and domestic violence of the elderly.* Washington, DC: Police Executive Research Forum and American Association of Retired Persons.

Quinn, M., & Tomita, S. (1997). *Elder abuse and neglect: Causes, diagnosis, and intervention strategies* (2nd ed.). New York: Springer.

Reis, M. (2000). The IOA screen: The abuse-alert measure that dispels myths. *Generations, 24*(11), 13–16.

Shibusawa, T. (2004, March 4). *Older women and abuse: A global research agenda.* Paper presented at the United Nations NGO Committee on Ageing, New York.

Somers, S. B. (2003). *Protective services for adults in New York state: Fighting adult abuse while restoring dignity and quality of life to New York's impaired adults.* Albany: New York State Office of Children and Families.

Tatara, T. (1995). Elder abuse. In R. L. Edwards (Ed.), *Encyclopedia of social work* (19th ed., pp. 834–842). Washington, DC: National Association of Social Workers.

Tatara, T., & Thomas, C. (1998). *National elder abuse incidence study: Final report.* Washington, DC: National Center on Elder Abuse at the American Public Human Services Organization in collaboration with Westat, Inc.

U.S. Administration on Aging. (2004). Older Americans Act History. Available from www.aoa.gov/aoa/pages/titlevii.html.

U.S. Census Bureau. (2002). *Census 2000 summary file 1. General Population Characteristics, United States.* Washington, DC: Government Printing Office.

U.S. House of Representatives, Select Committee on Aging. (1990). *Elder abuse: Decade of shame and inaction.* Washington, DC: Government Printing Office.

Wolf, R. (1988). Elder abuse: Ten years later. *Journal of the American Geriatrics Society, 36,* 758–762.

Wolf, R., & Pillemer, K. (1984). *Working with the abused elderly: Assessment, advocacy and intervention.* Wooster: University of Massachusetts Medical Center, University Center on Aging.

Zorza, J. (1999). Recent elder abuse findings. *Domestic Violence Report, 4*(4), 51–52.

Chapter 19

INSTITUTIONALIZATION AND RESIDENTIAL LIVING

MARY ANN OVERCAMP-MARTINI

What do we do for individuals who need more care than can be provided in their homes, or who do not have homes in which to receive care? Of all social problems, this remains our greatest quandary. Historically, the main residential strategies have been nursing facilities for those who are elderly with medical problems, state institutions and intermediate care facilities for those with mental retardation and developmental disabilities, and state and private psychiatric hospitals for those with serious mental illness. A brief review of this history demonstrates the embeddedness of our services in the structures of the past, even as we shift incrementally toward home and community services in the future.

Early in our history, we grappled with this complicated dilemma first by relocating people into poorhouses. Moving them out of poorhouses into institutions more suited to their particular needs was the progress marking the nineteenth century. At one point, effective treatment was characterized by the structure of the patient's day and the architectural structure of the facility, including the optimum size for a facility of about 200 (Grob, 1994; Wolfensberger, 1975). Although there were intense international discussions regarding the requirements for effective institutional treatment, the political economy of the United States was already such that the optimum size was quickly set aside. By the 1950s, institutions numbered in the thousands. For example, at the peak of the institutional period in 1955 there were an estimated 558,922 individuals with mental illness placed in institutional care nationally (National Institute of Mental Health, 1955).

As a result of multiple factors, a deinstitutionalization movement began for those in psychiatric hospitals and institutions for the developmentally disabled. These changes commenced with the introduction of the major tranquilizers in the 1950s, accelerated with the passage of Title XIX and Title XX of the Social

Security Act, and were supported and maintained by the disability rights movement. With even the minimal amount of money available for individuals under the Supplementary Security Income (SSI) and health insurance under Medicare and Medicaid, individuals were increasingly able to live in the home of parents or other relatives and in the evolving board and care home industry. Adding to these factors were the lawsuits on behalf of those who were institutionalized and the advocacy of family member coalitions. Alternatives to placement in large institutions have increased since that time, with subsequent decreasing numbers of U.S. citizens living in institutional care. Unfortunately, much of the deinstitutionalization was actually what Hollingsworth (1994) calls "trans-institutionalization," in which residents of institutions for those with mental illness or mental retardation were moved to placements in smaller institutions such as nursing homes, rather than into community-based placements designed specifically for their appropriate care and treatment.

For elderly needing residential assistance, the historical placement was the nursing home. Only recently has a separate trend among the elderly and those caring for the elderly led to a similar marked preference for services close to home and community and away from nursing home care. Although the bias toward institutional care remains in service systems and funding streams, the shift toward choice and empowerment of the elderly has linked with the goals of those advocating in the area of disabilities. The result is a momentous shift in the philosophy of care toward prevention of both institutionalization and residential placement. Because, in many cases, the residential alternatives have themselves been developed to prevent institutionalization, the focus in this chapter is largely on the development of a comprehensive continuum of care and treatment, describing the strategies useful in preventing people from reaching the institutional end of the continuum.

TRENDS AND INCIDENCE

Data from the National Health Interview Survey (NHIS) show that the 38 million noninstitutionalized people with disabilities in the United States claim a total of 61 million disabling conditions. For the purpose of the NHIS, disability is defined as a "limitation in social or other activity that is caused by a chronic mental or physical disorder, injury, or impairment" (LaPlante, 1996, p. 1). Disability rates have risen dramatically in the past 25 years, largely as a result of shifts in the nation's demographics. The shift toward an aging population accounts for a gradual rise in disabilities, but there has also been a recent rise in the numbers of young adults and children who are reported to have disabilities. For those 65 years and older the disability rate in 1994 was about 39% for women and 38% for men. Among younger adults (age 18 to 44), an increase from 8.7% for men and 8.9% for women in 1990 to 10.2% for men and 10.3% for women in 1994 occurred; orthopedic problems and mental and nervous disorders have also increased for this age group (LaPlante & Carlson, 1996).

Individuals with disabilities encompass such a wide variety of people and issues that it is difficult to provide a cohesive picture of problems or incidence. In general, there are three main categories of adults with disabilities: adults with developmental disabilities, adults (nonelderly and elderly) with physical, cognitive, or psychiatric disabilities, and adults with mental illness.

Adults with Developmental Disabilities

Adults whose serious disabling problems began at birth or in their developing years are said to have developmental disabilities. Because the disabling condition affects them in their developing years, it is assumed to have significantly affected their life course. By federal law, developmental disabilities are any severe, chronic disability that is

> caused by a mental or physical impairment or combination of mental and physical impairments and is evident before 22 years of age, is likely to continue indefinitely, and which results in substantial functional limitations in three or more of the following areas of major life activity: self-care, receptive and expressive language, learning, mobility, self-direction, capacity for independent living, or economic self-sufficiency.

These individuals are in need of treatment or care of a lifelong or extended period that is individually planned and coordinated. Between 1.2% and 1.65% of the U.S. population is considered developmentally disabled, representing between 3.2 and 4.5 million individuals (The Developmental Disabilities Assistance and Bill of Rights Act of 2000).

Adults with Physical, Cognitive, or Psychiatric Disabilities

This category comprises individuals whose disability occurred after age 22, or whose difficulties may have become more disabling to them over the course of a lifetime. This is the largest group of those considered disabled in this country, numbering some 52.6 million with some disability and 33 million with severe disabilities (U.S. Census Bureau, 2003). Most relevant to this discussion of risk of institutionalization or residential placement for adults are the individual's functional limitations caused by those disabilities, which increase the need for care by others. Although categorized in a variety of ways, functional limitations usually are determined by the number and interaction of disabling conditions affecting the ability to perform the activities of daily living (ADLs) and the instrumental activities of daily living (IADLs). ADLs are those skills basic to care of oneself, such as bathing, dressing, toileting, eating, and mobility. IADLs encompass those activities requiring mastery to maintain independence and self-sufficiency, such as food preparation, housekeeping skills, shopping, and money management. Difficulty or inability to perform ADLs or IADLs may affect individuals of any age. For the nonelderly population (age 18 to 64) living in the community in 1994, over 3.3 million or 2.1% received assistance of some kind. Of the 33 million elderly (age 65 and older) in 1994, almost 17% received assistance, with 11.8% living in the community and 4.9% living in institutional care (Spector, Fleishman, Pezzin, & Spillman, 2003).

Adults with Serious Mental Illness

Reporting the incidence of serious mental illness as a separate issue is important to understanding the use and prevention of institutional and residential care. For those with serious mental illness and accompanying potential for crisis, the risk of hospitalization or institutionalization rests with a different set of factors than with long-term physical disability. An estimate of the prevalence of mental illness is dependent on the configuration of diagnoses included, but usually the prevalence in the United States is considered to be between 10% and 20% (Chandler, 1990). The Epidemiologic Catchment Area program of the National Institute of Mental Health officially reported that 22% of the U.S. adult population has a mental disorder in a given 1-year period, with 2.8% of the population affected by a severe mental disorder, and 1.7% both affected by a severe mental disorder and actually using related mental health services.

Institutionalized Adults

Looking at those who are currently institutionalized, including in nursing facilities (1.6 million), institutions for those with mental retardation (106,000), and facilities for those with mental illness (57,000), an overall estimate is that 1.8 million U.S. citizens are housed in institutional settings at any given time (*Long-Term Care,* 2001). Given the cyclical nature of many mental illnesses, those being admitted and discharged repeatedly represent a core number of

100,000. A snapshot of the recent history of transinstitutionalization of those with mental illness may be helpful in describing the shift in placements.

While estimates of those institutionalized with mental illness in the United States have decreased from a peak of 558,922 in 1955 (National Institute of Mental Health, 1955) to 92,054 in 1990 (National Institute of Mental Health, 1990), this core number of the difficult state hospital clients (Goldman, Adams, & Taube, 1983) is expected to remain, with admissions no longer decreasing but, in fact, likely to increase (*Care of the Institutionalized,* 1985). Since deinstitutionalization, Isaac and Armat (1990) estimate that 800,000 individuals with Schizophrenia and Bipolar Disorder now live with relatives, mostly parents. By 1977, 100,000 state hospital patients had been transinstitutionalized to nursing home care, shifting some of the financial costs from the states to the federal budget (Department of Health and Human Services, 1980). Studies have consistently shown that approximately 35% of the homeless population has a serious mental illness, suggesting that about 150,000 people with serious mental illness lived on the streets in 1995. About 10% of those incarcerated in jails and prisons are also seriously mentally ill, numbering approximately 159,000 (Torrey, 1997). It is clear that along with the core 100,000 state hospital clients, those with serious mental illness have also been transinstitutionalized to nursing facilities, jails, and prisons, as well as being allowed to disengage from services altogether by entering the ranks of the homeless.

Individuals at Risk for Institutionalization

Clearly, the estimate of those at risk for institutionalization is more difficult to compute. The General Accounting Office recently defined this population as those having difficulty or inability to perform two ADLs and four IADLs, or three or more ADLs. Those living at home or in community-based residential settings in need of substantial assistance to perform two or more ADLs, an estimated 2.3 million individuals, are most at risk of institutionalization (*Long-Term Care,* 2001). Also at highest risk of institutionalization are those with multiple and interacting disabilities, those with behavioral dysfunctions, and those in psychiatric crisis or who are a danger to self or others.

RISK FACTORS

Any serious physical, cognitive, or psychiatric disability may act as a risk factor for residential or institutional placement. Each disability presents a separate picture of who is affected, how many, and what the risk factors are known to be. For the estimated 4.5 million individuals with Alzheimer's disease, for instance, this progressive disorder of the brain's nerve cells affects memory, thinking, and behavior, taking as long as 20 years to result in death. Risk factors for Alzheimer's disease are still largely undetermined, but include aging, family history, rare genetics, and possibly high cholesterol and high blood pressure. Only some of these factors are amenable to changes in lifestyle; others are seemingly beyond normal health changes (Alzheimer's Association, 2004). In contrast, the prevailing causes of traumatic brain injuries are traffic and firearm accidents, which may be preventable in the young males most affected through education, vocational opportunities, and access to substance abuse and mental health treatments (Forkosch, Kaye, & LaPlante, 1995).

However, it is not only the presence of a disabling condition or disorder that acts as a risk factor for placement in institutional or residential care. The lack of appropriate home and community-based services is currently the greatest risk factor for institutional or residential placement.

Disability

Functional disabilities occur because of chronic physical and mental disorders, impairments, and injuries. A brief description of these causal factors includes the following:

- Chronic physical health disorders are represented most commonly by heart disease, back problems, arthritis, orthopedic impairments, asthma, and diabetes (National Health Interview Survey, 1992).
- Serious mental disorders include (1) disorders with psychotic symptoms such as Bipolar Disorder, Schizophrenia, and Schizoaffective Disorder, and (2) the more severe forms of other disorders such as Unipolar Disorder, Panic Disorder, and Obsessive-Compulsive Disorder. Of these, Schizophrenia is the most common diagnosis among those with serious mental illness (National Advisory Mental Health Council, 1993).
- Impairments include deficits in vision, hearing, sensation, and speech, learning disabilities, paralysis, deformities, absence of anatomical structures such as limbs, and other orthopedic problems. They are considered to be "deficits of bodily structure or function, either congenital in origin or acquired from a past or ongoing disorder or injury" (LaPlante, 1996, p. 1).
- Injuries are included as impairments when they have caused the difficulty, but as a discrete category when they have not, creating some complication

in the presentation of the data. However, injuries causing a substantial limitation in activities account for about 1 million disabling conditions (LaPlante, 1996).

Lack of Home- and Community-Based Services

The greatest risk factor for residential or institutional placement is not the presence of a disabling disorder, impairment, or injury but the absence of the services and supports known to maintain people in their homes and communities. In other words, the greatest risk factor may well be someone's residency. For instance, the fact that 23 states do not provide any personal assistance services in the home under the Medicaid Home and Community-Based Waiver program means that in the absence of family caregiving, anyone in those states needing personal assistance may need to move to a higher level of care. Similarly, although all states provide some alternative services under the Home and Community-Based Waiver program under Medicaid, the services are "unevenly available within and across States, and reach a small percentage of eligible individuals" (Medicaid Community-Based Attendant Services and Supports Act of 2003).

In the same way, people are at risk for institutionalization in communities and states that lack access to the best practice models known to ameliorate people's difficulties so that they can continue to reside in home- and community-based settings. States or contracting agencies may not have adopted the models for use in their programs, or may have funded only a pilot program or one small program for an entire area. If the model programs are not available, they cannot provide the best known opportunity to prevent a greater level of residential placement or institutionalization.

EFFECTIVE UNIVERSAL PREVENTIVE INTERVENTIONS

Universal preventive interventions target the general public or a whole population group that has not been identified on the basis of individual risk. Universal preventive interventions relevant to the prevention of institutionalization or residential placement are those that are targeted to the general public to maintain physical health, cognitive health and development, and psychiatric health.

For each of the various disabling conditions, there is research suggesting linkage to genetic or hereditary conditions, prenatal care, and accidents. There is much that we do not know; however, improvements in prenatal and general health care generally decrease the incidence of disabling conditions. Similarly, early intervention and early education to ameliorate the child's disorder and to provide family education and supports may decrease the likelihood of later residential or institutional placement.

Prevention of injury and impairment through injury is another universal preventive intervention. Traffic accidents account for the largest number of cases of traumatic brain injuries, at about 31% of the estimated 1.9 million injuries a year. Therefore, preventing such accidents and their severity will lessen the occurrence of this type of disability. Similarly, strategies to decrease the number of firearm accidents and household and workplace accidents will also help to decrease the number of traumatic brain injuries sustained, particularly by young adults; about half of these are severe enough to cause significant short-term disability (Forkosch et al., 1995).

Just as middle-class status acts as a buffer against stress-related problems of abuse and neglect in families (Schorr & Schorr, 1989), economic stability can protect individuals and families from disabling conditions related to stress. In particular, public policy that protects families from the economic burdens of caring for their own members is public policy that can prevent unnecessary residential and institutional placements. A national health care policy incorporating economic strategies that protect families against the cost of long-term care is vital. Similarly, parity in insurance is necessary so that certain disabling conditions such as mental illness are not automatically ruled out of insurance coverage. Availability of housing under a state and national housing policy is also critical as a universal preventive intervention. Finally, a comprehensive family policy is needed, including economic and social supports for families providing care. Strategies such as economic allowances, tax breaks and incentives, and vouchers for services should be implemented for those providing the care that society would otherwise have to provide.

EFFECTIVE SELECTIVE PREVENTIVE INTERVENTIONS

For individuals who are at higher risk of being placed residentially, selective preventive interventions assist them to remain in their homes. These are generally individuals who are having difficulty performing ADLs without assistance. Currently, the main strategies for intervention are family caregiving and related supports, day care, personal care assistance, and assistive technology. Case management continues to be the main systemic strategy for brokering these various support services, sometimes becoming intensive in its implementation with individuals with disabilities and especially serious mental illness.

For instance, intensive case management is the backbone of the best practice model for individuals with serious mental illness most at risk for repeated (revolving door) hospitalization.

Family Caregiving

Social and economic support systems for family members providing care in the home is the frontline defense against out-of-home placements of all kinds. Family caregiving has historically been, and is currently, the mainstay of care of those with disabling conditions. Often, this involves the care activities of the spouse, allowing married people more opportunity to remain at home. Almost 66% of the 5.9 million caregivers providing informal care in 1994 were either spouses or children of the 3.6 million elderly recipients. Of all care providers, most were women, and most were the daughters of the elderly person (Spector et al., 2003).

There are few social situations more stressful than caregiving. According to the 1990 Pepper Commission, 2.4 million Americans living at home have such severe physical or mental impairments that they need full-time care. Caregivers often provide social and health services for periods of 10 years or more, saving the nation millions of dollars in the cost of alternative care. There are, however, costs to the individual caregiver—not only economic costs associated with working less or not working in the job market, but social costs such as depression, anxiety, and anger (Zarit, 1994). Formal support services for caregivers are fragmented and unevenly distributed, although nearly every state provides some assortment of these services. Until recently, support services for family members caring for those with disabilities were funded solely from state funds. Since 2000, the National Family Caregiver Support Program provides some federal funding to the states for education, training, counseling, respite care, and support groups.

Family Education

Education and skills training may involve both medical and social aspects of care for someone who is sick, who has a chronic health or mental health disorder, or who has been substantially injured. In the case of someone with medical disorders, this may involve education and skills training to perform medical care for the individual. It may also involve information regarding such issues as loss and grief, family communications, and techniques for alleviating stressors. For those caring for someone with a serious mental illness, family psychoeducation increases the effectiveness of drug therapy by stabilizing family dynamics and communications (Hogarty et al., 1991). Education may also involve valuable information regarding aspects of the social service system otherwise unknown to the family caregiver.

Respite Care

Respite care refers to formal substitute care that allows the caregiver time away from caregiving responsibilities. Substitute care may be provided in the individual's home or in a community-based or institutional setting for brief periods of time. Most respite care programs define those eligible for substitute care as caregivers who reside with the individual receiving care. For those caregivers who reside elsewhere, as is often the case with adult daughters, respite services are generally not available. Due to the prevalence of emotional problems for caregivers—one estimate is that more than 45% show symptoms of depression (Zarit, 1994) individual and family counseling as well as caregiver support groups are additional strategies for support. The importance of case management in increasing the utilization and coordination of support services is well documented. However, it remains difficult to encourage families to accept services early enough to be truly preventive. According to McConnell and Riggs (1994), the "more common situation is that of the caregiver who reaches the end of his or her rope before asking for help, by which time it may be too late to keep the family together" (p. 27).

Personal Care Assistance

Understandably, the use of formal care increases with greater disability levels in functional abilities. There is evidence that the overall use of formal care has also increased due to other factors, such as caregivers' higher level of education, economic ability to purchase services, and changing perceptions of the historical preference for social care provided by family, friends, or neighbors (Cantor & Gruland, 1993). In other words, the purchase or provision of formal support services such as personal assistance services has become for many a preferred or supplementary approach for personal or family member care.

Personal assistance services provide assistance with ADLs and IADLs. About 16% of Americans 65 and older require some personal assistance; of those, 80% live at home or in community-based alternatives. Among those 18 to 64, however, there has been a rise in the rates of those needing personal assistance due to substantial disabilities, from 2% in the 1980s to 2.7% in 1993 (Kaye, LaPlante, Carlson, & Wenger, 1996).

Assistive Technology and Home Adaptations

Assistive technology is any equipment that enhances the functional independence of people with disabilities. A few examples of the many types and variety of assistive technology are communication devices, environmental controls, personal care equipment, walking devices, mobility equipment, transportation vehicles, and computer hardware, software, and accessories. The ABLEDATA database (www.abledata.com), funded by the National Institute on Disability and Rehabilitation Research, provides comprehensive information on assistive technology and rehabilitation equipment. Universal design for housing and home modifications for a wide variety of disabling conditions is also becoming more prevalent and more readily accessible to the consumer.

Adult Day Services

Another alternative care service is adult day services. These are structured programs to provide part-time health, social, and other support services to individuals with functional impairments. Not only can these programs provide important medical and social services through individual care plans, they are also a form of indirect respite care for caregivers. Social interaction is a benefit for many recipients, as well as health monitoring, supervised therapeutic activities, and medication monitoring. Adult day services are available in many larger communities as specialized services for those who are elderly, who are developmentally disabled, and who have psychiatric illnesses. They usually are provided in conjunction with other selective preventive interventions.

Other Specialized Preventive Interventions

For nonelderly adults with developmental disabilities, physical disabilities, and serious mental illness, the past 25 years have witnessed a rapid shift in services to the home and community, with specialized services to meet the needs of these various groups. Because of the importance of work to this age group and the link between SSI benefits and disability, for instance, specialized work programs have become particularly important as a preventive measure. An ongoing problem for most individuals with serious mental illness, for instance, is the ability to maintain full-time employment, with estimates at only 8% to 15% involved in part-time or full-time employment (Anthony & Blanch, 1987; Braitman et al., 1995). In any increase from part-time to full-time employment, rising income can bar a disabled individual from the twin benefits of SSI and Medicaid, long considered a disincentive toward full employment. One recent addition to services is a program under Social Security called the Ticket to Work program. In 1999, the Ticket to Work and Work Incentives Improvement Act was passed, allowing disabled individuals who work or who wish to return to work at an income higher than previously allowed to buy into Medicaid coverage. With a Ticket to Work, individuals may now obtain employment, vocational rehabilitation, and other support services from an employment network of their choice during a transitional period in which they can retain economic and medical coverage. Economic and social stabilization can alleviate the stress related to decompensation and possibly prevent unnecessary hospitalization or higher-level care and treatment.

EFFECTIVE INDICATED PREVENTIVE INTERVENTIONS

Indicated preventive interventions are those directed at individuals with functional disabilities of any kind for whom preventive interventions may lessen the likelihood of institutional or residential placement. For people who have serious functional disabilities and are without caregiving or access to personal assistance or assistive technology, these preventive interventions may include such programs and services as adult foster care, group home care, assisted living, intensive supported living, or supported treatment services. Where this wide range of service alternatives is available, it is more the profound nature of multiple and interacting disabilities or other critical problems such as behavioral dysfunctions or psychiatric crisis that lead to institutional placement or a more structured residential placement. At the present time, we are also seeing a growing population of aging individuals with developmental disabilities and serious mental illness for whom established adult vocational and residential programs may no longer be adequate.

For individuals with severe disabilities without a home or family caregiving, housing with personal assistance services becomes the community-based alternative. The variety of alternatives has increased in the past couple of decades, including adult foster care, group homes, and other supported living arrangements. In community-supported living arrangements, an individual may live alone or with someone else in an apartment or other housing arrangement, with staff support for individually designed service provision for such needs as medication management, transportation, or budgeting and financial management.

For those at highest risk for placement in nursing homes, another alternative with increasing popularity is the assisted living facility, in which an individual can receive assistance in those areas of ADLs and IADLs at the level needed while living in a facility with other individuals. Presently, few states provide funding through Medicaid waiver programs, although some long-term insurance programs will provide for this level of service. There are about 1 million Americans in nearly 20,000 residences receiving some assisted living services.

For individuals with serious mental illness, psychiatric crisis often prompts hospitalization or institutionalization because of the gravity of the medical issue or the danger to self or others. Danger to self or others can also be a critical issue with individuals who do not have a serious mental illness but are involved in some other type of emotional crisis or behavioral dysfunction. At the time of crisis, the individual may be living independently or with few supportive services. While appropriate medication is generally the single most important treatment tool for mental illness, 60% of people generally relapse at some time. To strengthen the efficacy of medical intervention, psychosocial support systems can be built around the individual to buffer environmental stressors. Alleviating stressors through psychosocial interventions can reduce this hospitalization rate (National Advisory Mental Health Council, 1993). These support systems can take a variety of forms, and individuals who receive these specialized community services are substantially less likely to have psychiatric relapse.

To identify the range of services and supports recognized as vital to effective treatment for those with mental illness, the National Institute of Mental Health has developed a model of what it calls a "community support system." In this model, a case manager brokers services from a variety of agencies to meet the identified needs of the client. The greatest area of need, as with other populations, is housing; any systemic alternative to hospitalization inevitably includes some parts of the range of housing alternatives: family, adult foster care, board and care, group homes, nursing homes, hotel rooms, and homeless shelters (Fellin, 1996). The other nine components of this system include the following (Stroul, 1987):

- Outreach
- Assistance in meeting basic human needs
- Mental health care
- Twenty-four-hour crisis assistance
- Psychosocial and vocational services
- Consultation and education
- Natural support systems
- Protection of rights
- Case management

Although these support services can be brokered, programs that bundle them under one umbrella with intensive case management services have been found to be particularly effective with the 20% of clients at high risk of psychiatric readmission (Stein, 1990). The original model of intensive case management is the Program of Assertive Community Treatment (PACT) model. The PACT model attempts to establish a hospital without walls around the discharged client, what Hogarty (1991) calls a "therapeutic umbrella." Assertive outreach is crucial to the PACT approach, including mobile treatment teams for the more difficult-to-treat clients. Outcome studies suggest that PACT is particularly effective at lengthening community tenure for those at high risk for psychiatric readmissions as well as engaging and retaining clients in treatment (Herinckx, Kineey, Clarke, & Pauson, 1997; Stein & Test, 1985). Family advocacy and consumer groups have advocated for years for an increase in the number of PACT programs, which have stabilized many individuals without hospitalization or institutionalization.

PRACTICE AND POLICY IMPLICATIONS

Prevention of institutional and residential placement relies on the access and availability of alternative home- and community-based residential placements and services. Individuals with disabilities and their family members experience the fragility of the service system during times of cutbacks in funding for services as they struggle to maintain people in their homes and in their communities until there are no more options other than placement.

Along with access to and availability of services, there is an ongoing need for research in all areas of preventive interventions. With some groups, such as those with developmental disabilities and mental illness who are now aging out of adult vocational services, we have little descriptive information even in terms of projected utilization and service needs. With other groups, such as the elderly with disabilities, there is a strong knowledge base regarding utilization and service needs, but less understanding of the effectiveness of the variety of interventions (Spector, Shaffer, Hodlewsky, De La Mare, & Rhoades, 2002).

In particular, an insufficient level of service on the front end, within the home and family, is most common. For instance, involving caregivers of Alzheimer's patients in educational and supportive programs at the point of diagnosis rather than when they are reaching the end of their ability to provide may allow them to access supportive services more willingly throughout the course of their caregiving. In turn, willingness to access a variety of supportive services may extend their ability to maintain someone in the home or community.

The greatest need in the prevention of institutionalization is the continual implementation of effective models, with access and availability at the home and community levels. A national health care policy incorporating economic strategies that protect families against the cost of long-term care is vital to any preventive intervention policy. When public funding is involved, the increasing use of home- and community-based waivers under Medicaid is essential.

In each of these areas there are innumerable recommendations for policy and practice that the practitioner should further explore. To name a few of these:

- Practitioners should encourage supportive services as early as possible to family caregivers, while increasing the skills of family members to function as informal case managers for family members. Linkages between informal and formal case management systems should be developed and nurtured.

- Advocacy for access to personal assistance care should be increased, so that more individuals can remain in their homes and communities. Currently, there are 18 states still completely without a "personal care option" in their Medical Assistance State Plans (Medicaid). New are those states experimenting with the use of personal assistance services for those with psychiatric and cognitive disabilities, including reminders for medication compliance and safety assurance tasks, so that more individuals can live independently (Litvak, 1998). The preferred model for all adults with disabilities is now the independent living model, in which the individual with disabilities selects, trains, and manages the personal assistance worker (Batavia, 1998).

- PACT-type teams and assertive outreach activities for those who have disabilities or mental illness and who are homeless should be available in all communities.

- Extension of the Ticket to Work program, with both subsidization of individual's income and opportunities for work should be included in an overall plan for improved quality of life for those with both cognitive and physical disabilities.

- An interlocking of developmental disabilities policy, with its aggressive community-based alternatives, with resource development for the disabled elderly could lead to an overall improvement in service provision.

- Emphasis should be placed on quality of life issues in the process of developing home- and community-based services. Community inclusion can be accomplished in a variety of ways, but sometimes a more structured residential placement can provide continuity and security in ways most appropriate to the needs of the individual. In other words, the policy direction of services should not take precedence over the needs of the individual.

- Advocates will need to monitor the impact of a recent federal initiative, the Health Insurance Flexibility and Accountability Demonstration Initiative, that allows states to add uninsured individuals to Medicaid rolls but also allows them to hold spending to current levels. In effect, the states are now able to cut access to these community-based services used increasingly as preventive interventions for many of those who are elderly and disabled (Mathis, 2001).

- Cutbacks in mental health services and the fragmentation of services have increased the use of hospital emergency rooms for emergency holds for psychiatric patients. To decrease the practice of dumping patients without care, Congress passed the Emergency Medical Treatment and Active Labor Act (EMTALA) in 1986, requiring screening even for individuals with psychiatric symptomatology. Attempts to scale back the requirements of EMTALA should be monitored for implications regarding mental health care.

FUTURE DIRECTIONS

The future is choice. The disability rights, mental health consumer, and family advocacy groups and advocacy coalitions for the elderly have often worked separately toward the same goal. They are increasingly joining forces in their quest for greater choice and empowerment of the consumer and family member. This trend toward individuated services under the control of the consumer or family member as primary case manager seems to be the service philosophy of the future. Two important factors involved in this move are the *Olmstead* decision and the Medicaid waiver program as represented by proposed bills such as the Medicaid Community-Based Attendant Services and Supports Act (MiCASSA).

Olmstead Decision

The most impressive victory for preventive intervention services to date may have come with the *Olmstead* decision (*Olmstead v. L. C.,* 1999). This U.S. Supreme Court decision addressed issues regarding placement and care for individuals with disabilities. Brought on behalf of two women with mental illness and developmental disabilities in effect stuck in a psychiatric hospital by the lack of community-based services, *Olmstead* determined that states might be violating the Americans with Disabilities Act (ADA, 1990). The ADA requires that public entities provide services in "the most integrated setting appropriate to the needs of qualified individuals with disabilities" (ADA, 28 CFR § 35.130 (d)). The *Olmstead* decision has been interpreted to pertain to anyone at risk of institutionalization, not only those with developmental disabilities or mental illness.

The impact of the *Olmstead* decision remains unclear. The ruling does not require a wholesale revision of state care, but does require that reasonable progress be made in the development and implementation of state plans. In 2001, there were *Olmstead*-related lawsuits in about half the states. With the potential for ongoing legal filings, combined with a growing public expectation for community care, the push toward community-based care is likely to grow for all individuals whose ability to care for themselves has become impaired. That number is likely to increase as the boomer generation is affected by more mental and physical disabilities related to aging (U.S. General Accounting Office, 2001).

MiCASSA

A recent bill at the time of this writing, the 2003 MiCASSA is representative of the push for changes in services for the elderly and those with disabilities, and is indicative of the likely direction of future services. Currently, every state that receives Medicaid funding from Title XIX of the Social Security Act must provide nursing home services, while community- and home-based services remain optional; in fact, only 27 states provided personal care services under Medicaid in 2003. At the present time, the ratio of institutional dollars to community and home dollars nationally is 3 : 1; about 27% of long-term care funds under Medicaid pay for community- and home-based care nationally.

The ongoing bias toward institutional care has long been a rallying cry for advocacy groups. Despite this bias, the trend toward community- and home-based care is obvious as states move slowly in this direction. There are now 2 and ½ times more people receiving services in the home and community than in institutional settings. This bill would further shift the bias in favor of consumer choice, allowing the dollars to follow the person, regardless of age or disability, so that individuals or their representatives will choose how they receive services and supports. Allowing MiCASSA to speak for itself:

> (5) The goals of the Nation properly include providing families of children with disabilities, working-age adults with disabilities, and older Americans with—
> > (A) a meaningful choice of receiving long-term services and supports in the most integrated setting appropriate to their needs:
> > (B) the greatest possible control over the services received and, therefore, their own lives and futures; and
> > (C) quality services that maximize independence in the home and community, including the workplace. (MiCASSA, S971 IS, 108th Congress, 2003)

Under MiCASSA, two million Americans now placed in nursing facilities and other institutions will have choices as to where and how services they need to be as independent as possible will be obtained. As mentioned, advocates for those with serious mental illness are also seeking strategies to use the personal attendant services for the similar purpose of community tenure for those with cognitive and psychiatric disabilities, including use of personal attendants as prompts for medication compliance. In addition to choice on the part of the consumer, the MiCASSA bill provides states with financial capacity-building assistance to reconstruct comprehensive long-term service systems favoring consumer choice in the most integrated settings. Use of vouchers, cash payments, fiscal agents, and agency providers would be required to be consumer-controlled.

In addition to MiCASSA, another bill before Congress at the time of this writing is the Money Follows the Person Act, giving states resources to assist those who would like to leave a nursing facility or institution for a home- or community-based setting (www.ADAPT.org). The direction of service provision in the future would seem to be clear, regardless of the length of the advocacy challenge and struggle. Future services should allow greater choice and freedoms to those with functional disabilities of all kinds, allowing them to assume control and management of their service provision. Preventive interventions are the choice of today's health care consumer.

REFERENCES

Alzheimer's Association. (2004). *About Alzheimer's.* Available from www.alz.org /statistics/asp.

Americans with Disabilities Act of 1990, 42 U.S.C. §   12101 (1990).

Anthony, W. A., & Blanch, A. (1987). Supported employment for persons who are psychiatrically disabled: An historical and conceptual perspective. *Psychosocial Rehabilitation Journal, 11*(2), 5–23.

Batavia, A. I. (1998). Prospects for a national personal assistance services program: Enhancing choice for people with disabilities. *American Rehabilitation, 24*(4), 2–9. Retrieved February 2, 2004, from Academic Search Elite.

Braitman, A., Counts, P., Avenport, R., Zurlinden, B., Rogers, M., Clauss, J., et al. (1995). Comparison of barriers of employment and employed clients in a case management program: An exploratory study. *Psychiatric Rehabilitation Journal, 19*(1), 3–8.

Cantor, M. H., & Gruland, B. (1993). *Growing older in New York city in the 1990s.* New York: New York Community Trust, New York Center for Policy on Aging.

Care of the institutionalized mentally disabled persons: Joint hearings before the Subcommittee on the Handicapped, Committee on Labor and Human Resources, Subcommittee on Labor, Health and Human Services and Education, and Related Agencies of the Committee on Appropriations, U.S. Senate 99th Cong., 1st Sess. 1 (1985) (testimony of Carol Sands).

Chandler, S. M. (1990). *Competing realities: The contested terrain of mental health advocacy.* New York: Praeger.

Department of Health and Human Services. (1980). *Toward a national plan for the chronically mentally ill* (DHHS Publication No. ADM 1-1077). Washington, DC: Public Health Service.

Developmental Disabilities Assistance and Bill of Rights Act of 2000, 42 U.S.C. 15002 § 102 (2000).

Fellin, P. (1996). *Mental health and mental illness: Policies, programs, and services.* Itasca, IL: Peacock Press.

Forkosch, J. A., Kaye, H. S., & LaPlante, M. P. (1995). *The incidence of traumatic brain injury in the United States* (Disability Statistics Abstract No. 14). Washington, DC: U.S. Department of Education, National Institute on Disability and Rehabilitation Research.

Goldman, H. H., Adams, N. H., & Taube, C. A. (1983). Deinstitutionalization: The data demythologized. *Hospital and Community Psychiatry, 34*(2), 129–134.

Grob, G. N. (1994). *The mad among us: A history of the care of America's mentally ill.* New York: Free Press.

Herinckx, H. A., Kineey, R. F., Clarke, G. N., & Pauson, R. I. (1997). Assertive community treatment versus usual care in engaging and retaining clients with severe mental illness. *Psychiatric Services, 48*(10), 1297–1306.

Hogarty, G. E. (1991). *Drug and psychosocial treatment of schizophrenia: The state of the art.* Pittsburgh, PA: University of Pittsburgh.

Hogarty, G. E., Anderson, C. M., Reiss, D. J., Kornblith, S. J., Greenwald, D. P., Ulrich, R. F., et al. (1991). Family psychoeducation, social skills training, and maintenance chemotherapy in the aftercare treatment of schizophrenia. *Archives of General Psychiatry, 48,* 340–347.

Hollingsworth, E. J. (1994). Falling through the cracks: Care of the chronically mentally ill in the United States. In J. R. Hollingsworth & E. J. Hollingsworth (Eds.), *Care of the chronically and severely ill: Comparative social policies* (pp. 145–172). New York: Aldine de Gruyter.

Isaac, R. J., & Armat, V. C. (1990). *Madness in the streets: How psychiatry and the law abandoned the mentally ill.* New York: Free Press.

Kaye, H. S., LaPlante, M. P., Carlson, D., & Wenger, B. L. (1996). *Trends in disability rates in the United States, 1970–1994* (Disability Statistics Abstract No. 17). Washington, DC: U.S. Department of Education, National Institute on Disability and Rehabilitation Research.

LaPlante, M. P. (1996). *Health conditions and impairments causing disability* (Disability Statistics Abstract 16). Washington, DC: U.S. Department of Education, National Institute on Disability and Rehabilitation Research.

LaPlante, M. P., & Carlson, D. (1996). *Disability in the United States: Prevalence and causes, 1992* (Disability Statistics Report No. 6). Washington, DC: U.S. Department of Education, National Institute on Disability and Rehabilitation Research.

Litvak, S. (1998). Personal assistance service policy: Where we have been and where we are going. *American Rehabilitation, 24*(4), 9–15. Retrieved February 2, 2004, from Academic Search Elite.

Mathis, J. (2001, November/December). Community integration of individuals with disabilities: An update on Olmstead implementation. *Journal of Poverty Law and Policy,* 395–410. Retrieved February 22, 2004, from www.povertylaw.org /legalresearch/articles/index.

McConnell, S., & Riggs, J. A. (1994). A public policy agenda: Supporting family care-giving. In M. H. Cantor (Ed.), *Family caregiving: Agenda for the future.* San Francisco, CA: American Society on Aging.

Medicaid Community-Based Attendant Services and Supports Act of 2003, § 971 IS, 108th Cong. (2003).

National Advisory Mental Health Council. (1993). Health care reform for Americans with severe mental illnesses: Report of the National Advisory Mental Health Council. *American Journal of Psychiatry, 150*(10), 1447–1465.

National Center for Health Statistics. (1992). National Health Interview Survey. Hyattsville, MD: U.S. Department of Health and Human Services.

National Institute of Mental Health. (1955). *Patients in mental institutions, 1950–1955.* Bethesda, MD: Author.

National Institute of Mental Health. (1990). *Additions and resident patients at end of year, state and county mental hospitals, by age and diagnosis, by state, United States, 1990.* Bethesda, MD: Author.

Olmstead v. L. C., 527 U.S. 581 (1999).

Pepper Commission. (1990). *A call for action: Final report for Bipartisan Committee on Comprehensive Health Care.* Washington, DC: U.S. Government Printing Office.

Schorr, L. B., & Schorr, D. (1989). *Within our reach: Breaking the cycle of disadvantage.* NY: Anchor Books.

Spector, W. D., Fleishman, J. A., Pezzin, L. E., & Spillman, B. C. (2003). *Characteristics of long-term care users* (Agency for Health Care Research and Quality [AHRQ] research report). Retrieved January 10, 2004, from www.ahcpr.gov/research /ltcusers/index.html.

Spector, W. D., Shaffer, T. J., Hodlewsky, R. T., De La Mare, J. J., & Rhoades, J. A. (2002). *Future directions for community-based long-term care health services research* (AHRQ Publication No. 02-0022). Washington, DC: U.S. Department of Health and Human Services, Public Health Service.

Stein, L. I. (1990). Comments by Leonard Stein. *Hospital and Community Psychiatry, 41,* 649–651.

Stein, L. I., & Test, M. A. (1985). The evolution of the Training in Community Living model. In L. I. Stein & M. A. Test (Eds.), *The training in community living model: A decade of experience* (pp. 7–16). San Francisco: Jossey-Bass.

Stroul, B. A. (1987). *Crisis residential services in a community support system.* Rockville, MD: National Institute of Mental Health.

Torrey, E. F. (1997). *Out of the shadows: Confronting the mental illness crisis.* New York: Wiley.

U.S. Census Bureau. (1997). Survey of income and program participation. Retrieved March 1, 2004, from http://www.census.gov/hhes/www/disable/sipp/disable97.html.

U.S. General Accounting Office. (2001, September 24). *Long-term care: Implications of Supreme Court's Olmstead decision are still unfolding.* Testimony by the U.S. General Accounting Office before the Special Committee on Aging, U.S. Senate (testimony of Kathryn G. Allen, Director, Health Care—Medicaid and Private Health Insurance Issues).

Wolfensberger, W. (1975). *The origins and nature of our institutional models.* Syracuse, NY: Human Policy Press.

Zarit, S. H. (1994). Research perspectives on family caregiving. In M. H. Cantor (Ed.), *Family caregiving: Agenda for the future.* San Francisco, CA: American Society on Aging.

Chapter 20

ECONOMIC INSTABILITY

SONDRA J. FOGEL

According to Cauthen and Lu (2003), "Economic security includes: (1) stable, predictable income, (2) savings and assets that can help families survive crises and plan for the future, and (3) human and social capital (e.g., education, skills, and support systems) that help families improve their financial status" (p. 2). In the United States today, too many families lack at least one, if not all, of these. This situation has led to rising levels of economic instability in the country, with a related increase in psychological and physical hardship for many.

Typically, the adult wage-earning years extend from age 18 to retirement. Until recently, retirement age was 65, but, due to recent changes in the Federal Social Security program, workers currently 55 or younger can now expect to work until age 67, and perhaps longer. This change means that individuals will now have the opportunity, on paper, to work well over 45 years during their lifetime. In spite of this lengthy wage-earning period, the majority of Americans will experience at least one period of poverty (as defined by the U.S. Bureau of the Census guidelines) in their lifetime (Devine & Wright, 1993; Rank & Hirschl, 1999).

Based on these findings, it is clearly important to establish and promote interventions aimed at averting poverty. Such interventions, which can be classified as "universal, selective, or indicated" (Gordon, 1983, p. 110), must be fluid, however. For many interventions, the exact form they take will be affected by such factors as the social, economic, and political climate of the country, governmental assistance programs, global conditions, and the circumstances of the individuals involved. (Please see previous chapters in Part 4 for more information about individual circumstances.)

Beyond this, the definition of economic stability needs to be clarified. Dooley and Catalano (2003) point out that much of the research on economic stability has focused on how an individual's status as employed or unemployed affects their mental and physical status. They go on to assert that this dichotomous view ignores the continuum of economic stages between the two states, thus overlooking a range of possible work conditions in which individuals may find themselves. This gap is filled by Jensen and Slack's (2003) overview of categories increasingly used to describe these intermediate stages. Based on the Labor Utilization Framework proposed by Hauser (1974), these are:

- *Subunemployed or discouraged workers:* Individuals who are not currently working, and who did not look for work during the previous 4 weeks because they felt no jobs were available.
- *Unemployed workers:* Those not looking for work, but who have looked for work during the previous 4 weeks, or who are currently laid off.
- *Underemployed by low hours or involuntary part-time employment:* This follows the official definition of those who are working "part-time for economic reasons."

  —It includes those individuals who are working less than 35 hours because they can not find full-time employment.
- *Underemployed by low-income, or the "working poor":* This includes those individuals whose adjusted earnings for the year prior were less than 125% of the official poverty line for an individual living alone.
- *Underemployed by occupational mismatch, or overeducated for the position held:* This includes those individuals whose educational level (measured in years of schooling) is greater than one standard deviation above the mean education for workers with the same occupation (Jensen & Slack, 2003, pp. 23–24).

This taxonomy guides the growing literature supporting Dooley and Catalano's (2003) claim that more needs to be known about what lies between employment and unemployment as increasingly more researchers are using these categories to investigate trends, risk factors, and protective factors associated with economic instability. Furthermore, this schema is helpful in elucidating the universal, selective, and indicated measures that could be used to address the range of situations that may contribute to adult economic insecurities. This, then, is the terminology used throughout this chapter.

TRENDS AND INCIDENCE

For much of the history of the United States, economic self-sufficiency, usually achieved through work, has been the predominant value used to assess the worthiness of a person (Piven & Cloward, 1971; Segal & Kilty, 2003). In accordance with cultural and religious values, able-bodied individuals were expected to work to support themselves and their families. Failure to do so was seen as a deviation from the social order and as a sign of personal deficiency. It was only relatively recently, during the Great Depression era, that economic and societal conditions became acceptable alternative explanations for a person's joblessness or state of economic instability (Jensen & Slack, 2003).

The origin and subsequent elaboration of the official definition of poverty also needs consideration. Originally conceptualized in 1955, it was based on an "economy food plan," put forth by the Department of Agriculture (Mangum, Mangum, & Sum, 2003). According to this definition, it was the ability to feed oneself and one's family on a thrift plan budget that determined whether one was considered poor. In 1969, as the War on Poverty continued, Mollie Orshansky, a senior official in the Social Security Administration, used this basic concept to develop the official poverty level. By using a basic family meal plan and multiplying this amount by three, a minimal income was established for individuals and families, adjusting for the number in the household. This minimal income measure was adopted by the federal government as the absolute measure of poverty. The gauge, known as the "poverty threshold," is updated annually by the U.S. Census Bureau, using the Current Population Survey (CPS). (This information is available on the Census web site at www.census.gov.) For a family of four in 2003, the poverty threshold was set at $18,660.

A similar measure of poverty is used by the federal government to determine eligibility requirements for federal programs such as Head Start, food stamps, and the Low Income Home Energy Assistance Program. Referred to as "poverty guidelines," these measures are announced each year in the Federal Register by the Department of Health and Human Services (HHS). In 2004, the HHS poverty guideline for a family of four living in one of the 48 contiguous states or DC was set at $18,850. (For more information, see http://aspe.hhs.gov/poverty.)

To begin to comprehend the complexity of adult economic instability and identify prevention measures, it is essential to reflect on how individuals are classified with regard to economic stability. Following the Orshansky scheme, the ability to purchase food on a thrift plan is the data source used to identify poverty levels. However, the validity of this method has been challenged. It does not, for instance, take into account transportation, child care or housing costs, or regional differences in the cost of living (Mangum et al., 2003). Therefore, this method underestimates the number of individuals who are struggling economically. It is no surprise, then, that a growing interest among researchers and policy makers concerns the plight of the working poor, a visible phenomenon that is escalating throughout this country (Meyers & Lee, 2003).

It was, however, the "invisible poor," as identified by Harrington (1962), that reawakened America's concern with adult economic problems. Earlier government interventions, coupled with a strong post-World War II economy, had returned many individuals to the workplace. For example, in response to the Great Depression in the 1930s, numerous programs, such as the National Youth Administration, the Civilian Conservation Corps, the Public Works Administration, and the Works Progress Administration, were created as part of the New Deal. These programs provided employment to approximately 5% of the population. In addition, federal programs were created that offered various social and health benefits tied to work hours and established assistance to female-headed households with children (Levitan, Mangum, Mangum, & Sum, 2003).

In the early 1960s, fostered by growing media outlets and through the writings of numerous social activists and commentators, public awareness of income inequities, the impact of regional conditions on industries, and personal stories of poverty grew and made possible the political will to declare a War on Poverty (Mangum et al., 2003). Harrington's (1962) estimate of almost 50 million adults living in poverty at this time helped fuel President Lyndon Johnson's commitment to help the poor. Again, government programs were created with the aim of alleviating the distressed living conditions of those unable to sustain themselves in the marketplace. These programs were primarily based on the assumption that individuals could be drawn into or returned to the workforce through training, education, and the elimination of workplace discrimination. The Vietnam War and a robust economy enhanced the success of these antipoverty efforts. Indeed, in 1973, the number of persons considered poor in the United States was about 23 million, representing 11.1% of the population, down from 40 million (22.4%) in 1959 (Levitan et al., 2003, p. 4). This represents the lowest rate of poverty in U.S. history.

Throughout the 1970s, 1980s, and much of the 1990s, it was the economy, rather than government programs, that helped adults escape economic instability. The percentage of persons living in poverty, however, rose from 11.1% to a high of 15.1% during the 1991 recession. It then slowly declined to 11.3%, representing 31.1 million individuals, by 2000 (Levitan et al., 2003, p. 5).

The decline in the number of families in poverty was more dramatic. In 1973, family poverty was estimated at 8.8% of the population. This was a historic low. Yet, the number of families in poverty changed according to economic conditions over the next 27 years, dramatically increasing during the recessions in the 1980s and 1990s. However, in 2000, only 8.6% or 6.2 million families were poor. This number represents the new historic low for families (Levitan et al., 2003, pp. 5–6). Yet, the number of individuals working full time and still considered poor, that is, the working poor, grew throughout the 1980s and 1990s (Meyers & Lee, 2003).

Concurrent with business conditions, confidence in the marketplace and political and social forces reaffirmed the value of economic self-sufficiency. This ideology produced significant changes in the administration of federal programs and people's belief that government should care for the poor and working poor (Stricker, 2003). State and local governments were granted increased authority over the management of federal programs, a change that has led to variation of services and requirements (Anderson, Halter, & Gryzlak, 2002). In addition, challenges to fundamental guidelines in social programs to assist the deserving poor began to slowly emerge in legislation. For example, the Family Support Act of 1988 targeted mothers with children receiving federal aid for training and education programs to assist them toward economic self-sufficiency through participation in the workforce (Simmons, Bok, Churchill, & Pritchard, 2001).

Further changes occurred in 1996 with the adoption of the Personal Responsibility and Work Opportunity Reconciliation Act (PRWORA, Pub. L. 104-103). This drastically altered government aid to the poor, particularly for immigrants and women with children receiving aid. New guidelines replaced Aid to Families with Dependent Children with the Temporary Assistance for Needy Families program (TANF). Utilization of this aid program was contingent on the able-bodied adult preparing for or entering the workforce. In addition, a 2-year time limit for accomplishing this goal was set, with a further limit of five years for total program participation. Individual states, however, retain flexibility over this time requirement (Cheng, 2002).

Through the end of the 1990s and on into the twenty-first century, a new framework for governmental assistance has emerged for those individuals and families in need of some help regardless of whether they are working, part of the working poor, or below the poverty line. It is during this time that general assistance programs have also been reduced (Anderson et al., 2002). While there are many reports of declining TANF rolls, research on the effectiveness of the TANF program has produced mixed results due to a variety of political and methodological issues (Anderson & Gryzlak, 2002). And, once again, the economy is volatile, creating economic instability for many individuals and families who are trying to enter the labor force, retrain for the new market conditions, or just maintain their position (Stricker, 2003). Those attempting to identify prevention activities for adult economic instability must be cognizant of labor market conditions as well as personal characteristics and issues that may have an impact on economic stability. The interplay of these variables affects all prevention efforts.

RISK FACTORS

Research has repeatedly identified low educational attainment as the strongest predictor of economic instability and poverty (Meyers & Lee, 2003). Age is also a factor; young people are more likely to be economically insecure (Mosisa, 2003). Gender (women), race (non-White), martial status (single with children), and nationality (non-American) are other individual characteristics that influence economic self-sufficiency. In addition, physical and mental health conditions and place of residence (urban poverty neighborhood, rural, industry-dependant local) also influence economic self-sufficiency. Any combination of these issues increases the likelihood of economic instability. The implications of these will be discussed briefly.

Gender

Women are disproportionately economically insecure due to multiple factors. To begin with, despite record numbers of women in the workforce, women typically do not earn the same wage as men for the same or comparable job. This discrimination can be found at all levels in the marketplace (Christy-McMullin, 2002; Ozawa & Yoon, 2003; Segal & Kilty, 2003; Stricker, 2003). In concert with this are the types of work in which women are more likely to participate than men. These include "part-time work, contract work, temporary work, and contingency work," especially in "service-oriented industries" (Ozawa & Yoon, 2003, p. 117).

A woman's martial status also has an impact on her level of economic security, more so than for men. A divorced woman or a woman heading a household is more likely to experience low levels of economic security than a married woman. The number of children a woman has and is caring for in her home is also associated with her level of economic security (Ozawa & Yoon, 2003).

Race, though a risk factor for both men and women, has a greater impact on a woman's economic instability. With the exception of Asian American women, a non-White woman is more likely to be poor than a non-White man (Meyers & Lee, 2003; Segal, Kilty, & Kim, 2002). Specifically, according to Caiazza (2004), in 1999, the percentage of women of color below the poverty line was 23.5% for African American women, 22.2% for Native American women, 22.4% for Hispanic women, and 10.9% for Asian American women. The percentage for White women during the same year was 8.5% (p. 43).

Citizenship Status

Closely linked to race, immigration status can determine whether someone can legally work in this country and therefore has obvious implications for economic stability. As Belanger (2001) points out, legal immigration is controlled by sociopolitical factors such as war and the need for cheap labor. Those individuals who enter this country to work illegally are more at risk for economic instability and poverty. Despite various legislative measures intended both to deter employers from hiring these individuals and to increase opportunities for immigrants to legally work, little has changed to alleviate the low wages and irregular employment of these individuals (Belanger, 2001; Lim & Resko, 2002). Language barriers and discrimination further exacerbate this condition (Segal et al., 2002).

Employment Setting and Regional Area

Opportunities for employment vary greatly in this country; certain types of industry are more prevalent in some parts of the country than others. Regional industries, such as auto manufacturing and steel and fabric mills, created towns and their supporting economies. When such industries folded, towns were left with huge numbers of people without work, some remaining unemployed for a very long time. Those formerly employed in manufacturing industries remain unemployed the longest, according to Allegretto and Stettner (2004). In the 1980s, many individuals who once held manufacturing positions saw components of their industry move to other parts of the world, leaving few local opportunities for comparable work and wages.

Residents in rural areas are also affected by declining economic prospects and reductions in social organizations to support personal and employment distress caused by lack of employment opportunities (Parisi, McLaughlin, Grice, Taquino, & Gill, 2003). At the same time, poor urban inner-city living areas typically do not have the types of jobs, for example, retail jobs, that can use the available labor pool in these neighborhoods. As Coulton (2003) states, "Place-based disparities in opportunity structures and social and institutional resources affect labor market success," particularly for those individuals using federal programs (p. 159).

In summary, there are numerous descriptive characteristics, personal choices, and environmental conditions that may impede an individual's ability to remain economically stable over his or her work lifetime. Many of these risk factors are further complicated by social networks and other extenuating circumstances. Certainly, the events of September 11, 2001, continue to affect the daily lives of all individuals in this country. New regulations regarding travel, privacy, and documents used for employment are now in place. Foreign student educational opportunities, as well as employment prospects, have changed dramatically. In addition, economic conditions continue to be volatile, responding to issues such as ethics scandals in businesses, technology changes and challenges, and decreased union and labor market protections (Stricker, 2003). Given these factors, it is no surprise that the numbers of working poor continue to grow in the twenty-first century (Meyers & Lee, 2003). Prevention measures to correct this situation must address a broad range of systemic issues at multiple levels as well as individual conditions.

INTERVENTIONS

Any discussion of intervention activities in this area has to begin by stating assumptions about the economy. For adults to be financially stable, there have to be jobs available in a variety of industries in various areas that match the desires, interests, talents, and availability of individuals. However, this is not a condition that will likely return to this country for some time. The market situation in the early twenty-first century in the United States reflects a slow recovery from a recession, a decrease in technology and manufacturing positions, an increase of outsourcing production to other countries, and an increased gap in wages between the rich and the poor. Therefore, the following prevention activities are provided with an eye toward a growing economy, with noted limitations by industry and region.

Effective Universal Preventive Interventions

Gordon's (1983) use of "universal" as a category in his prevention model suggests that these activities should, or could, be practical for the general public, as well as cost-effective. There are two cost-effective and efficient strategies that would help all adults avoid the perils of economic instability: quality education and implementation of a mandatory living wage.

Education

"Education and a strong base in literacy and numeracy proficiencies have become widely recognized as the primary means of prevention of and escape from poverty in the United States" (Levitan et al., 2003, p. 167). While race, gender, age, and the state of the economy influence the impact of education on earnings, in general, college graduates and those with higher degrees are less likely to be poor than other groups. However, providing access to quality education for all students, from grade school through high school, remains a long-standing, unrealized goal in the United States.

Federal initiatives to promote effective learning opportunities for young people have taken many forms, including legislation to establish programs to support individuals and groups at high risk for poverty (Head Start, Title I of the Elementary and Secondary Education Act of 1965, No Child Left Behind), federal funds for magnet and charter schools, grant programs to remove obstacles to higher education, such as TRIO and GEAR-UP, and postsecondary grants, loans, and work opportunities. However, many of these and other programs are not funded adequately. As Levitan et al. (2003, p. 176) point out, pressure to balance state budgets resulted in pervasive cuts in educational expenditures in 2002. Therefore, while a solid education is well-recognized as an effective weapon against adult economic problems, the challenge for one system (education) to provide this basic necessity appears to be too great. Projects at the local level are emerging to coordinate school, work, and citizenship preparation to prepare young people for the transition to the workforce (Gore, Kadish, & Aseltine, 2003). Research is needed on this new "youth development initiative" to assess how effective it is in preparing young adults for future economic success.

Living Wage

The concept of a living wage has been promoted since the turn of the twentieth century (Francoeur, 1999). Political and social turbulence in the early 1900s led to many legislative acts seeking to control rising rates of unemployment and poverty and the militancy of those seeking relief (Piven & Cloward, 1971). It was in this historical context that the need for a laborer's wage to be "large enough to meet ordinary family needs adequately" was promoted by Catholic religious leaders as a matter of social justice (Francoeur, 1999, p. 12). In addition, it was recognized that lack of wages can have a demoralizing effect on individuals.

The link between mental and physical health and job and socioeconomic status must be introduced. Higher socioeconomic status has been shown to be associated with better physical and emotional health (Belanger, 2001; Lynch, Kaplan, & Salonen, 1997). While the relationship of unemployment and health has been well documented (Dooley & Catalano, 2003), the relationship between underemployment, or employment status, and physical and mental health has increasingly come under study due to a growing awareness of the employment continuum mentioned earlier. Dooley (2003), in a review of the literature on the topic of underemployment, found that mental health concerns and problems among the underemployed were similar to those of individuals who had suffered a job loss. Friedland and Price (2003) suggest that underemployment is a constant stressor. From their longitudinal investigation of 1,429 adults, underemployed adults' experience lower levels of psychological well-being, with some related health concerns. Therefore, even those who are working but can be classified as underemployed, working poor, or underemployed by occupational mismatch may be predisposed to physical or mental health conditions that could be prevented, or at least reduced, with the institution of a national living wage standard.

The current federal minimum wage is $5.15 per hour, although some states can set a higher wage. What constitutes a living wage is determined by the amount needed to support a family above the federal poverty line. This wage is adjusted for regional differences. Currently, over 70 counties have passed living wage ordinances for those who work in government or have a government contract. This obviously affects only a very limited number of individuals. There is growing evidence that urban workers receiving a living wage do slightly reduce their poverty level (Cauthen & Lu, 2003; Neumark & Adams, 2000). A living wage should be provided to all workers regardless of employment status or employer. The current reliance on the federal minimum wage standard (which has not been raised for 6 years) is not adequate for the majority of low-skilled and underemployed workers to support themselves or their family (see www.epinet.org).

Effective Selective Preventive Interventions

Selective interventions, according to Gordon (1983), are recommended "only when the individual is a member of a subgroup of the population distinguished by age, sex, occupation, or other obvious characteristics whose risk of becoming ill is above average" (p. 108). In terms of economic instability, subgroups of the American population particularly at risk are the working poor, which includes discouraged workers, underemployed or subunemployed workers, and those working in regional or service industries. In 2001, those most likely to be classifiable as working poor included women, members of female-headed households, members of families with a larger number of children than average, individuals with less than a high school education, minority young adults, and those who live in rural communities and distressed urban areas (Jensen & Slack, 2003; Mosisa, 2003). (The U.S. Department of Labor, Bureau of Labor Statistics maintains a comprehensive data collection site with information about these variables and others at www.bls.gov.)

The working poor are the most disadvantaged group in American society (Meyers & Lee, 2003). Often making too much to qualify for federal assistance programs such as food stamps, medical insurance, or housing assistance programs, this group suffers numerous daily challenges in order to work. Working costs money for this group (Macarov, 2003). Transportation, child care, and taxes are just a few of the expenses that approximately 6.8 million working poor individuals in 2001 had to pay in order to work (Allegretto & Stettner, 2004, p. 18).

There are other drawbacks as well. Meyers and Lee (2003), after comparing the needs of working poor families with those of nonworking poor and nonpoor families living in New York City, found that working poor families were "one-third more likely to experience living in over-crowded housing, one-sixth lived with serious structural inadequacies, one-third described their neighborhood as unsafe, and nearly two-thirds had one or more uninsured family members at some point in the year" (p. 195).

Because of the multifactorial nature of the problem at this level, multiple forms of selected preventive measures are called for. As indicated earlier, mental and physical health problems such as depression and low self-esteem are associated with the various employment situations that the working poor are in (Dooley, 2003). Individual interventions should consider this. However, two broad areas will be discussed here: a revision of how the working poor are taxed and increased financial support during times of unemployment.

Taxes

Levitan et al. (2003) emphasize the need to expand cash support programs and to adjust the tax rate for the working poor. For example, the Earned Income Tax Credit of 1975 has been expanded several times to adjust for inflation (Baeg-Eui & Ozawa, 2003). Its basic approach is to reduce the tax liability of low-income workers, especially those with children. Workers whose tax credit exceeds their liability receive a refund if they file their yearly tax forms. There are limits to how much credit a worker can claim. However, this assistance program is not well-known among the working poor (Levitan et al., 2003). Therefore, its effectiveness is reduced. Greater efforts must be made to educate eligible workers about this assistance, and the tax credit limit must be increased.

Another tax issue impacting the working poor is the regressive payroll tax. This tax, established by the Federal Insurance Contributions Act, pays for Social Security and unemployment insurance. It begins with the first earned dollar for all but the lowest-paid workers and continues up to a specified wage limit (Levitan et al., 2003). This tax structure ensures that the working poor experience a disproportionate reduction of their income through taxation. Reversing this tax structure would substantially assist millions of low-wage workers.

Unemployment Insurance

At the beginning of the twenty-first century, the impact of the 1993 recession and changing business practices such as increased privatization and global outsourcing dramatically changed the opportunities of the working poor to find improved salary conditions and also created substantial changes in their demographics. Suddenly, those with specialized skills, especially in the manufacturing, technology, health, and education industries, college graduates, and those older than 45, found themselves entering into extended periods of unemployment, lasting 6 months or more (Allegretto & Stettner, 2004; Macarov, 2003). The predominant safety net for most of this group, as well as low-wage workers, is unemployment insurance. In the current economic climate—a jobless recovery—the average duration of unemployment insurance has not been suffi-cient to sustain workers through their time of unemployment. This led Congress to extend the period of eligibility for collection of unemployment insurance for most workers. However, at the end of 2003, Congress did not reauthorize the ex-tension of this benefit. Instead, they allowed the Temporary Extended Unem-ployment Compensation to expire, leaving millions of former workers with no federal support to maintain a household in a jobless labor market (Allegretto & Stettner, 2004). This program needs to be extended again to forestall an increase in the number of skilled workers entering into long-term economic instability (Cauthen & Lu, 2003).

Overall, the tax structure in the United States is a complicated system that continuously changes; currently, it benefits those with the most wealth (Mac-arov, 2003). Incremental interventions, like the ones suggested here, as well as job-retraining programs, adult education, housing assistance, and expansion of federal aid programs targeted to this broad range of workers are needed to assist working adults and those temporarily out of the workforce with additional in-come to combat life's daily challenges (Cheng, 2002). More drastic actions, such as reconfiguring poverty thresholds to capture the large number of working poor, removing income as the primary gauge for vast governmental assistance, and ceasing to think that work is the answer to poverty and economic instability may be the best strategies for helping individuals who fall into the selective pre-vention category (Macarov, 2003; Mangum et al., 2003; Stricker, 2003).

Effective Indicated Preventive Interventions

Indicated prevention measures, according to Gordon (1983), are directed at indi-viduals who are at high risk for the problem; they are not "totally benign or mini-mal in cost" (p. 108). Throughout this chapter, the continuum between employed and unemployed has been used to capture the range of labor and market condi-tions that impact the economic solvency of adults. For both universal and selected preventions, factors such as gender, youth, race, and industry type and location have been shown to affect an individual's economic security. There is no question that these characteristics also come into play in situations calling for more aggres-sive federal efforts to prevent economic instability. Long-term unemployment and welfare use are two situations that require indicated prevention measures.

Long-Term Unemployment

As suggested earlier, the availability of jobs is often influenced by situations out-side an individual's control. Such factors include market conditions, privatization, and regional industry conditions. Thus, long-term unemployment may not be a consequence of personal "deviance" but simply situational and outside the control of the individual. Losing a job and the benefits associated with the position may add to personal distress (Allegretto & Stettner, 2004; Dooley, 2003; Dooley & Catalano, 2003).

Strategies to bring these workers back into the labor force often focus on vocational training and education programs (Mangum et al., 2003). However, traditional employment training programs have had questionable impact on returning individuals to the labor market (Macarov, 2003). In part, this may be due to the changing demographics of the long-term unemployed. Included in this group now are college graduates, workers 45 years and older, and those formerly in manufacturing and well-paid professional and business sector industries (Allegretto & Stettner, 2004, p. 2). Current training programs may not be prepared to match the skills and education levels already acquired by this group or the needs of the job market. This is a problem in need of further study.

In addition, as previously stated, evidence suggests that unemployment and underemployment are associated with increased mental and physical health concerns (Dooley & Catalano, 2003). Therefore, extension of health insurance benefits to cover predictable as well as preexisting conditions is a necessary prevention activity to forestall further economic decline in this group. Providing affordable access to health care is one of the most important prevention services for this group of workers.

Welfare Use

To some degree, the enactment of PRWORA attempts to bring the most economically vulnerable individuals back into the labor market. However, the philosophical underpinnings of this legislation assume that self-sufficiency is obtainable through work and that individuals should be held accountable (or punished) for any behavior that may lead to economic instability (Lee & Curran, 2003; Macarov, 2003). Although not specifically targeted at women, the new welfare legislation has significantly changed federal and state monetary and service support for women with children. Therefore, indicated prevention measures must address the numerous conditions that render women more vulnerable to and that tend to keep them in a state of economic instability. These include domestic violence, marital breakups and divorce, child care costs, nonenforcement of child support payments, disrupted employment histories, underemployed and part-time labor in service industries, discrimination based on race, nationality, immigration status, and age, sexual harassment, and unequal earnings compared to men (Anderson-Butcher, Khairallah, & Race-Bigelow, 2004; Mangum et al., 2003; Segal & Kilty, 2003; Simmons et al., 2001).

Given the numerous environmental, situational, and personal factors that affect individuals using welfare, it is extremely unlikely that one program can address them all to successfully assist this population out of their economic condition. According to Sommerfeld and Reisch (2003), nonprofit groups have responded to the new demands on welfare recipients by changing program focuses to meet outcomes associated with PRWORA. Nevertheless, financial support for emergency services and mental and physical care continues to be under financed, despite increased need.

In addition, many recipients (and caseworkers) are not aware of the various tax, in-kind, and financial support programs that can be bundled to assist with daily living expenses (Winicki, 2003). Due to changing regulations and documentation requirements for programs such as food stamps, WIC, and cash assistance, this is not a surprise. Efforts should be made to better educate individuals (and social workers) in the efficient use of these resources.

Furthermore, efforts should be made to create specialized, intensive programs to move adults toward work by providing individualized wraparound assistance. Exemplifying this approach is the growing number of community-based programs representing public-private collaborations and faith-based initiatives aimed at groups at high risk for economic instability. These programs include individual development accounts (IDAs), microenterprise development, and entrepreneurial job training programs for women and youth, home ownership programs, workplace awareness, youth mentoring, and literacy programs, as well as incentives for local community development corporations to reinvest in distressed communities. These initiatives look very promising (Clohesy Consulting, 2002); however, there is a need for more outcome research on these programs to assess their impact on the lives of those most at risk for economic instability.

In summary, the federal and state patchwork of official services for this indicated group continues to promote the idea that work can solve the multitude of problems that persist with these individuals and in these families (Lee & Curran, 2003). Increasingly, there is evidence to argue that this approach is not working (Stricker, 2003). For example, many states are changing the regulations and time restrictions of PRWORA to adapt to the present weak economy; the result is an increase in family problems, revolving employment patterns, homelessness, hunger, and mental and health emergencies. There is also a growing awareness that patterns of poverty and economic instability have lasting repercussions for the children and adults in these environments (Jackson, 2003a, 2003b; Kost & Smyth, 2002).

Welfare users and others who are unemployed for extended periods of time have found a way to adapt to their situation by using a coordinated and at times informal system to acquire the help they need to survive (Anderson-Butcher et al., 2004; Stack, 1974). For example, Zippay (2002) investigated the common but rarely studied use of "income packaging" among displaced steelworkers over a 10-year period. This strategy, used by many working poor adults, combines "paid employment, unreported odd jobs, social services, and other sources to make ends meet" rather than total reliance on governmental programs (p. 291). Learning from their experiences and the growing success of private-public partnership models, it is apparent that indicated prevention initiatives for high-risk groups must be intensive, systems-oriented, community-based, and available to help for an extended period of time.

PRACTICE AND POLICY DIRECTIONS

It is imperative for human service workers, medical and mental health personnel, and researchers to recognize the range of employment situations that contribute to economic instability for individuals and their families, and the risk factors for long-term joblessness. Determination of an individual's status on the working continuum, and whether gender, race, ethnicity, or age, for example, are affecting this status, are important assessments to make. From there, a professional can construct, refer to, or provide a variety of educational or other resources to address the economic instability. Examples of interventions include financial literacy programs to encourage individuals to save and reduce staggering credit card debt, and education for financial preparation for retirement, especially for younger workers. Mental health professionals must also consider ways to be available to those who are without health insurance. Evidence suggests that these individuals are often in crisis situations without support just when they need it (Dooley & Catalano, 2003).

In addition, more research is needed that identifies effective and efficient practice approaches for the range of work patterns that are emerging. A recent example of such research is that of Lee and Curran (2003), who question the use of clinical knowledge in the current configuration of TANF programs. They point out that mental health services and pharmacological interventions have been used to assist many individuals back into the workforce. The assumption that these interventions will work with those in severe economic conditions has yet to be tested; however, there are increasing calls for mental health screenings for TANF users. Anderson-Butcher et al. (2004) suggest from their study on long-term welfare users that mutual support groups can be an effective practice approach.

In the current economic climate, increased advocacy efforts on behalf of the economically insecure are needed. Shifting of the financial burden of programs from the federal to the state level, coupled with federal and state budget cuts, continue to reduce the amount of assistance to those who are economically insecure. Social work has a long history of incorporating advocacy efforts into practice activities. It is imperative that social workers act to reinvigorate this tradition and, either individually or jointly, through established government policy or issue-specific groups, lobby to educate and influence policy and legislation decisions affecting work and work benefits.

FUTURE DIRECTIONS

Gordon's (1983) three-tiered model of prevention activities encourages one to recognize the costs and consequences of an issue, and its remedy, to society as a whole. The topic of economic instability is a confounding one because it is so large and has such varied manifestations in our society. To cover all the elements of this issue requires a book in itself. Of necessity, some issues have been left out of this discussion. For example, the need for affordable and decent housing for all and the impact of a disability on economic stability could have been included in this chapter. Homelessness was not discussed because it represents the total failure of every system (governmental, private, and family) to arrest its progression.

However, there are several emerging issues that need further research to inform prevention activities and practice interventions for mental health and health professionals. These are (1) the array of needs of the growing number of individuals who are underemployed or working and poor; (2) the array of needs of the growing number of working men and women who also serve as caretakers for aging parents and who may also be raising children; (3) examples of successful local private-public community-based partnerships for combating economic instability and neighborhood distress; and (4) grassroots organizations and citizen efforts that are seeking to address economic inequalities.

As rampant consumerism, personal debt, globalization, and privatization are expected to continue to increase during the twenty-first century, the economic solvency of individuals will repeatedly be tested over the course of their working years. More individuals, even those with a strong educational background, will find themselves classified as nearly, or actually, part of the working poor. Yet, this reality does not seem to be accepted by the general public. Perhaps, then, this is the best place to start, with a universal preventive intervention educating adults that economic instability, or even a time in poverty, is a very real possibility for all.

REFERENCES

Allegretto, S., & Stettner, A. (2004, March). Educated, experienced and out of work. *Economic Policy Institute Issue Brief, 198,* 1–10.

Anderson, S. G., & Gryzlak, B. M. (2002). Social work advocacy in the post-TANF environment: Lessons from early TANF research studies. *Social Work, 47*(3), 301–314.

Anderson, S. G., Halter, A. P., & Gryzlak, B. M. (2002). Changing safety net of last report: Downsizing general assistance for employable adults. *Social Work, 47*(3), 249–258.

Anderson-Butcher, D., Khairallah, A. O., & Race-Bigelow, J. (2004). Mutual support groups for long-term recipients of TANF. *Social Work, 49*(1), 131–141.

Baeg-Eui, M. N., & Ozawa, H. (2003). The effects of EITC and children's allowances on the economic well-being of children. *Social Work Research, 27*(3), 163–179.

Belanger, K. (2001). Social justice in education for undocumented families. *Journal of Family Social Work, 6*(4), 61–73.

Caiazza, A. B. (2004). *The status of women in the states* (4th ed.). Washington, DC: Institute for Women's Policy Research.

Cauthen, N. K., & Lu, H. (2003). *Living at the edge* (Research Brief No. 1). New York: Columbia University, National Center for Children in Poverty.

Cheng, T. (2002). Welfare recipients: How do they become independent? *Social Work Research, 26*(3), 159–170.

Christy-McMullin, K. (2002). Designing policies that address the relationship between woman abuse and economic resources. *Journal of Sociology and Social Welfare, 29*(3), 109–124.

Clohesy Consulting. (2002, April). *A review of community development and poverty intervention projects and strategies.* Waterloo, IA: OpportunityWorks.

Coulton, C. J. (2003). Metropolitan inequities and the ecology of work: Implications for welfare reform. *Social Service Review, 77*(2), 159–190.

Devine, J. A., & Wright, J. D. (1993). *The greatest of evils: Urban poverty and the American underclass.* New York: Aldine De Gruyter.

Dooley, D. (2003). Unemployment, underemployment, and mental health: Conceptualizing employment status as a continuum. *American Journal of Community Psychology, 32*(1/2), 9–20.

Dooley, D., & Catalano, R. (2003). Introduction to underemployment and its social costs. *American Journal of Community Psychology, 32*(1/2), 1–7.

Francoeur, R. B. (1999). In pursuit of a living wage: The ethical and economic thought of Father John A. Ryan from the late 1890's until the New Deal. *Social Thought, 19*(1), 1–14.

Friedland, D. S., & Price, R. H. (2003). Underemployment: Consequences for the health and well-being of workers. *American Journal of Community Psychology, 32*(1/2), 33–45.

Gordon, R. (1983). An operational classification of disease prevention. *Public Health Reports, 98*(2), 107–109.

Gore, S., Kadish, S., & Aseltine, R. H., Jr. (2003). Career centered high school education and post-high school career adaptation. *American Journal of Community Psychology, 32*(1/2), 77–88.

Harrington, M. (1962). *The other America.* New York: Macmillan.

Hauser, P. M. (1974). The measurement of labor utilization. *Malayan Economic Review, 19,* 1–17.

Jackson, A. P. (2003a). The effects of family and neighborhood characteristics on the behavioral and cognitive development of poor black children: A longitudinal study. *American Journal of Community Psychology, 32*(1/2), 175–187.

Jackson, A. P. (2003b). Mothers' employment and poor and near poor African-American children's development: A longitudinal study. *Social Service Review, 77*(1), 93–103.

Jensen, L., & Slack, T. (2003). Underemployment in America: Measurement and evidence. *American Journal of Community Psychology, 32*(1/2), 1–7.

Kost, K. A., & Smyth, N. J. (2002). Two strikes against them? Exploring the influence of a history of poverty and growing up in an alcoholic family and alcohol problems and income. *Journal of Social Service Research, 28*(4), 23–52.

Lee, R., & Curran, L. (2003). Serving the "hard to serve": The use of clinical knowledge in welfare reform. *Journal of Sociology and Social Welfare, 30*(3), 59–80.

Levitan, S. A., Mangum, G. L., Mangum, S. L., & Sum, A. M. (2003). *Programs in aid of the poor* (8th ed.). Baltimore: Johns Hopkins University Press.

Lim, Y., & Resko, S. M. (2002). Immigrants' use of welfare after welfare reform: Cross-group comparison. *Journal of Poverty, 6*(4), 63–82.

Lynch, J. W., Kaplan, G. A., & Salonen, J. T. (1997). Why do poor people behave poorly? Variation in adult health behaviours and psychosocial characteristics by stages of the socioeconomic lifecourse. *Social Science Medicine, 44*(6), 809–819.

Macarov, D. (2003). *What the market does to people: Privatization, globalization and poverty.* Atlanta, GA: Clarity Press.

Mangum, G. L., Mangum, S. L., & Sum, A. M. (2003). *The persistence of poverty in the United States.* Baltimore, MD: Johns Hopkins University Press.

Meyers, M. K., & Lee, J. M. (2003). Working but poor: How are families faring? *Children and Youth Services Review, 25*(3), 177–201.

Mosisa, A. T. (2003, November/December). The working poor in 2001. *Monthly Labor Review,* 13–19.

Neumark, D., & Adams, S. (2000). *Do living wage ordinances reduce urban poverty?* (Working Paper No. 7606). Cambridge, MA: National Bureau of Economic Research.

Ozawa, M. N., & Yoon, H. S. (2003). Gender differences in the economic well-being of nonaged adults in the United States. *Journal of Poverty, 7*(1/2), 97–122.

Parisi, D., McLaughlin, D. K., Grice, S. M., Taquino, M., & Gill, D. A. (2003). TANF participation rates: Do community conditions matter? *Rural Sociology, 64*(4), 491–512.

Piven, F. F., & Cloward, R. A. (1971). *Regulating the poor: The functions of public welfare*. New York: Random House.

Rank, M. A., & Hirschl, T. A. (1999). The likelihood of poverty across the American adult life span. *Social Work, 44*(3), 201–216.

Segal, E. A., & Kilty, K. M. (2003). Political promises for welfare reform. *Journal of Poverty, 7*(1/2), 51–67.

Segal, E. A., Kilty, K. M., & Kim, R. Y. (2002). Social and economic inequality and Asian Americans in the United States. *Journal of Poverty, 6*(4), 5–21.

Simmons, L., Bok, M., Churchill, N., & Pritchard, A. (2001). Urban economic development: What's welfare-to-work got to do with it? *Journal of Poverty, 5*(2), 87–114.

Sommerfeld, D., & Reisch, M. (2003). The "other America" after welfare reform: A view from the nonprofit sector. *Journal of Poverty, 7*(1/2), 69–95.

Stack, C. B. (1974). *All our kin: Strategies for survival in a Black community*. New York: Harper & Row.

Stricker, F. (2003). Staying poor in the Clinton boom: Welfare reform and the nearby labor force. *Journal of Poverty, 7*(1/2), 23–49.

Winicki, J. (2003). Children in homes below poverty: Changes in program participation since welfare reform. *Children and Youth Services Review, 25*(8), 651–668.

Zippay, A. (2002). Dynamics of income packaging: A 10-year longitudinal study. *Social Work, 47*(3), 291–300.

PART V

Conclusion

Chapter 21

THE FUTURE OF PREVENTION

MATTHEW T. THERIOT and WILLIAM D. LEMLEY

To bring a sense of closure to such an important handbook, this final chapter reflects on the previous chapters. Rather than review each section separately, though, the focus is on the true strength of this book: the sum of the parts. Alone, each chapter covers one problem in a diverse collection of physical, mental, and social disorders, with topics ranging from obesity to domestic violence, diabetes, suicide, ineffective parenting, and heart disease. A quick glance at the table of contents might lead one to worry that this book is stretched too broadly, being nothing more than a bound anthology of unrelated topics and pages. Yet, as this last chapter now unfolds and all of the preceding chapters have been read, it is clear that this multidisciplinary assemblage of subjects and authors yields a remarkably rich mixture of viewpoints and ideas. Drawing on experts in medicine and nursing, social work, psychology, public health, and other social sciences, this handbook has something to offer professionals from a variety of helping professions. It has utility as an educational tool, a reference book, and a guide for program development.

Though such a multidisciplinary approach strengthens this handbook, the real significance of the book does not come from those differences contained herein, but rather from the ribbon of similarity that binds the chapters together. Each chapter promotes the use of prevention efforts with adults and then highlights examples of such efforts that are bolstered by strong empirical evidence. Thus, despite the seemingly divergent chapter topics, the authors demonstrate again and again that prevention plays a key role in alleviating or eliminating many different physical and mental health conditions.

437

TOWARD A COMMON LANGUAGE FOR PREVENTION

At this point in the book, Gordon's (1983, 1987) model of prevention has already been fully defined and described. Repeating such here would be redundant and superfluous, especially as effort is better spent now emphasizing why Gordon's model was so appropriate for use in this book. In each chapter, prevention programs and efforts have been organized around Gordon's model and defined using Gordon's terminology and examples have been given for each of Gordon's three categories.

Numerous *universal* preventive interventions are noted throughout this book. The same is true for *selective* preventive interventions and *indicated* preventive interventions. Moreover, most chapters include several examples in illustration of each level of prevention. The appropriateness of Gordon's model is thus evident in each chapter as well as stretched across the book. Quite simply, the ease and relevance with which Gordon's model is used to structure prevention for the myriad different problems described in the preceding chapters speaks to both its appropriateness for use in this book as well as its general utility in the helping professions.

By fostering a shared terminology, Gordon's model has the potential to promote and advance interdisciplinary collaboration. This could then lead to the sharing of techniques, increased learning about different or complementary disciplines, and better linkage of researchers with practitioners (Keefe, Buffington, Studts, & Rumble, 2002). All of these improvements would benefit the entire health care field (Keefe et al., 2002).

IDENTIFYING THE FUTURE OF PREVENTION

The future of prevention is the continued development and expansion of preventive interventions for adults. In the opening chapter of this book, the authors state that prevention efforts have traditionally targeted children and adolescents, to the negligence of adults. While it is true that many behaviors associated with adult health problems do begin in childhood or adolescence (Smith, Kendall, & Keefe, 2002), this does not excuse inattention to adult preventive interventions. Poor dietary habits acquired in childhood, for example, will certainly increase one's risk for a number of health problems in adulthood. Yet, this person is not doomed to later suffering and illness because the cessation of such harmful behavior at any time in life has significant health benefits. By improving on these poor dietary habits in adulthood, persons can still dramatically reduce their risk for many possible health problems. For this reason, researchers and health care professionals have started (quite appropriately) to value prevention and health across the life span (Smith et al., 2002). This contrasts with the somewhat fatalistic beliefs that have contributed to the past neglect of adult prevention. It also supports the continued development and study of preventive approaches for adults.

THE ECONOMICS OF PREVENTION

This movement to view prevention across the life span has perhaps never been more timely or necessary. The rising costs of health care services, longer life expectancies, and an aging trend in the general population make economic affairs an important consideration in health care practice and research (Smith et al., 2002). The frequent introduction of expensive new medical tests, devices, and treatments further contributes to rising health care costs (Smith et al., 2002).

Furthermore, the provision of health care is absolutely impacted by national economic trends. The factors listed earlier in conjunction with sluggish or slow gross domestic product growth could lead to a scenario in which an increasing proportion of economic resources are consumed by health care costs and expenses (Heffler et al., 2001). Perhaps, then, our modern landscape of scarce funding and limited resources has set the stage for adult preventive measures to assume a more prominent role in health and health care. Emerging research and mounting evidence show that many comprehensive prevention programs are highly cost-effective (Tovian, 2004). Concrete examples of such are cited throughout this book.

Measures of cost-effectiveness are compelling and highly influential for obtaining funding in a cost-conscious environment (Rice, Hodgson, & Kopstein, 1985). When confronted with limited resources, those programs that produce a ratio of high net health benefits to low net health care costs hold greater promise than those programs not supported by such a ratio. Cost-effectiveness analysis is the computation of this ratio, wherein, for prevention research, health benefits may be operationalized to be *estimated cases of disease prevented, years of life saved,* or *quality-adjusted life years saved* (Yates & Taub, 2003). Hence, the demonstrated cost-effectiveness of preventive interventions for adults should make them especially appealing to those people charged with making difficult resource-allocation decisions (Weinstein & Stason, 1977).

To fully appreciate the promise of cost-effective adult prevention programs, one must consider the full economic burden of illness and disease. The economic costs of caring for the sick or disordered extend beyond the value of those resources allocated for diagnostics and treatment. Beyond these direct costs, one must also account for the indirect costs of illness. These include lost wages and lost work productivity resulting from bad health or disability as well as lost future earnings due to premature death (Rice et al., 1985). Because successful prevention programs lower both direct and indirect costs, they not only are cost-effective but also contribute to lessening the national burden of disease.

THE PREVENTION OF SHARED RISK FACTORS

Reflecting again on the chapters contained in this book, one notices that none of the various physical, mental, or social problems possesses a unique and exclusive list of risk factors. Some risk factors are associated with many different disorders, and some disorders are themselves risk factors for other disorders. This concept was introduced briefly in the first chapter, but can be further developed here using concrete examples.

An attempt to unravel the complex web of risk factors proves to be futile. Obesity, for example, emerges as a risk factor for several other serious health problems: heart disease, cancer, hypertension, and diabetes, among others. One might postulate that the lack of mobility, social isolation, and chronic health problems resulting from extreme obesity will then be associated with an increased risk for depression, unemployment, and even suicide. These conditions pose an increased risk for unresolved grief, substance abuse, sexual dysfunction, sleep disorders, and ineffective parenting, which, in turn, may all contribute to the development of the unhealthy habits that lead to obesity. Thus, the interplay of risk factors and disorders becomes increasingly murky.

In light of such muddy entanglements, the future of prevention should include sustained actions that develop and evaluate prevention approaches targeting these shared risk factors. For instance, a *universal* preventive intervention aiming to reduce obesity would subsequently lower people's risk for many of the other life-threatening health problems listed in the previous paragraph. In a like example, a *selective* preventive intervention directed to women may help to raise awareness on a number of problems specific to this group, including breast cancer and partner violence. Similar programs could also be developed for different age groups. By targeting such shared risk factors with effective and evidence-based prevention programs, it stands to reason that gains will be made in the fight against several different problems. Such programs would be not only cost-effective but instrumental in improving the overall quality of life.

This latter outcome is consistent with a new movement in medicine that is gaining significant momentum. Whereas the traditional focus of medical care has been on the diagnosis and treatment of the specific disease, some are now stating that this approach is outdated and potentially harmful (Tinetti & Fried, 2004).

Instead, it is argued, treatment should be based on achieving a patient's individual goals and on providing a more comprehensive level of care intended to improve the patient's quality of life (Sullivan, 2003; Tinetti & Fried, 2004). According to Sullivan, "The physicians' job description will be changed to focus on patients' lives rather than patients' bodies" (p. 1595). Moreover, "the definitive evaluations of medical effectiveness will occur within patients' lives rather than within doctor's hospitals" (p. 1595). This move to incorporate the patient's perspective and values results in a more patient-centered and subjective approach to health care. It is a dramatic shift away from the more objective and narrowly focused disease-amelioration methods that have driven traditional medical practice.

SUMMARY AND CONCLUSIONS

Despite traditional thinking about prevention, this book clearly shows that prevention is a valuable and necessary approach to health care with adults. Preventive tactics have the potential to reduce health care costs and improve the overall quality of life for a large portion of the population. The current economic climate also favors expanding such prevention efforts, which are often more cost-effective than standard treatment approaches.

In making such measurements, it should be remembered that cost-effectiveness analyses compare costs to benefits. Accordingly, determinations about the worthiness of a specific program or intervention should not be based solely on costs. An inexpensive intervention, for example, is not automatically cost-effective; low costs may simply produce small or negligible benefits. On the contrary, an expensive intervention may be very cost-effective, requiring great costs but yielding even greater health benefits.

This value on health benefits is extremely important because it helps to ensure that health care will not be dictated entirely by money-saving practices, but by the most efficient use of resources while still effectively and ethically improving health and wellness. Accordingly, in health practice, the measurement of benefits and effectiveness should be outcome-oriented (Weinstein & Stason, 1977), and it is important to select appropriate outcomes (Keefe et al., 2002). As there is little consensus on what constitutes meaningful improvement (Keefe et al., 2002), outcome measures should be selected based on the stated goals of the particular prevention intervention.

Above all, though, cost-effectiveness analyses should be just one part of a more comprehensive battery of research and assessment measures used to evaluate the success or failure of the prevention activity. As preventive interventions targeting adults expand, so too should the research and evidence base informing their practice. The development of cost-effective *and* evidence-based approaches will accelerate the movement of prevention to the forefront of health care for adults in the United States.

REFERENCES

Gordon, R. (1983). An operational classification of disease prevention. *Public Health Reports, 98,* 107–109.

Gordon, R. (1987). An operational classification of disease prevention. In J. A. Steinberg & M. M. Silverman (Eds.), *Preventing mental disorders* (pp. 20–26). Rockville, MD: U.S. Department of Health and Human Services.

Heffler, S., Levit, K., Smith, S., Smith, C., Cowan, C., Lazenby, H., et al. (2001). Health spending growth up in 1999: Faster growth expected in the future. *Health Affairs, 20*(2), 193–203.

Keefe, F. J., Buffington, A. L. H., Studts, J. L., & Rumble, M. E. (2002). Behavioral medicine: 2002 and beyond. *Journal of Consulting and Clinical Psychology, 70*(3), 852–856.

Rice, D. P., Hodgson, T. A., & Kopstein, A. N. (1985). The economic costs of illness: A replication and update. *Health Care Financing Review, 7*(1), 61–80.

Smith, T. W., Kendall, P. C., & Keefe, F. J. (2002). Behavioral medicine and clinical health psychology: Introduction to the special issue, a view from the decade of behavior. *Journal of Consulting and Clinical Psychology, 70*(3), 459–462.

Sullivan, M. (2003). The new subjective medicine: Taking the patient's point of view on health care and health. *Social Science and Medicine, 56,* 1595–1604.

Tinetti, M. E., & Fried, T. (2004). The end of the disease era. *American Journal of Medicine, 116,* 179–185.

Tovian, S. M. (2004). Health services and health care economics: The health psychology marketplace. *Health Psychology, 23*(2), 138–141.

Weinstein, M. C., & Stason, W. B. (1977). Foundations of cost-effectiveness analysis for health and medical practices. *New England Journal of Medicine, 296*(13), 716–721.

Yates, B. T., & Taub, J. (2003). Assessing the costs, benefits, cost-effectiveness, and cost-benefit of psychological assessment: We should, we can, and here's how. *Psychological Assessment, 15*(4), 478–495.

Author Index

Subject Index